D1568398

Clinical Guide to the Use of Antithrombotic Drugs in Coronary Artery Disease

Edited by

Dominick J Angiolillo MD PhD
University of Florida College of Medicine, Jacksonville
Jacksonville, FL
USA

Adnan Kastrati MD
Deutsches Herzenntrum Munchen
Munchen
Germany

Daniel I Simon MD
Case Western Reserve University School of Medicine
Cleveland, OH
USA

informa
healthcare

© 2008 Informa UK Ltd

First published in the United Kingdom in 2008 by Informa Healthcare, Telephone House, 69-77 Paul Street, London EC2A 4LQ. Informa Healthcare is a trading division of Informa UK Ltd. Registered Office: 37/41 Mortimer Street, London W1T 3JH. Registered in England and Wales number 1072954.

Tel: +44 (0)20 7017 5000
Fax: +44 (0)20 7017 6699
Website: www.informahealthcare.com

A CIP record for this book is available from the British Library.
Library of Congress Cataloging-in-Publication Data

Data available on application

ISBN-10: 1 84184 639 2
ISBN-13: 978 1 84184 639 2

Distributed in North and South America by
Taylor & Francis
6000 Broken Sound Parkway, NW, (Suite 300)
Boca Raton, FL 33487, USA

Within Continental USA
Tel: 1 (800) 272 7737; Fax: 1 (800) 374 3401
Outside Continental USA
Tel: (561) 994 0555; Fax: (561) 361 6018
Email: orders@crcpress.Com

Book orders in the rest of the world
Paul Abrahams
Tel: +44 (0) 207 017 4036
Email: bookorders@informa.com

Composition by Exeter Premedia Servies Private Ltd., Chennai, India
Printed and bound in India by Replika Press Pvt Ltd.

Contents

iv **Contents**

Contributors

Fernando Alfonso MD PhD
Cardiovascular Institute
Hospital Clínico San Carlos
Madrid
Spain

Dominick J Angiolillo MD PhD
Division of Cardiology
University of Florida College of Medicine, Jacksonville
Jacksonville, FL
USA

Elliott M Antman MD
Cardiovascular Division
Brigham and Women's Hospital
Harvard Medical School
Boston, MA
USA

Lina Badimon MD
Cardiovascular Research Center
Barcelona
Spain

Theodore A Bass MD
Division of Cardiology
University of Florida College of Medicine, Jacksonville
Jacksonville, FL
USA

Nicolas von Beckerath MD
Department of Cardiology
Deutsches Herzzentrum
Technische Universität München
Munich
Germany

Joshua A Beckman MD MS
Cardiovascular Division
Brigham and Women's Hospital
Harvard Medical School
Boston, MA
USA

Peter B Berger MD
Center for Clinical Studies
Geisinger Clinic
Danville, PA
USA

Esther Bernardo BSc
Cardiovascular Institute
San Carlos University Hospital
Madrid
Spain

Deepak L Bhatt MD FACC FSCAI FESC FACP
Department of Cardiovascular Medicine
Cleveland Clinic Foundation
Cleveland, OH
USA

Piera Capranzano MD
Division of Cardiology
University of Florida College of Medicine, Jacksonville
Jacksonville, FL
USA

Raffaele De Caterina MD PhD
Institute of Cardiology
"G. d'Annunzio" University – Chieti
Ospedale San Camillo de Lellis
Chieti
Italy

Wai-Hong Chen MBBS
Division of Cardiology
The University of Hong Kong
Hong Kong
China

Marco A Costa MD PhD
Division of Cardiology
University of Florida College of Medicine, Jacksonville
Jacksonville, FL
USA

Raphaelle Dumaine MD
Institute de Cardiologie
Pitié-Salpêtrière University Hospital
Paris
France

John W Eikelboom MBBS MSc FRACP
Department of Medicine
McMaster University
Hamilton, Ontario
Canada

Francisco Fernández-Avilés MD
Servicio de Cardiología
Hospital General Universitario Gregorio Marañón
Madrid
Spain

Antonio Fernández-Ortiz MD
Cardiovascular Institute
San Carlos University Hospital
Madrid
Spain

Andrew L Frelinger III PhD
Center for Platelet Function Studies
University of Massachusetts Medical School
Worcester, MA
USA

Desmond Fitzgerald MD
Institute of Biomolecular and Biomedical Research
University College Dublin
Belfield, Dublin
Ireland

Rajeev Garg MD
Division of Cardiology
University of Missouri-Columbia
Columbia, MO
USA

Meinrad Gawaz MD
Eberhard Karls Universität Tübingen
Medizinische Klinik III
Tübingen
Germany

Robert P Giugliano MD SM
Cardiovascular Division
Brigham and Women's Hospital
Harvard Medical School
Boston, MA
USA

Luis A Guzman MD
Division of Cardiology
University of Florida College of Medicine, Jacksonville
Jacksonville, FL
USA

Howard C Herrmann MD
Interventional Cardiology and Cardiac
Catheterization Laboratories
University of Pennsylvania School of Medicine
Philadelphia, PA
USA

Steven Jain MD
University Hospitals Care Medical Center
Case Western Reserve School of Medicine
Cleveland, OH
USA

Joseph Jozic MD
Division of Cardiovascular Medicine
Gill Heart Institute
University of Kentucky
Lexington, KY
USA

Neal Kleiman MD
Cardiac Catheterization Laboratory
Methodist DeBakey Heart Center
Houston, TX
USA

Adnan Kastrati MD
Department of Cardiology
Deutsches Herzzentrum Muenchen
Munich
Germany

Ken Kozuma MD PhD
Division of Cardiology
Teikyo University School of Medicine
Tokyo
Japan

Takaaki Isshiki MD PhD
Division of Cardiology
Teikyo University School of Medicine
Tokyo
Japan

Eli Lev MD
Cardiology Department
Rabin Medical Center
Petah-Tikva
and the Sackler Faculty of Medicine
Tel-Aviv University
Tel-Aviv
Israel

Lori-Ann Linkins MD MSc FRCPC
Department of Medicine
McMaster University
Hamilton, Ontario
Canada

Carlos Macaya MD PhD
Cardiovascular Institute
San Carlos University Hospital
Madrid
Spain

Alan D Michelson MD
Center for Platelet Function Studies
University of Massachusetts Medical School
Worcester, MA
USA

Shamir R Mehta MD MSc FRCPC FACC
Department of Medicine
McMaster University
Hamilton, Ontario
Canada

David J Moliterno MD
Department of Cardiovascular Medicine
University of Kentucky
Lexington, KY
USA

Gilles Montalescot MD
Institute Cardiologie
Pitié-Salpêtrière University Hospital
Paris
France

David A Morrow MD MPH
Cardiovascular Division
Brigham and Women's Hospital
Harvard Medical School
Boston, MA
USA

Sahil A Parikh MD
Cardiovascular Division
Brigham and Women's Hospital
Harvard Medical School
Boston, MA
USA

Karthik Reddy MD
Interventional Cardiology and Cardiac
Catheterization Laboratories
University of Pennsylvania School of Medicine
Philadelphia, PA
USA

Giulia Renda MD PhD
Institute of Cardiology
"G. d'Annunzio" University – Chieti
Ospedale San Camillo de Lellis
Chieti
Italy

Christian T Ruff MD
Cardiovascular Division
Brigham and Women's Hospital
Harvard Medical School
Boston, MA
USA

Manel Sabaté MD PhD
Interventional Cardiology Unit
Hospital de Sant Pau
Barcelona
Spain

Pedro L Sánchez MD
Servicio de Cardiología
Hospital General Universitario Gregorio Marañón
Madrid
Spain

Melchior Seyfarth MD
Department of Cardiology
Deutsches Herzzentrum München
Technische Universität München
Munich
Germany

Dirk Sibbing MD
Department of Cardiology
Deutsches Herzzentrum München
Technische Universität München
Munich
Germany

Daniel I Simon MD
Heart and Vascular Institute
Case Western Reserve University School of Medicine
Cleveland, OH
USA

Peter R Sinnaeve MD
Department of Cardiology
Gasthuisberg University Hospital
University of Leuven
Leuven
Belgium

Alexander G Turpie MD FRCPC
General Division
Hamilton Health Sciences
Hamilton, Ontario
Canada

Gemma Vilahur MD
Cardiovascular Research Center
Barcelona
Spain

Theodore E Warkentin MD
Hamilton Regional Laboratory Medicine Program
Hamilton Health Sciences
Hamilton, Ontario
Canada

Jeffrey I Weitz MD
Departments of Medicine and Biochemistry
McMaster University
Hamilton, Ontario
Canada

Frans J Van de Werf MD PhD
Department of Cardiology
Gasthuisberg University Hospital
University of Leuven
Leuven
Belgium

Stephen D Wiviott MD
Cardiovascular Division
Brigham and Women's Hospital
Harvard Medical School
Boston, MA
USA

Marco Zimarino MD PhD
Institute of Cardiology
"G. d'Annunzio" University – Chieti
Ospedale San Camillo de Lellis
Chieti
Italy

Foreword

In his classic textbook *The Principles and Practice of Medicine* published in 1892, William Osler established clearly the pathologic link between thrombotic coronary occlusion and myocardial infarction. Early in the Twentieth Century, Obraztov and Stazhenko in Russia and Herrick in the United States reported that coronary thrombosis was not always immediately fatal. For decades the terms 'coronary thrombosis' and 'myocardial infarction' were used interchangeably. We now know that coronary thrombi – occlusive and non-occlusive – cause an important clinical syndrome, an acute coronary syndrome, that has a wide spectrum of presentations and that its prevalence is the highest of any cardiovascular condition requiring hospital admission.

The deposition of platelets and fibrin are of such importance in the development and progression of atherosclerosis that this condition is now frequently referred to as 'atherothrombosis'. Both platelets and the coagulation system are also responsible for the conversion of chronic coronary artery disease to acute coronary syndrome. Powerful antiplatelet agents and anticoagulants have been developed to prevent or halt this conversion. In addition, fibrinolytic agents have become available to lyse fresh thrombi. Clinicians must use these drugs both with understanding and care. Understanding, because they act on different aspects of the thrombotic process and their pharmacology must be understood, and care, because when given inappropriately or in excessive dosage they can cause severe – occasionally fatal – bleeding. Indeed up to now we have never "gotten a free lunch" as increased bleeding has always been the price of reduced thrombosis.

The *Clinical Guide to the Use of Antithrombotic Drugs in Coronary Artery Disease* is more than its name implies. It is not a 'cookbook', but provides a detailed, contemporary review of platelet function, coagulation and fibrinolysis. It then describes, systematically and with clarity, the pharmacology of antiplatelet drugs, anticoagulants and fibrinolytic agents, as well as the clinical trials on which their use is based. The editors, Drs. Angiolillo, Kastrati and Simon bring great complementary strengths to this effort. They and their authors have provided an authoritative, yet eminently practical and readable book that will be especially useful to clinicians.

Within the specialty of cardiology a number of important subspecialties have developed; these include, among others, interventional cardiology, electrophysiology, heart failure, cardiac imaging, and preventive cardiology. To these, we can now add *thrombocardiology* and it may be appropriate to add the subtitle: *A Textbook of Thrombocardiology* to the title of *Clinical Guide to the Use of Antithrombotic Drugs in Coronary Artery Disease*.

Eugene Braunwald MD
Hersey Distinguished Professor of Theory and
Practice of Medicine
Chairman, TIMI Study Group
Brigham and Women's Hospital
Harvard Medical School
Boston, MA
USA

Preface

The understanding of the importance of platelets and coagulation factors in atherothrombotic events has led to the widespread use as well as continuous development of new antithrombotic agents. This field of cardiovascular pharmacology has advanced at a very rapid rate. Understanding the basic principles of atherothrombosis as well as the pharmacological agents currently available or under clinical development are key to health care professionals treating patients with atherothrombotic manifestations, in particular coronary artery disease.

In *Clinical Guide to the Use of Antithrombotic Drugs in Coronary Artery Disease* we have created chapters which describe a) the basic concepts of atherothrombosis, b) the pharmacological principles, indications for use, and pitfalls of antithrombotic agents most commonly utilized in treating patients with coronary artery disease, and c) special clinical scenarios which may imply a multi-pharmacological approach or which represent undesired effects of antithrombotic agents.

We would like to thank the contributors who responded with great enthusiasm to our quest to create a current and practical textbook.

Dominick J Angiolillo
Adnan Kastrati
Daniel I Simon

Color plate

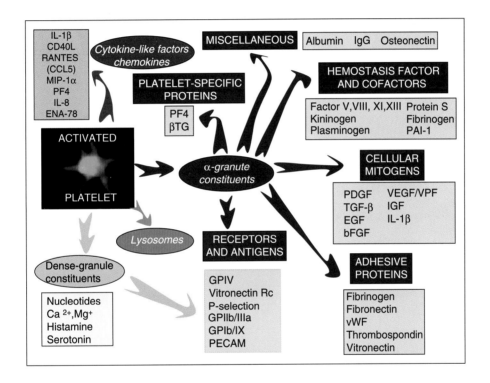

Figure 1.2

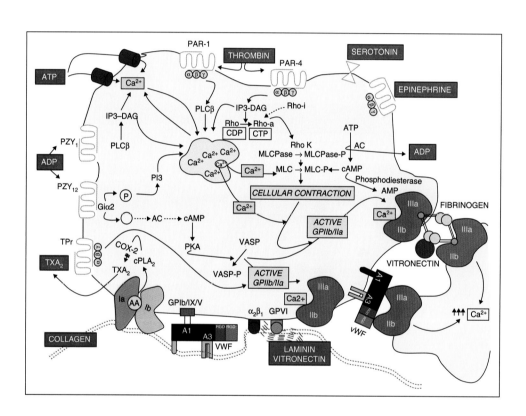

Figure 1.3

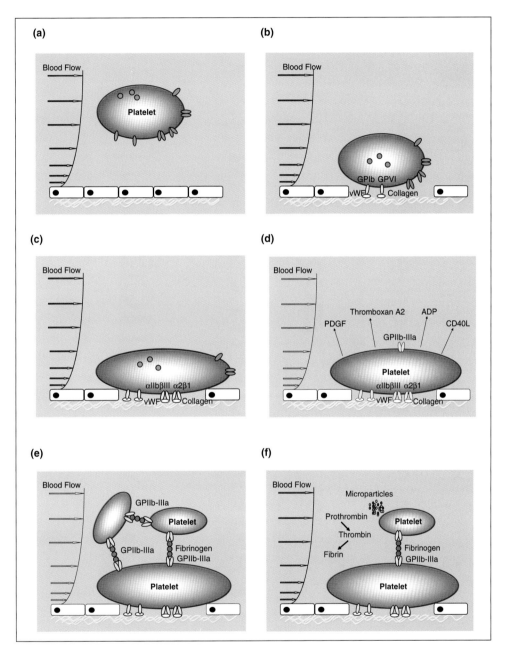

Figure 2.3
Under physiological conditions, platelets do not adhere to intact endothelium. (b) If the endothelial monolyer is disrupted, subendothelial matrix proteins are exposed, including collagen and von Willebrand factor (vWF). Platelets initiate initial contact with the subendothelium via their membrane adhesion receptors GPIb and GPVI. (c) This contact results in activation of platelet integrins $\alpha_{IIb}\beta_3$ (fibrinogen receptor) and $\alpha_2\beta_1$ (collagen receptor). Interaction of $\alpha_{IIb}\beta_3$ and $\alpha_2\beta_1$ with extracellular matrix proteins leads to 'spreading' and firm adhesion of platelets. (d) Subsequently, platelets secrete mediators and recruit other circulating platelets. (e) Platelets form microaggregates via a fibrinogen bridging mechanism between two GPIIb/IIIa receptors. (f) Formation of microparticles in the microenvironment of platelet aggregates catalytes thrombin and subsequently fibrin generation, which stabilizes the growing thrombus.

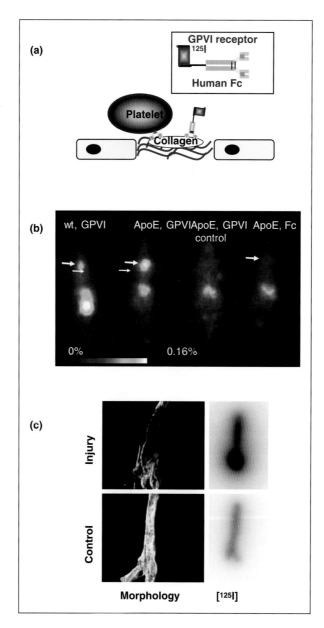

Figure 2.4
Detection of vulnerable plaques by soluble GPVI. (a) A soluble dimeric form of human platelet GPVI conjugated to an Fc fragment, radiolabeled with iodine-125 (^{125}I) was used. GPVI is essential to establish the first interaction of platelets with an exposed collagen surface. Therefore, we made use of this natural mechanism to detect thrombogenic, and thus vulnerable, plaques. (b) Gamma-camera images of wild-type (wt) and *ApoE$^{-/-}$* mice with and without (control animals) experimental carotid injury. Images were aquired 24 hours after administration of 7.4 MBq [^{125}I]GPVI or [^{125}I]Fc-fragment (control compound). The imaging time was 20 minutes. The arrow indicates the area of carotid injury. (c) Representative photomicrographs of injured and control carotid arteries of wild-type mice and the corresponding ex vivo autoradiographs.

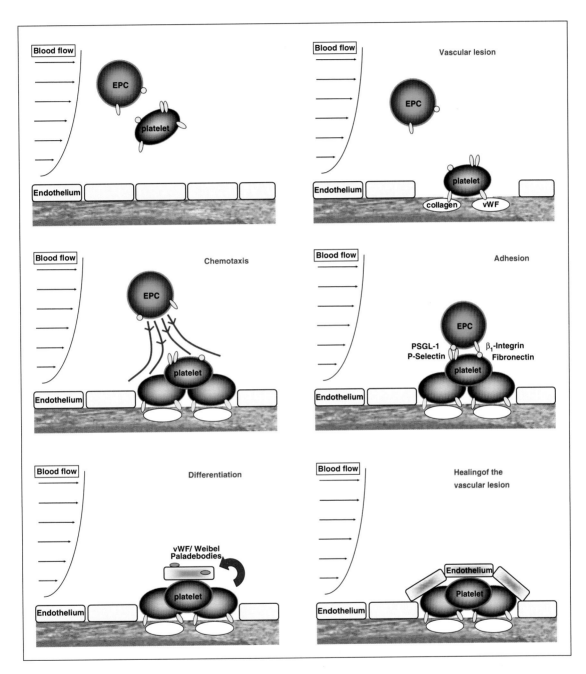

Figure 2.5
Schematic overview of the processes involved in platelet-mediated endothelial progenitor cell (EPC) recruitment to vascular lesions with exposed subendothelial matrix, finally resulting in differentiation to endothelial cells – a process that could initiate and sustain healing of vascular lesions.

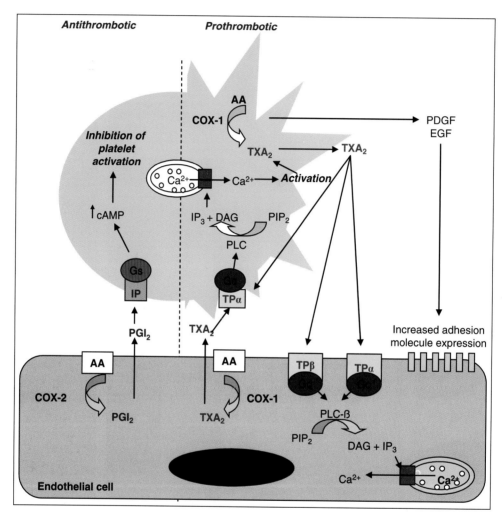

Figure 4.2
Schematic representation of the role of COX-1 and COX-2 on the vasculature. Endothelial cells express both COX-1 and COX-2, resulting in the generation of PGI_2 and TXA_2, respectively. Conversely, platelets express only COX-1. PGI_2 and TXA_2 mediate opposing effects on the platelet. TXA_2 is a potent platelet activator, whereas PGI_2 is a platelet inhibitor. In atherosclerosis, PGI_2 generation inhibits TXA_2-induced platelet activation and aggregation. Administration of a non-selective non-steroidal anti-inflammatory drug (NSAID) decreases generation of both TXA_2 and PGI_2, leading to reduced platelet aggregation. However, selective inhibition of COX-2 decreases PGI_2 without a concomitant inhibition of TXA_2, and hence increases platelet aggregation. AA, arachidonic acid; PDGF, platelet-derived growth factor; EGF, epidermal growth factor; cAMP, cyclic adenosine monophosphate; IP_3, inositol trisphosphate; DAG, diacylglycerol; PIP_2 phosphatidylinositol biphosphate; PhC, phospholipase C.

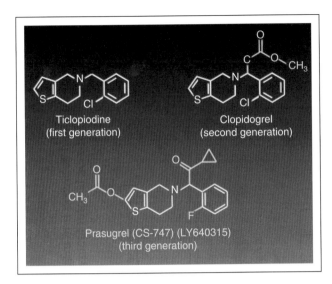

Figure 9.1
Structures of thienopyridine antiplatelet agents.

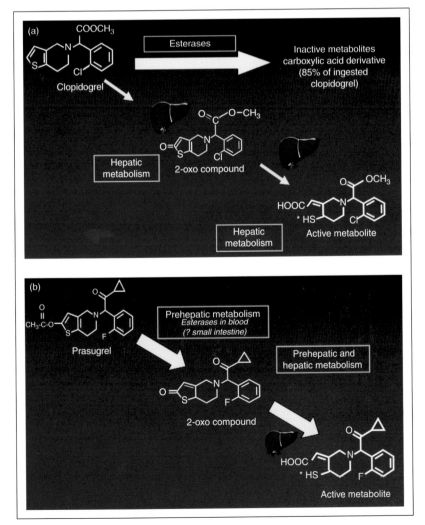

Figure 9.2
Schematics of the metabolism of clopidogrel (a)
and prasugrel (b).

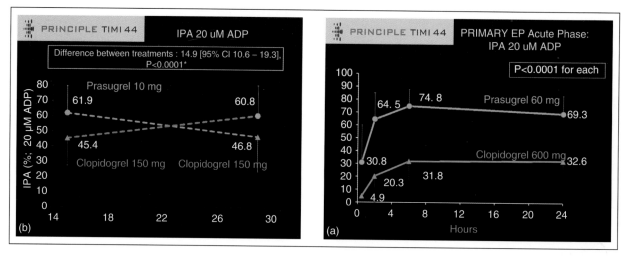

Figure 9.3

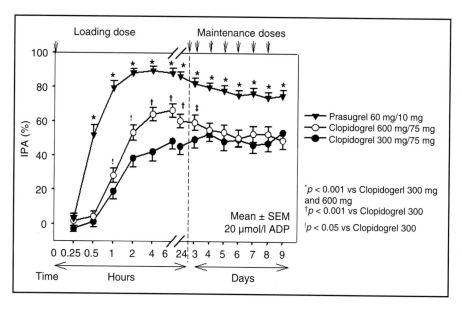

Figure 9.5
Inhibition of platelet aggregation (IPA) among healthy subjects receiving prasugrel or two dosing regimens of clopidogrel.[6]

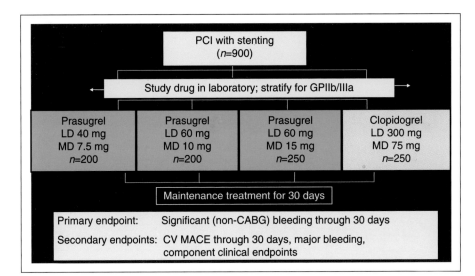

Figure 9.6
Design of the JUMBO–TIMI 26 trial.[8] PCI, percutaneous coronary intervention; GPIIb/IIIa, glycoprotein IIb/IIIa; LD, loading dose; MD, maintenance dose; CABG, coronary artery bypass surgery; MACE, major adverse cardiovascular events.

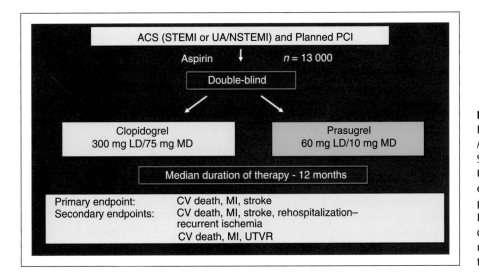

Figure 9.7.
Design of the TRITON–TIMI 38 trial.[10] ACS, acute coronary syndrome; STEMI, ST-elevation myocardial infarction; UA/NSTEMI, unstable angina/non-ST-elevation myocardial infarction; PCI, percutaneous coronary intervention; LD, loading dose; MD, maintenance dose; CV, cardiovascular; MI, myocardial infarction; UTVR, urgent target vessel revascularization.

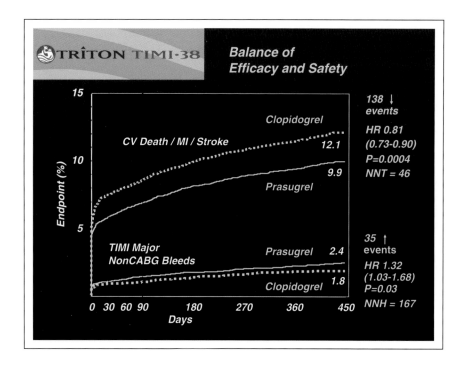

Figure 9.8

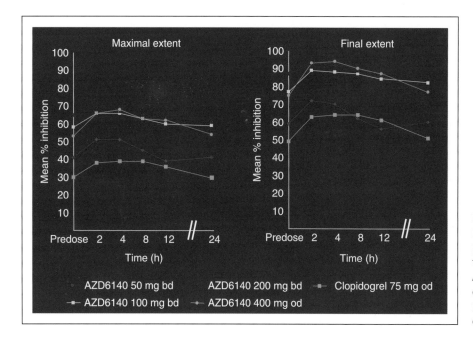

Figure 10.3
Mean inhibition of ADP-induced platelet aggregation on maximum and final response by different dosages of AZD6140 and clopidogrel standard dosage after 14 days of therapy in patients with stable atherosclerotic disease.

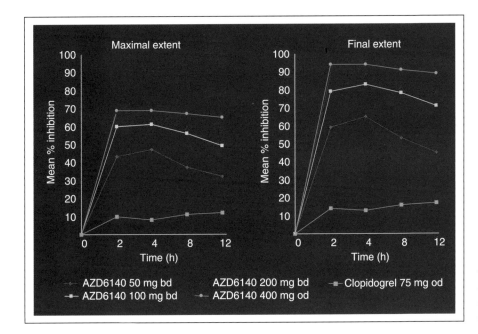

Figure 10.4
Mean inhibition of ADP-induced platelet aggregation on maximum and final response following one single oral dosage of AZD6140, 50–400 mg and clopidogrel 75 mg in patients with stable atherosclerotic disease.

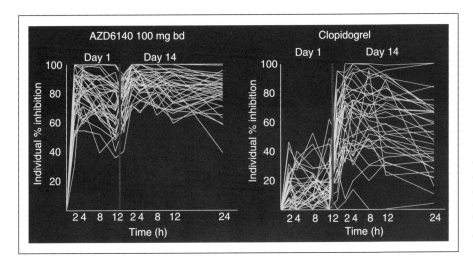

Figure 10.5
Individual inhibitory effect on response to ADP-induced platelet aggregation by AZD6140, a direct acting, reversible $P2Y_{12}$ receptor antagonist, 100 mg twice daily and clopidogrel 75 mg daily in patients with stable atherosclerotic disease after one single dosage and after 14 days of therapy.

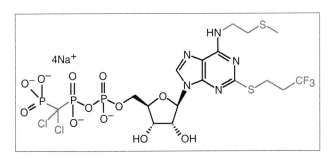

Figure 14.2
The inhibitory effects of cangrelor come from its molecular structure, which is analogous to that of the competitive antagonist ATP. During development, cangrelor was referred to as AR-C69931MX, where MX stands for the tetrasodium salt.

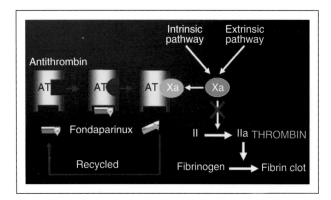

Figure 17.1
Mechanism of action fondaparinux. (Adapted from Turpie AG et al. N Engl J Med 2001;344:619–25.[12])

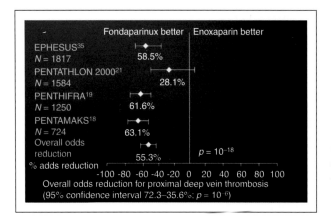

Figure 17.2
Overall efficacy of fondaparinux versus enoxaparin in prevention of versus thromboembolism: meta-analysis of trials in patients undergoing orthopedic surgery. (Adapted from Turpie AG et al. Arch Intern Med 2002;162:1833–40.[23])

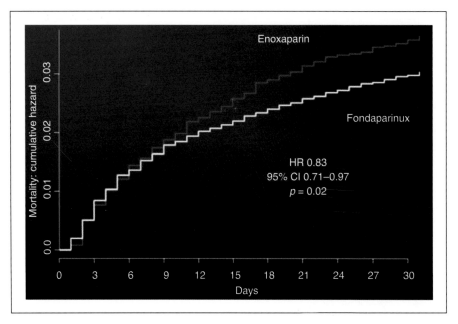

Figure 17.3
Fondaparinux reduces all-cause mortality compared with enoxaparin in patients with NSTE ACS.

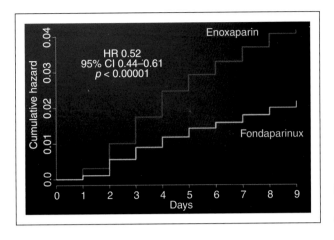

Figure 17.4
Fondaparinux reduces major bleeding substantially compared with enoxaparin in patients with NSTE ACS.

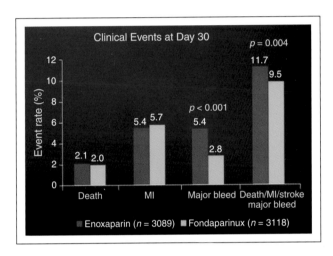

Figure 17.5
In patients undergoing PCI in OASIS-5, efficacy outcomes were similar between the enoxaparin and fondaparinux groups, but there was a large reduction in major bleeding in the latter, resulting in a significant net clinical benefit with fondaparinux.

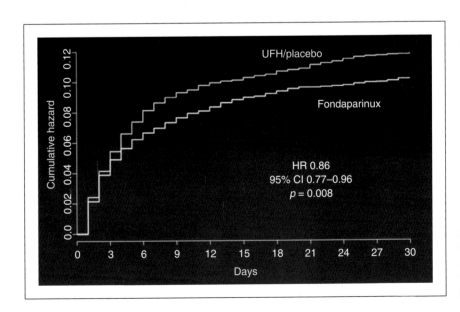

Figure 17.6
OASIS 6: fondaparinux reduces death or MI compared with standard care in STEMI. (Reproduced from Yusuf S et al. JAMA 2006;295:1519–30.[33])

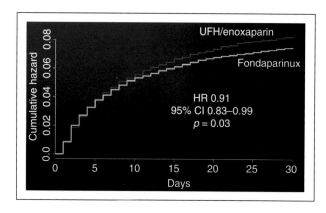

Figure 17.7
Combined analysis of OASIS-5 and -6 showing superiority of fondaparinux compared with UFH or enoxaparin.

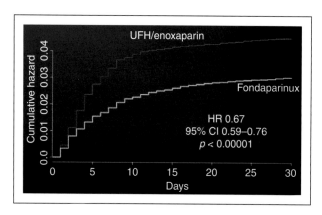

Figure 17.8
Combined analysis of OASIS-5 and -6 showing major bleeding at 30 days: fondaparinux versus UFH/enoxaparin.

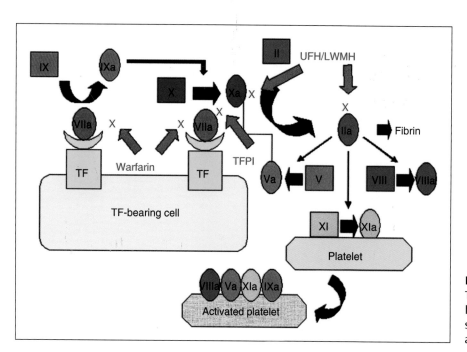

Figure 18.1
The role of the coagulation cascade leading to platelet activation and the sites of action of various anticoagulants. See text for details.

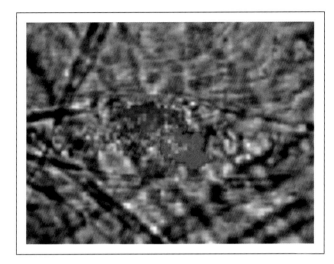

Figure 18.2
Tissue factor, platelet, and fibrin deposition during thrombus formation. Using color-coded antibodies during the experimental induction of thrombi in mice, the constituents of a growing thrombus (25% of maximum size) includes predominantly platelets (red), tissue factor (green), fibrin (blue), tissue factor + platelets (yellow), with lesser amounts of fibrin (turquoise) and platelets + fibrin (magenta). (Adapted with permission from ref.[50])

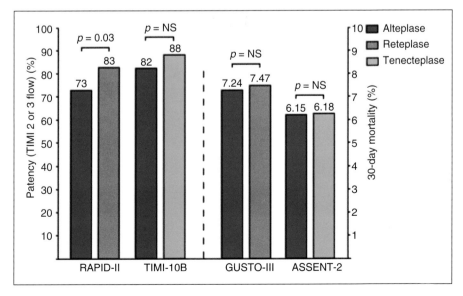

Figure 19.2
Patency rates (TIMI flow grade 2 or 3) and mortality rates with reteplase or tenecteplase versus alteplase.

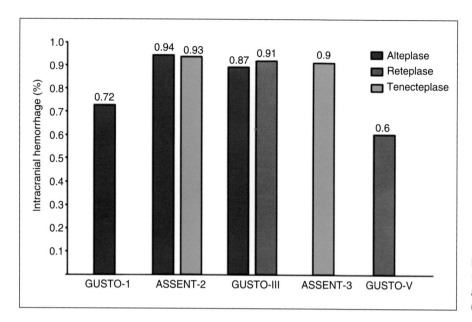

Figure 19.3
Rates of intracranial hemorrhage after alteplase, reteplase or tenecteplase (UFH groups only).

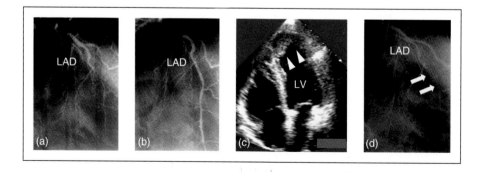

Figure 28.1
In a patient admitted for ST-segment-elevation myocardial infarction (STEMI) after 5 hours from symptom onset, an urgent coronary angiogram (a) showed that the left anterior descending (LAD) coronary artery was occluded in its distal segment (asterisk). A successful primary percutaneous coronary intervention (PPCI) was performed, with implantation of a bare metal stent (b). An echocardiogram (c) documented a left ventricular (LV) apical aneurysm with a thrombotic formation (arrowheads). The patient was discharged with aspirin (100 mg) indefinitely, clopidogrel (75 mg) for 30 days and warfarin for 6 months, aiming at an INR in the range 2–3. The patient prematurely discontinued clopidogrel after 14 days, and was admitted after further 7 days for a recurrent episode of STEMI (on day 21 from the first episode). Repeat angiography documented a thrombotic occlusion (arrows) of the previously deployed stent (d).

Section I

Basic concepts of atherothrombosis

1. Fundamentals of the thrombosis cascade: interaction between platelets and the coagulation cascade

2. Platelet receptors and their role in atherothrombosis

3. Laboratory assessment of platelet function and coagulation

1

Fundamentals of the thrombosis cascade: interaction between platelets and the coagulation cascade

Lina Badimon, Antonio Fernández-Ortiz, and Gemma Vilahur

Introduction

Arterial thrombosis comprises three basic pathways: platelet activation and aggregation, blood coagulation with fibrin formation, and fibrinolysis. Platelet activation and blood coagulation are complementary, mutually dependent processes in hemostasis and thrombosis. Indeed, platelets interact with several coagulation factors, while the coagulation product thrombin is a potent platelet-activating agonist.[1–3] Additionally, inflammatory pathways can aggravate the atherothrombotic process.

This chapter highlights the molecular machinery used by platelets and coagulation components in order to interplay and thus initiate and acccelerate the thrombotic process, as well as discussing the mechanisms involved in clot dissolution.

Platelet involvement in thrombus formation

The endothelium is a dynamic autocrine and paracrine organ that regulates contractile, secretory, and mitogenic activities in the vessel wall and the hemostatic process within the vessel lumen by producing several locally active substances. Indeed, under physiological conditions, endothelial cells exhibit antithrombotic properties such as (a) exposure of negatively charged heparin-like glycosaminoglycans and of neutral phospholipids in the external layer of the cell membrane; (b) synthesis, exposure, or secretion of platelet inhibitors (prostacyclin, nitric oxide, and ectoADPase), coagulation inhibitors (thrombomodulin, protein S, tissue factor pathway inhibitor, and glycosaminoglycans), and fibrinolysis activators (tissue-type plasminogen activator and urokinase-type plasminogen activator). When activated by damage, endothelial cells shift from antithrombotic to prothrombotic, characterized by exposure of anionic phospholipids on the outer leaflet of the cell membrane, secretion of platelet-activating agents, exposure of coagulation factor receptors or cofactors, and secretion of inhibitors of fibrinolysis. Endothelial damage also exposes the subendothelial layer, which contains highly thrombogenic components such as collagen, von Willebrand factor (vWF), and other molecules (e.g., fibronectin and laminin) that bind to platelet receptors, promoting platelet attachment (Figure 1.1).[4,5] Under high-shear-rate conditions, circulating vWF may also interact with the exposed collagen, providing a further substrate for platelet adhesion. Besides platelet receptors, platelet membranes include phospholipids that play a key role in platelet function since they act as second messengers, and as cofactors for platelet procoagulant activity. The platelet cytosol is mainly constituted by a complex membrane system, cytoskeletal structures (microtubules and microfilaments), and granules (dense granules, α-granules, and lysosomes), all of which are actively involved in thrombus formation. Cytoskeletal structures are essential in shape changes after activation, whereas granules contain active components that are excreted upon platelet activation,[6] thus promoting thrombus formation, atherosclerotic plaque progression (e.g., local release of growth factors), and the inflammatory process itself (Figure 1.2).

As already mentioned, collagen and vWF are the main substrates for platelet adhesion although a role of fibronectin and laminin has also been described.[7,8] However, platelets adherent to fibronectin are easily detached under increased shear stress compared with platelets adherent to vWF or collagen, indicating that platelet adhesion to fibronectin is less stable when compared with adhesion to vWF and/or collagen. As depicted in Figure 1.3 fibronectin and laminin bind to glycoprotein (GP) VI; collagen binds to the platelets' GPIa/IIa receptor complex; and vWF binds to the GPIb/IX/V receptor complex. vWF transiently

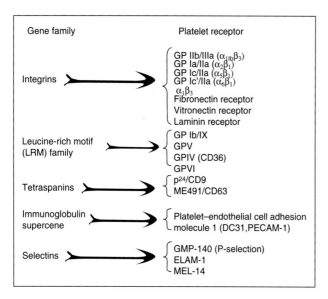

Gene family	Platelet receptor
Integrins	GP IIb/IIIa ($\alpha_{IIb}\beta_3$) GP Ia/IIa ($\alpha_2\beta_1$) GP Ic/IIa ($\alpha_5\beta_1$) GP Ic'/IIa ($\alpha_6\beta_1$) $\alpha_1\beta_3$ Fibronectin receptor Vitronectin receptor Laminin receptor
Leucine-rich motif (LRM) family	GP Ib/IX GPV GPIV (CD36) GPVI
Tetraspanins	p24/CD9 ME491/CD63
Immunoglobulin supercene	Platelet–endothelial cell adhesion molecule 1 (DC31,PECAM-1)
Selectins	GMP-140 (P-selection) ELAM-1 MEL-14

Figure 1.1
Recepetors on the platelet surface. GP, glycoprotein.

bridges the platelet GPIb/IX/V receptor either with other platelet GPIb/IX/V receptors or with vessel wall constituents (collagen I, III, and VI), thereby tethering the platelet to the vessel surface.[9] The GPIb/IX complex consist of two disulfide-linked subunits (GPIbα and GPIbβ) tightly (not covalently) complexed with GPIX in a 1:1 heterodimer. GPIbβ and GPIX are transmembrane glycoproteins and form the larger globular domain. The major role of GPIb/IX is to bind immobilized vWF on the exposed vascular subendothelium and initiate adhesion of platelets. GPIb does not bind soluble vWF in plasma; apparently it undergoes a conformation change upon binding to the extracellular matrix and then exposes a recognition sequence for GPIb/IX. The vWF-binding domain of GPIb/IX has been narrowed to amino acids 251–279 on GPIbα. The GPIbα-binding domain of vWF resides in a tryptic fragment extending from residue 449 to residue 728 of the subunit that does not contain an RGD (arginine–glycine–aspartate) sequence.[10] The cytoplasmic domain of GPIb/IX has a major function in linking the plasma membrane to the intracellular actin filaments of the cytoskeleton and functions to stabilize the membrane and to maintain the platelet shape. Moreover, through a mechanism that is not yet understood, the engagement of vWF with GPIb/IX/V, specifically under high shear, initiates platelet signalling mechanisms, as evidenced by an influx of calcium ions, the secretion of granule contents,[11] and the formation of active IIb/IIIa complexes. In contrast, GPVI binding to matrix collagen, although characterized by a slower binding kinetics, once initiated promotes a firm adhesion of platelet to the vessel surface.

In addition to vessel-induced platelet attachment, platelets can also be vaguely and/or powerfully activated by interacting with circulating agents with different induction activity such as epinephrine (adrenaline), thrombin, serotonin, thromboxane A$_2$ (TXA$_2$), and adenosine diphosphate (ADP) via specific platelet surface receptors (Figures 1.3 and 1.4). Once activated, intracellular Ca^{2+} increase causes discoid platelets to become spherical, pseudopodia to appear, and granules to become centralized and come into contact with membrane invaginations, leading to the secretion of active substances. These active substances themselves amplify the process by increasing platelet adhesion and aggregation (ADP, vWF, fibrinogen, and thrombospondin), by participating in plasma coagulation (factor V and fibrinogen), by enhancing vascular tone and by vascular contraction (serotonin), and by promoting cell proliferation and migration (platelet-derived growth factor, PDGF). Platelet activation also induces phospholipase A$_2$ (PLA$_2$) activation, which triggers arachidonic acid metabolism. Platelet cyclooxygenase-1 (COX-1) catalyzes the conversion of arachidonic acid to prostaglandin (PG) G$_2$/H$_2$, and the latter is converted to TXA$_2$. These substances can bind to specific receptors on other platelet membranes, leading to new platelet recruitment (Figure 1.3). An essential process in platelet recruitment is the exposure and activation of the integrin receptors GPIIb/IIIa ($\alpha_{IIb}\beta_3$) on the platelet surface. This activation allows the binding of these receptors to adhesive proteins (primarily fibrinogen) favoring platelet–platelet interaction (i.e., the aggregation process) (Figure 1.3).[12] About 50 000 GPIIb/IIIa receptors are randomly distributed on the surfaces of resting platelets. The heterodimeric complex is composed of one molecule of GPIIb (disulfide-linked heavy and light chains) and one of GPIIIa (single polypeptide chain). It is a Ca^{2+}-dependent heterodimer, non-covalently associated on the platelet membrane.[13] Ca^{2+} is required for maintenance of the complex and for binding of adhesive proteins. On activated platelets, the GPIIb/IIIa is a receptor not only for fibrinogen, but also to a lesser extent, for fibronectin, vWF, vitronectin, and thrombospondin. The receptor recognition sequences are localized to small peptide sequences (RGD) in the adhesive proteins. Fibrinogen contains two RGD sequences in its α-chain: one near the N-terminus (residues 95–97) and a second near the C-terminus (residues 572–574). Fibrinogen has a second site of recognition for GPIIb/IIIa, which is a 12-amino acid sequence located at the C-terminus of the γ-chain of the molecule. This dodecapeptide is specific for fibrinogen and does not contain the RGD sequence, but competes with RGD-containing peptides for binding to GPIIb/IIIa.[14] At the same time as GPIIb/IIIa activation, platelet membrane phospholipids translocate, leading to exposition of negatively charged phosphatidylserine (PS) at the outer part of the membrane. PS forms a critical catalytic surface for coagulation factor activity.[3] Accumulation of PS also induces emission of microvesicles, which probably play a major role in disseminating platelet procoagulant activity.[15] Since PS-expressing platelets enhance coagulation, and, in turn, the coagulation product

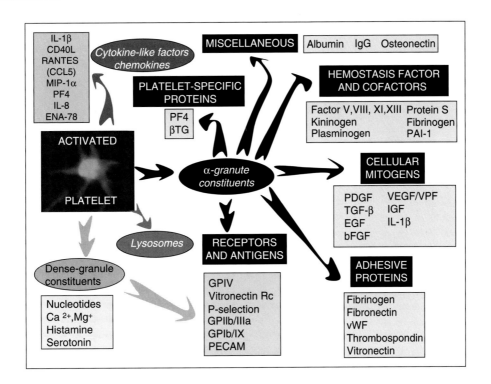

Figure 1.2
(see color plate)

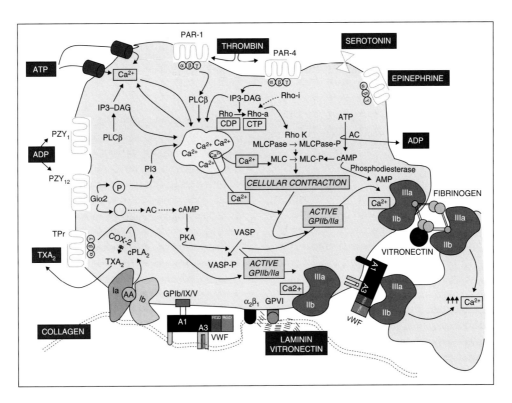

Figure 1.3
(see color plate)

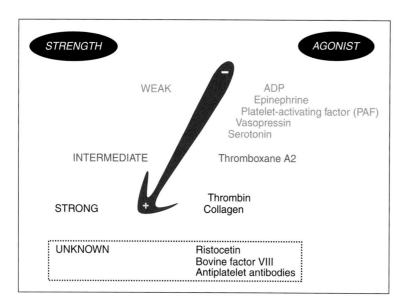

Figure 1.4

thrombin stimulates platelets, both processes are in a strong positive-feedback loop, which can have a control function in hemostasis and thrombosis.[16] In fact, thrombin generation measurements with platelets in plasma indeed demonstrate synergistic activity of PS-expressing platelets and the coagulant system.[16]

Coagulation cascade
Clot formation

Thrombin is one of the most potent known agonists for platelet activation and recruitment and constitutes a bridge between platelets and the coagulation cascade.

The blood coagulation system involves a sequence of reactions integrating zymogens (proteins susceptible to activation by enzymes via limited proteolysis) and cofactors (non-proteolytic enzyme activators) in three groups: (i) contact activation (generation of activated factor XI (FXIa) via the Hageman factor (FXII), (ii) the conversion of FX to FXa in a complex reaction requiring the participation of factors IX and VIII, and (iii) the conversion of prothrombin to thrombin and fibrin formation (Figure 1.5). Clotting factors are synthesized mainly in the liver and circulate in the bloodstream, except tissue factor (TF) and FV, FXI, and FXIII, which are also found in extravascular cells and platelets. The clotting enzymes do not collide and interact on a random basis in the plasma, but interact in complexes in a highly efficient manner on platelet and endothelial surfaces. In fact, the major regulatory events in coagulation (activation, inhibition, and generation of anticoagulant proteins) occur on membrane surfaces.

The so-called intrinsic pathway (i.e., contact activation) plays a minor role in physiological haemostasis. Vessel wall sulfatides and glycosaminoglycans have been suggested to be the in vivo triggers of the intrinsic pathway. However, the physiological role of this system is unclear, because absence of Hageman factor (FXII), prekallikrein, or high-molecular-weight kininogen (HMWK) does not impair normal hemostasis, although they induce a prolongation of the activated partial thromboplastin time (aPTT). Once activated, FXII, prekalikrein, and HMWK result in FXI activation, which in turn induces the activation of FIX in the presence of Ca^{2+}. FIX is a vitamin K-dependent enzyme, as are FVII, FX, prothrombin, and protein C. Thereafter, FIXa forms a catalytic complex with FVIII on the membrane surface and efficiently activates FX in the presence of Ca^{2+}. FVIII forms a non-covalent complex with vWF in plasma, and its function in coagulation is the acceleration of the effects of FIXa on the activation of FX to FXa. Absence of FVIII or IX produces the hemophilic syndromes, whereas FXI deficiency is associated with abnormal bleeding.

The initiating event for the activation of the extrinsic coagulation pathway is the exposure of TF to flowing blood. TF, also known as thrombokinase, thromboplastin, CD142, and FIII, is a 47 kDa membrane glycoprotein that consists of a large extracellular domain with two fibronectin type III modules joined by a hinge region, a single transmembrane domain, and a short cytoplasmic tail.[17,18] The two modules in the extracellular domain are important for TF function in coagulation.

Ruptured plaque, damaged vessels, and dysfunctional endothelium express TF on their surfaces, although TF may also be carried by leukocytes, lymphocytes, and (as recently detected) activated platelets.[19–21] Furthermore, non-functional or encrypted TF present in microparticles (MPs) from monocytes and neutrophils is present in blood from healthy subjects, and the term bloodborne TF was introduced for such TF.[19] The concept of bloodborne TF was corroborated by Chou et al[22] in elegant experiments using in vitro microscopy for studying thrombus formation in

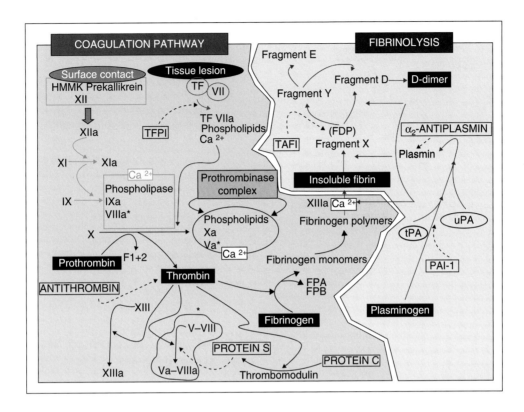

Figure 1.5

living mice. It was found that low-TF mice (1%) in contrast to wild-type mice developed very small platelet thrombi lacking TF or fibrin. Furthermore, wild-type and low-TF mice were then given transplants of bone marrow from wild-type or low-TF mice to produce chimera. Arterial thrombi in wild-type bone marrow/low-TF chimeric mice showed decreased platelet thrombus size but normal TF and fibrin levels, whereas low-TF bone marrow/wild-type chimera had decreased thrombus size and decreased TF and fibrin levels. It was therefore concluded that bloodborne TF associated with MPs derived from hematopoietic cells contributes to thrombus propagation in the microvascular system. Nevertheless, the occurrence of circulating TF-containing MPs,[23] elevated levels of TF antigen measured in patients with acute coronary syndromes,[24] neutrophil-associated TF, and platelet-associated TF are all phenomena that raise new questions regarding the role and potential of TF in inflammation, thrombosis, and haemostasis.

Once TF is exposed to the circulation, it forms a complex with FVII or FVIIa (about 1% of the FVII protein is normally present in an activated form in the circulation)[25] on the surface of the TF-bearing cell.[26] There is a disulfide bond in the membrane-proximal domain of TF that links adjacent strands in the same β-sheet; this has been called a cross-strand bond. This cross-strand bond is reduced in cryptic TF, but not in the active form. The high-affinity

($K_d < 10$ pmol/l) binding between exposed TF and circulating FVII/VIIa creates a reactive vessel surface that proteolytically cleaves FIX and FX. The rate of this surface-bound reaction depends not only on biochemical factors (number and surface density of TF/VIIa complexes, intrinsic kinetic activity, and local phospholipid composition)[27] but also on the rate at which the substrates FIX and FX are transported by the flowing medium to the reactive surface[28] and the rate at which product is removed.[29] Moreover, the local accumulation of reaction product may be critical in overpowering endogenous inhibitors and successfully initiating coagulation. Nevertheless, once coupled, the TF/FVIIa complex activates FIX and FX, generating low amounts of FXa (initiation phase). Eventually, the final step of the initiation phase of the hemostatic process is the formation of a limited amount of thrombin that not only causes back-activation of FV, FVIII, and FXI but also influences a wide range of physiological responses, as illustrated in Figure 1.6.[30,31]

The role of thrombin in platelet activation and aggregation involves protease-activated receptor (PAR)-1 and PAR-4 at much lower concentrations than those needed to produce its coagulant effect. Once cleaved, PAR-1 rapidly transmits a signal across the plasma membrane to internally located G-proteins, culminating in the formation of platelet–platelet aggregates.[32] PAR-1-dependent formation of platelet–platelet aggregates through GPIIb/IIIa tends to be transient unless strengthened by additional inputs from the

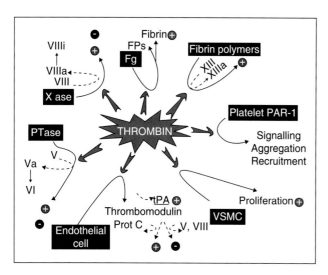

Figure 1.6

P2Y$_{12}$ ADP receptor or from the PAR-4 receptor. Conversely, thrombin signalling through PAR-4 is quite distinct from that through PAR-1. PAR-4 is cleaved and signals more slowly, but, despite its slower response, generates a large intracellular calcium flux that does not require additional input from the P2Y$_{12}$ ADP receptor to form stable platelet–platelet aggregates.[33]

It has been proposed that during the initial stage of coagulation, where a low level of thrombin is generated, the plasma inhibitors antithrombin III (ATIII) and TF pathway inhibitor (TFPI) can prevent the formation of fibrin. ATIII is present in plasma at high concentrations; it binds thrombin and other activated clotting factors and inhibits their enzyme activities, whereas TFPI binds to FXa first, and the TFPI/FXa complex then binds to and inhibits FVIIa/TF activity.

The second phase – the propagation phase – occurs on the surface of the thrombin-activated platelet through complex formation between FIXa and FVIIIa (the tenase complex) and between FXa and FVa (the prothrombinase complex). As a result, a full burst of thrombin is generated on the thrombin-activated platelet surface.[34–36] In turn, thrombin is capable of cleaving fibrinopeptides A and B from fibrinogen, yielding insoluble fibrin, which effectively anchors the evolving thrombus.[37] FXIII, once activated by thrombin, stabilizes the fibrin plug by creating covalent links between fibrin monomers. The resulting fibrin mesh holds the platelets together and contributes to the attachment of the thrombus to the vessel wall. If fibrinolysis is impaired, this platelet/fibrin clot can propagate rapidly, resulting in an occlusive thrombus and the subsequent acute clinical event.

In vitro microscopy has provided evidence that plasma fibronectin may be a substitute for fibrinogen to occlude the injured vessel and play a significant role in platelet thrombus formation under high-shear conditions.[38] Fibronectin is a glycoprotein dimer of 250 kDa subunits that is present in a soluble form in plasma and other body fluids and in an insoluble form in tissues.[39] Moreover, plasma fibronectin has been demonstrated to be a substrate for FXIIIa, thereby becoming incorporated into fibrin clots.[40] Fibrin crosslinked to fibronectin by FXIIIa constitutes a three-dimensional matrix that increases adhesion and spreading of fibroblasts compared with fibrin alone, and thus causes altered shear moduli and denser fibrin clots.[41]

Aside from altering the structure of the fibrin network, a possible role of fibronectin in blood clots is to mediate interactions between cells or platelets and fibrin. Thus, as described above, fibronectin as well as fibrin may interact with platelet GPIIb/IIIa during clot retraction, a function that is deficient in Glanzmann's thrombasthenia.[42]

Physiological pathways involved in clot dissolution

Fibrinolysis is the enzymatic process leading to fibrin clot solubilization by plasmin originating from fibrin-bound plasminogen (Figure 1.5). Plasmin is also able to proteolyze FVIII, FV, vWF, and FXIII, as well as selected components of the extracellular matrix. Proteolysis of fibrin by plasmin induces generation of fibrin degradation products (FDP). The most specific of stabilized FDP are D-dimers. Elevated plasma levels of D-dimers are a marker for increased thrombin formation and fibrin degradation turn-over.

Plasminogen is synthesized by hepatocytes and has a high affinity for fibrin through peptidic loops called 'kringles'. The principal plasminogen activator is tissue-type plasminogen activator (tPA), which also exhibits two 'kringle' loops with a high affinity for fibrin. tPA is synthesized mainly by endothelial cells, and is secreted locally after stimulation of the endothelium by histamine, epinephrine, thrombin, FXa, and hypoxia. The second plasminogen activator is urokinase-type plasminogen activator (uPA), which is synthesized by numerous cell types, including fibroblasts, epithelial cells, and placental cells, and plays a minor role in physiological fibrinolysis. The native form of uPA is pro-urokinase, a single-chain protein, which is turned into a two-chain protein by plasmin or the contact factors (FXII, prekallikrein, and HMWK).

Under physiological conditions, thrombin also plays a pivotal role in maintaining the complex balance of initial prothrombotic events and subsequent endogenous anticoagulant and thrombolytic pathways. Thrombin generated at the site of injury binds to thrombomodulin, an endothelial surface membrane protein, initiating activation of protein C, which in turn (in the presence of protein S) inactivates FVa and FVIIIa (Figure 1.5). Thrombin stimulates successive release of both tPA and plasminogen activator inhibitor type 1 (PAI-1) from endothelial cells, thus initiating endogenous lysis through plasmin generation from plasminogen by tPA, with subsequent modulation through PAI-1.[43] PAI-1 is present in large excess in flowing blood, and prevents inappropriate plasmin generation by forming an inactive covalent complex with tPA and uPA. PAI-1 plasma levels are increased in inflammatory states, insulin resistance syndromes, and obesity. Finally, besides PAI-1, another regulator of fibrinolysis is thrombin-activatable fibrinolysis inhibitor (TAFI), which is synthesized by hepatocytes and is able to decrease plasminogen binding to fibrin.[44] TAFI circulates as an inactive protein, which is activated by the thrombin/thrombomodulin complex and then eliminates the arginine and lysine residues exposed on the surface of fibrin.

Summary

Thrombosis is the final step in the clinical complication of atherosclerotic plaque progression, and is therefore a common process in the presentation of coronary artery disease, cerebrovascular disease, peripheral artery disease, and revascularization procedures. In addition to platelets, coagulation and fibrinolysis, inflammatory pathways are also activated within a growing thrombus and can participate in the clinical complication of silent atherosclerosis. Plaque–platelet–fibrin–leukocyte interactions are currently under intensive investigation in order to evaluate their real impact in clinical thrombosis. Advances in the cellular and molecular characterization of all the partners participating in the process might open up new possibilities to reduce or inhibit the impact of this highly relevant problem for patients with high cardiovascular risk.

References

1. Badimon L, Chesebro JH, Badimon JJ. Thrombus formation on ruptured atherosclerotic plaques and rethrombosis on evolving thrombi. Circulation 1992;86(6 Suppl):III74–85.
2. Badimon L, Fuster V, Corti R et al. Coronary thrombosis: local and systemic factors. In: Fuster V, ed. Hurst's the Heart, 11th edn. New York: McGraw-Hill, 2004;1141–51.
3. Heemskerk JW, Bevers EM, Lindhout T. Platelet activation and blood coagulation. Thromb Haemost 2002;88:186–93.
4. Siljander PR, Munnix IC, Smethurst PA et al. Platelet receptor interplay regulates collagen-induced thrombus formation in flowing human blood. Blood 2004;103:1333–41.
5. Denis CV, Wagner DD. Platelet adhesion receptors and their ligands in mouse models of thrombosis. Arterioscler Thromb Vasc Biol 2007;27:728–39.
6. Rendu F, Brohard-Bohn B. The platelet release reaction: granules' constituents, secretion and functions. Platelets 2001;12:261–73.
7. Cho J, Mosher DF. Role of fibronectin assembly in platelet thrombus formation. J Thromb Haemost 2006;4:1461–69.
8. Bastida E, Escolar G, Ordinas A et al. Fibronectin is required for platelet adhesion and for thrombus formation on subendothelium and collagen surfaces. Blood 1987;70:1437–42.
9. Canobbio I, Balduini C, Torti M. Signalling through the platelet glycoprotein Ib–V–IX complex. Cell Signal 2004;16:1329–44.
10. Ware J. Molecular analyses of the platelet glycoprotein Ib–IX–V receptor. Thromb Haemost 1998;79:466–78.
11. Chow TW, Hellums JD, Moake JL et al. Shear stress-induced von Willebrand factor binding to platelet glycoprotein Ib initiates calcium influx associated with aggregation. Blood 1992;80:113–20.
12. Andrews RK, Berndt MC. Platelet physiology and thrombosis. Thromb Res 2004;114:447–53.
13. Schwarz M, Meade G, Stoll P et al. Conformation-specific blockade of the integrin GPIIb/IIIa: a novel antiplatelet strategy that selectively targets activated platelets. Circ Res 2006;99:25–33.
14. Kamata T, Takada Y. Platelet integrin $\alpha_{IIb}\beta_3$-ligand interactions: What can we learn from the structure? Int J Hematol 2001;74:382–9.
15. Basse F, Gaffet P, Rendu F et al. Translocation of spin-labeled phospholipids through plasma membrane during thrombin- and ionophore A23187-induced platelet activation. Biochemistry 1993;32:2337–44.
16. Beguin S, Kumar R. Thrombin, fibrin and platelets: a resonance loop in which von Willebrand factor is a necessary link. Thromb Haemost 1997;78:590–4.
17. Ruf W, Edgington TS. Structural biology of tissue factor, the initiator of thrombogenesis in vivo. FASEB J 1994;8:385–90.
18. Eilertsen KE, Osterud B. Tissue factor: (patho)physiology and cellular biology. Blood Coagul Fibrinolysis 2004;15:521–38.
19. Giesen PL, Rauch U, Bohrmann B et al. Blood-borne tissue factor: another view of thrombosis. Proc Natl Acad Sci U S A 1999;96:2311–15.
20. Panes O, Matus V, Saez CG et al. Human platelets synthesize and express functional tissue factor. Blood 2007;109:5242–50.
21. Osterud B, Bjorklid E. Sources of tissue factor. Semin Thromb Hemost 2006;32:11–23.
22. Chou J, Mackman N, Merrill-Skoloff G et al. Hematopoietic cell-derived microparticle tissue factor contributes to fibrin formation during thrombus propagation. Blood 2004;104:3190–7.
23. Nieuwland R, Berckmans RJ, McGregor S et al. Cellular origin and procoagulant properties of microparticles in meningococcal sepsis. Blood 2000;95:930–5.
24. Suefuji H, Ogawa H, Yasue H et al. Increased plasma tissue factor levels in acute myocardial infarction. Am Heart J 1997;134:253–9.
25. Wildgoose P, Nemerson Y, Hansen LL et al. Measurement of basal levels of factor VIIa in hemophilia A and B patients. Blood 1992;80:25–8.
26. Rapaport SI, Rao LV. Initiation and regulation of tissue factor-dependent blood coagulation. Arterioscler Thromb 1992;12:1111–21.
27. Hathcock J. Vascular biology - the role of tissue factor. Semin Hematol 2004;41(1 Suppl 1):30–4.
28. Contino PB, Andree HA, Nemerson Y. Flow dependence of factor X activation by tissue factor–factor VIIa. J Physiol Pharmacol 1994;45:81–90.
29. Hathcock JJ, Rusinova E, Gentry RD et al. Phospholipid regulates the activation of factor X by tissue factor/factor VIIa (TF/VIIa) via substrate and product interactions. Biochemistry 2005;44:8187–97.
30. Vu TK, Hung DT, Wheaton VI et al. Molecular cloning of a functional thrombin receptor reveals a novel proteolytic mechanism of receptor activation. Cell 1991;64:1057–68.
31. Leger AJ, Covic L, Kuliopulos A. Protease-activated receptors in cardiovascular diseases. Circulation 2006;114:1070–7.
32. Leger A, Lidija C, Kuliopulos A. Protease-activated receptors in cardiovascular diseases. Circulation 2006;114:1070–7.
33. Covic L, Gresser A, Kuliopulos A. Biphasic kinetics of activation and signaling for PAR1 and PAR4 thrombin receptors in platelets. Biochemistry 2000;39:5458–67.
34. Hedner U. Mechanism of action of factor VIIa in the treatment of coagulopathies. Semin Thromb Hemost 2006;32(Suppl 1):77–85.

35. Monroe DM, Hoffman M, Roberts HR. Platelets and thrombin generation. Arterioscler Thromb Vasc Biol 2002;22:1381–9.

36. Kempton CL, Hoffman M, Roberts HR et al. Platelet heterogeneity: variation in coagulation complexes on platelet subpopulations. Arterioscler Thromb Vasc Biol 2005;25:861–6.

37. Pechik I, Yakovlev S, Mosesson MW et al. Structural basis for sequential cleavage of fibrinopeptides upon fibrin assembly. Biochemistry 2006;45:3588–97.

38. Ni H, Yuen PS, Papalia JM et al. Plasma fibronectin promotes thrombus growth and stability in injured arterioles. Proc Natl Acad Sci U S A 2003;100:2415–19.

39. Cho J, Mosher DF. Enhancement of thrombogenesis by plasma fibronectin cross-linked to fibrin and assembled in platelet thrombi. Blood 2006;107:3555–63.

40. Mosher DF. Cross-linking of cold-insoluble globulin by fibrin-stabilizing factor. J Biol Chem 1975;250:6614–21.

41. Bereczky Z, Katona E, Muszbek L. Fibrin stabilization (factor XIII), fibrin structure and thrombosis. Pathophysiol Haemost Thromb 2003/4;33:430–7.

42. Jelenska M, Kopec M, Breddin K. On the retraction of collagen and fibrin induced by normal, defective and modified platelets. Haemostasis 1985;15:169–75.

43. Collen D, Lijnen HR. Tissue-type plasminogen activator: a historical perspective and personal account. J Thromb Haemost 2004;2:541–6.

44. Bouma BN, Mosnier LO. Thrombin activatable fibrinolysis inhibitor (TAFI) at the interface between coagulation and fibrinolysis. Pathophysiol Haemost Thromb 2003/4;33:375–81.

2

Platelet receptors and their role in atherothrombosis

Harald Langer and Meinrad Gawaz

Introduction

Unlike other cells, Figure 1 platelets lack a nucleus and therefore cannot adapt rapidly to their microenvironment with extensive de novo protein synthesis, although evidence for protein synthesis from mRNA in platelets has been described.[1] Thus, platelets need to be equipped with a sufficient supply of pre-existing molecules ready to react properly and efficiently within seconds to different (patho)physiological requirements. One of the predominant characteristics of platelets is the presence of a wide range of receptors, which are either constitutively expressed on the platelet surface or partially stored in storage granules and rapidly brought to the surface upon activation. Although the 'original' role of platelets is primary hemostasis, they express many receptors not directly involved in the thrombotic process. Thus, besides their role in hemostasis/thrombosis, platelets are significantly involved in various pathophysiological mechanisms, including inflammation, immunomodulation, tumor progression, and atherogenesis.[2–4] The border between physiological hemostasis and initiation or progression of diseases mediated by platelets is narrow and shifting. This chapter gives an overview of the central role of platelet receptors in platelet function, and focuses on their role receptors in atherothrombosis.

Platelet receptors

The mechanisms of hemostasis and thrombosis require close interplay between platelets, endothelium, plasma coagulation factors, and the structures of the vessel wall (extracellular matrix). Adhesion processes regulated by numerous specific adhesion receptors play a major role in these mechanisms. Platelets express glycoproteins (GPs) on their membranes that mediate the interactions of the platelets among themselves (GPIIb/IIIa) as well as with the subendothelial matrix (von Willebrand factor (vWF) receptors

and collagen receptors), with plasma coagulation factors (von Willebrand receptor), and with endothelial cells (GPIIb/IIIa) and leukocytes (P-selectin). Besides adhesion receptors, platelets possess a variety of signal transduction receptors that respond primarily to soluble agonists such as adenosine diphosphate (ADP) and thrombin and play a major role in platelet activation.

Platelet adhesion receptors are classified into four groups according to their characteristic molecular structures: *integrins, leucine-rich glycoproteins, selectins,* and *receptors of immunoglobulin type* (Figure 2.1). The function of many platelet receptors has been elucidated, although the physiological role of various other receptors remains obscure. In this chapter, the focus is on platelet receptors that are already or will become pharmacological targets for antithrombotics in the treatment of cardiovascular diseases (Figure 2.1).

Integrins

Integrins are adhesion receptors that link structures of the cytoskeleton with the extracellular matrix.[5] They are noncovalently linked heterodimers consisting of α- and β-subunits, interact with numerous glycoproteins (e.g., collagen, fibronectin, fibrinogen, laminin, thrombospondin, vitronectin and vWF), mediate platelet aggregation, and contribute to tissue differentiation and development. Five different integrins have been described on platelets: three of the β_1 class and two of the β_3 class. The β_1 and β_3 integrins recognize the arginine–glycine–aspartate (RGD) amino acid sequence – a sequence found in extracellular matrix proteins, including fibrinogen.

Leucine-rich receptors

The leucine-rich family is represented in platelets by the GPIb/IX/V complex, the second most common receptor on

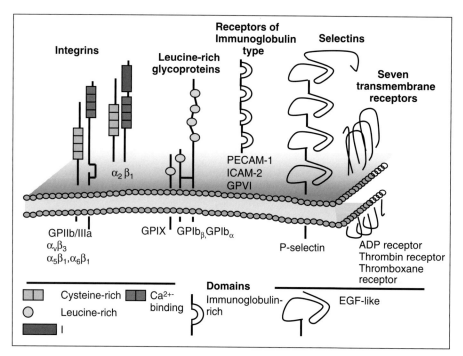

Figure 2.1
Central platelet membrane receptors involved in atherothrombosis. GP, glycoprotein; PECAM, platelet–endothelial cell adhesion molecule; ICAM, intercellular adhesion molecule, EGF, epidermal growth factor.

platelets (after $\alpha_{IIb}\beta_3$ integrin). It forms an adhesion complex for vWF and plays a central role in primary hemostasis. Despite the high shear forces that exist in arterial flow, it is capable of establishing a firm contact to vWF immobilized in collagen fibrils. Its absence or deficiency leads to Bernard–Soulier syndrome, the second most common bleeding disorder linked to a platelet receptor.

Receptors of immunoglobulin type

The role of the immunoglobulin-type receptor family is currently under intense investigation. Next to intercellular adhesion molecule 2 (ICAM-2) and platelet–endothelial cell adhesion molecule 1 (PECAM-1), which are involved in the interaction of platelets with leukocytes, GPVI, one of the two major platelet collagen receptors, has been recognized as playing a central role in platelet function, and may be a potential therapeutic target for cardiovascular diseases.[6,7] Therefore, this receptor and its implications in atherothrombosis are discussed in detail below.

Selectins

The selectins are an important group of adhesion receptors present on platelets (P-selectin), endothelium (E- and P-selectin), and lymphocytes (L-selectin). Following platelet activation, P-selectin is rapidly released and surface-expressed. Selectins mediate multiple transient weak interactions with ligands, thereby facilitating the establishment of stable binding via other involved receptors.

Seven transmembrane receptors

The major agonist receptor family is represented by the seven transmembrane receptors, including thrombin receptors, the prostaglandin family receptors, and the ADP receptors. By binding of thrombin, platelets can be activated via a G-protein-linked pathway. Platelet activation by ADP plays a key role in the development and pathogenesis of atherothrombosis, and therefore these mechanisms are of particular pharmacological and medical interest.[8] Platelets are presently the only cells known to express ADP-specific purinoreceptors, including the $P2Y_1$ and $P2Y_{12}$ receptors.

Role of platelets in early atherosclerosis

Atherosclerosis is a systemic inflammatory disease characterized by the accumulation of monocytes/macrophages and lymphocytes in the intima of large arteries.[9] Rupture or erosion of the advanced lesion initiates platelet activation and aggregation on the surface of the disrupted atherosclerotic plaque. Thrombotic vascular occlusion is associated with ischemic episodes, including acute coronary syndromes and cerebral infarction. While it is widely accepted that platelets play a significant role in thromboembolic complications of advanced atherosclerotic lesions, their involvement in the initiation of the atherosclerotic process has received scant attention. In the last few years, however, it has become increasingly evident that endothelial denudation is not an absolute prerequisite for platelet attachment to the arterial wall.[10] The intact, non-activated endothelium normally prevents platelet adhesion to the extracellular matrix. Under inflammatory conditions, platelets can adhere to the intact, but activated, endothelial cell monolayer.[11–13] Even under high shear stress, platelet adhesion to the intact endothelium occurs in vivo and is coordinated in a multistep process that involves platelet tethering, followed by rolling and subsequent firm adhesion to the vascular wall.[14,15] These processes involve receptor interactions via selectins, integrins, and immunoglobulin-like receptors, which induce receptor-specific activation signals in both platelets and the respective adhesive cell type.

The initial loose contact between circulating platelets and vascular endothelium ('platelet rolling') is mediated by selectins, present on both endothelial cells and platelets.[14,16–19] P-selectin is rapidly expressed on the endothelial surface in response to inflammatory stimuli by translocating from membranes of storage granules (Weibel–Palade bodies) to the plasma membrane within seconds. Endothelial P-selectin has been demonstrated to mediate platelet rolling in both arterioles and venules in acute inflammatory processes.[14,16] E-selectin, which is also expressed on inflamed endothelial cells, allows a loose contact between platelets and endothelium in vivo, too.[16] In line with the concept of endothelial inflammation as a trigger for platelet accumulation, the process of platelet rolling does not require previous platelet activation, since platelets from mice lacking P- and/or E-selectin roll as efficiently as wild-type platelets.[15]

GPIIb/IIIa ($\alpha_{IIb}\beta_3$) is the major integrin on platelets and plays a key role in platelet accumulation on activated endothelium. In the presence of soluble fibrinogen, $\alpha_{IIb}\beta_3$ mediates heterotypic cell adhesion to $\alpha_v\beta_3$-expressing cells, including endothelial cells.[13,20] Moreover, platelets adhere firmly to activated endothelial cells via $\alpha_{IIb}\beta_3$, a mechanism that can be blocked by antagonists of β_3 integrins.[13] In vivo, firm platelet adhesion to the endothelium can be inhibited by anti-$\alpha_{IIb}\beta_3$ monoclonal antibodies, and platelets defective in $\alpha_{IIb}\beta_3$ do not adhere firmly to activated endothelial cells.[21] Taken together, these data indicate that, apart from mediating platelet aggregation, the platelet fibrinogen receptor $\alpha_{IIb}\beta_3$ is of paramount importance in mediating firm attachment of platelets to the vascular endothelium. Recently, a new receptor for platelet $\alpha_{IIb}\beta_3$, ADAM15, has been identified, which is able to mediate platelet adhesion to endothelial cells, activation of platelets, and thrombus formation.[22]

Among the integrins expressed on the luminal side of endothelial cells, the vitronectin receptor ($\alpha_v\beta_3$) appears to play a crucial role in promoting platelet adhesion. The vitronectin receptor is upregulated in response to endothelial cell activation, for example by interleukin (IL)-1β or thrombin.[13,23] Inhibition of $\alpha_v\beta_3$ attenuates platelet–endothelial cell interaction.[13] Hence, both platelet $\alpha_{IIb}\beta_3$ and endothelial $\alpha_v\beta_3$ are involved in mediating firm platelet adhesion to activated endothelial cells. However, direct binding of $\alpha_{IIb}\beta_3$ to endothelial $\alpha_v\beta_3$ has not been reported so far. In fact, heterotypic cell adhesion through $\alpha_{IIb}\beta_3$ and $\alpha_v\beta_3$ requires the presence of fibrinogen, which bridges the platelet fibrinogen receptor to the endothelial vitronectin receptor.[20] The affinity of platelet $\alpha_{IIb}\beta_3$ for its ligand underlies strict regulation and increases with platelet activation ('inside-out integrin signaling'). During adhesion, platelets are activated and release proinflammatory cytokines and chemoattractants (e.g., IL-1 and RANTES (CCL5)) and surface-express CD40 ligand (CD40L). Interaction of platelets with endothelial cells triggers secretion of chemokines and expression of adhesion molecules, and promotes adhesion of leukocytes. In this manner, the adhesion of platelets to the endothelial surface might generate signals for recruitment and extravasation of monocytes during atherosclerotic plaque formation, a process of paramount importance for atherogenesis. In vivo experiments in *ApoE−/−* mice in the early and advanced stages of atherosclerosis showed that platelets adhere to the arterial wall in vivo in the absence of endothelial cell denudation. Inhibition of this interaction significantly reduced atherosclerosis formation, indicating that platelet adhesion plays a critical role in the initiation of atherosclerosis.[24]

In summary, platelet–endothelial cell interactions involve a multistep process, in which selectins, integrins, and immunoglobin-like adhesion receptors play a predominant role. These receptor-dependent platelet–endothelial cell interactions allow transcellular communication via soluble mediators and therefore play an important role in the initiation and progression of vascular inflammation and atheroprogression (Figure 2.2).

Activated platelets roll along the endothelial monolayer via GPIb/P-selectin or P-selectin glycoprotein ligand 1 (PSGL-1)/P-selectin. Thereafter, platelets adhere firmly to vascular endothelium via β_3 integrins, release proinflammatory compounds (IL-1β and CD40L), and induce a proatherogenic phenotype of endothelial cells (chemotaxis: monocyte chemotactic protein 1: (MCP-1); adhesion: (ICAM-1). Subsequently, adherent platelets recruit circulating leukocytes, bind them, and activate them by receptor interactions and paracrine pathways, thereby initiating leukocyte transmigration and foam cell formation. Thus, platelets provide the inflammatory basis for plaque formation before physically occluding the vessel by thrombosis upon plaque rupture.

Platelet adhesion to vascular lesions (Figure 2.3)

At the site of vascular lesions, rupture of an atherosclerotic plaque results in discontinuity of the endothelial barrier, with exposure of thrombogenic subendothelial matrix proteins. Platelets are the first cellular components to cover

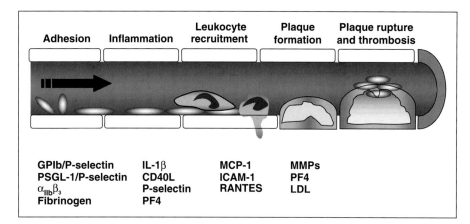

Figure 2.2
Model of atherogenesis triggered by platelets. GP, glycoprotein; PSGL, P-selectin glycoprotein ligand; IL, interleukin; PF, platelet factor; MCP, monocyte chemotactic protein; ICAM, intercellular adhesion molecule; MMP, matrix metalloproteinase; LDL, low-density lipoprotein.

such a defect by a complex cascade with distinct interacting mechanisms.[25]

Numerous studies have shown that the initial contact of circulating platelets with the vascular lesion is mediated via interaction of platelet GPIb/V/IX with collagen-bound vWF. Recent data have revealed that a further membrane glycoprotein, the platelet collagen receptor GPVI, plays a critical role in the adhesion process. Fibrillar collagen is the major extracellular matrix protein. Inhibition of interaction of GPVI with collagen by anti-GPVI monoclonal antibodies or soluble dimeric GPVI attenuates thrombosis at arterial lesions in vivo.[26] In contrast to GPIb/V/IX, it directly mediates adhesion to subendothelial collagen and the activation of other adhesion receptors such as GPIIb/IIIa and $\alpha_2\beta_1$. These integrins are essential for firm adhesion of platelets. While $\alpha_2\beta_1$ binds directly to collagen, the GPIIb/IIIa receptor mediates irreversible adhesion through binding to an RGD sequence in the C1 domain of vWF. The firm integrin-mediated adhesion results in activation and change in shape of platelets. During this process, platelets form pseudopodia, which allow effective coverage of the injured vessel wall. The adhesive and activated platelets produce thromboxane A_2 (TXA_2) from arachidonic acid (AA), which strengthens the activation process by binding to the specific thromboxane receptor. Following TXA_2, ADP is released from platelets and intensifies the process of adhesion, activation, and finally aggregation.

Platelet aggregation and thrombus formation (Figure 2.3)

Aggregation is the amplification step that, within minutes, leads to the accumulation of platelets into the hemostatic thrombus. It is mediated by adhesive substrates bound to the membranes of activated platelets. After platelets have established contact with the thrombogenic substrate, the interaction of further platelets from the circulation with already-adherent platelets is mediated via the activated GPIIb/IIIa receptor. A principal outcome of platelet activation is a change in the ligand-binding function of $\alpha IIb\beta III$. During the initial phase (primary aggregation), platelets are connected to each other only by 'loose' fibrinogen bridges. Seconds to minutes later, this contact is followed by an irreversible stabilization of the fibrinogen bridges at the GPIIb/IIIa complex. Furthermore, platelets are shedding microparticles from their cell membrane, which catalyze fibrin formation and stabilization of the thrombus. Stability of the aggregate is as important as its rate of growth, determining whether a thrombus will occlude an artery. CD40L, another recently described receptor expressed on platelets, seems to be crucial for stabilization of the aggregates. Table 2.1 gives an overview of the main receptor/ligand interactions involved in the process of thrombus formation, from the initiation of adhesion to thrombus formation.

Depending on the extent of thrombus formation within coronary vessels, this process determines the extent of clinical manifestations, ranging from asymptomatic coronary heart disease to fatal myocardial infarction.[27]

Perspectives
Plaque imaging

At late stages, there are sufficient modalities to measure the extent of atherosclerotic disease and therapeutic success, including clinical parameters, laboratory markers such as troponin and creatinine kinase, and imaging techniques such as coronary angiography and computed tomograph (CT). However, in the early stage of atherosclerosis, there are to date no practicable facilities to image patients with vulnerable atherosclerotic plaques, which are prone to plaque rupture with subsequent thrombosis. In recent studies, we have made use of the platelet collagen receptor GPVI to detect vulnerable atherosclerotic lesions. Using a soluble dimeric form of human GPVI conjugated to an Fc fragment

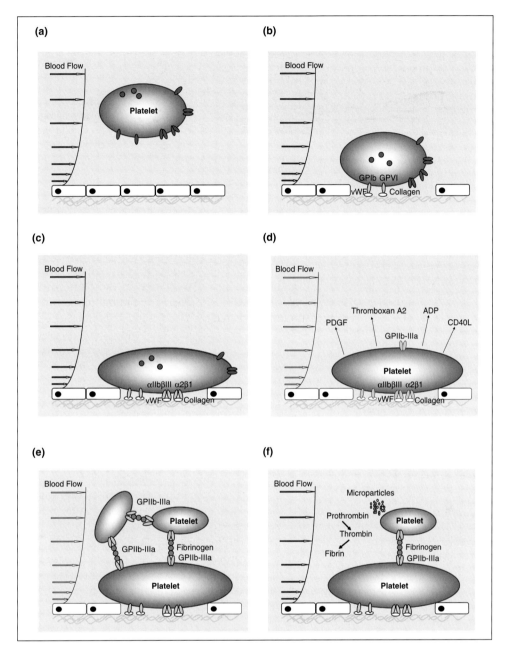

Figure 2.3
Under physiological conditions, platelets do not adhere to intact endothelium. (b) If the endothelial monolyer is disrupted, subendothelial matrix proteins are exposed, including collagen and von Willebrand factor (vWF). Platelets initiate initial contact with the subendothelium via their membrane adhesion receptors GPIb and GPVI. (c) This contact results in activation of platelet integrins $\alpha_{IIb}\beta_3$ (fibrinogen receptor) and $\alpha_2\beta_1$ (collagen receptor). Interaction of $\alpha_{IIb}\beta_3$ and $\alpha_2\beta_1$ with extracellular matrix proteins leads to 'spreading' and firm adhesion of platelets. (d) Subsequently, platelets secrete mediators and recruit other circulating platelets. (e) Platelets form microaggregates via a fibrinogen bridging mechanism between two GPIIb/IIIa receptors. (f) Formation of microparticles in the microenvironment of platelet aggregates catalytes thrombin and subsequently fibrin generation, which stabilizes the growing thrombus. (see color plate)

that was radioiodinated, we were able to visualize lesions of injured carotic arteries in mice by ex vivo and in vivo imaging (Figure 2.4).[28] As an experimental model for vulnerable plaques in atherosclerosis, *ApoE−/−* knockout mice were used and wire-induced injury of the carotid artery was per-

formed. In general, the thrombogenity of atherosclerotic plaques is one of the most promising approaches to detect vulnerable plaques, and is currently being evaluated using new imgaging modalities such as positron emission tomography (PET)-CT.

Table 2.1 *Receptors and agonists involved in thrombus formation*

Phase of thrombus formation	Agonist	Receptor
Adhesion	vWF	GPIb/V/IX
	Collagen	$\alpha_2\beta_1$, GPVI
	Fibrinogen	$\alpha_{IIb}\beta_3$
	Fibronectin	$\alpha_5\beta_1$
	Laminin	$\alpha_6\beta_1$
Activation	α-thrombin	PAR-1, PAR-4
		GPIb/V/IX
	ADP	$P2Y_1$
		$P2Y_{12}$
	TXA_2	TP
Aggregation	Fibrinogen, vWF	$\alpha_{IIb}\beta_3$ (activated)
	P-selectin	PSGL-1, GPIb/V/IX
	CD40L	$\alpha_{IIb}\beta_3$ (activated)

vWF, von Willebrand factor; GP, glycoprotein; PAR, protease-activated receptor; PSGL, P-selectin glycoprotein ligand.

Prevention of atherothrombosis by application of soluble GPVI

Future approaches to the treatment or prevention of atherosclerosis and its complications may include techniques for the inhibition of platelet receptors, other than those already established. One very attractive candidate is the platelet collagen receptor GPVI, as it is crucial for the central processes leading to atherothrombosis. It has recently been shown that local delivery of soluble GPVI can prevent thrombosis in mice and rabbits.[29] Therefore, local or systemic application of soluble GPVI may be a potential new modality for therapy of atherothrombosis.

Role of platelets in regenerative medicine

Emerging evidence suggests that circulating endothelial progenitor cells (EPCs) home to sites of endothelial denudation[30,31] and that EPCs recruited at the site of a vascular lesion accelerate reendothelization and lesion repair.[32] Recently, stem cell therapy has been introduced into the treatment of ischemic cardiac diseases. In the three largest trials using progenitor cells, which were administered by intracoronary injection during myocardial infarction, stem cell treatment was associated with an increase in neovascularization and global left ventricular ejection fraction.[33,34] The exact mechanisms responsible for the homing of progenitor cells to the sites of vascular lesions are not yet well understood. A new mechanism has recently been identified, by which platelets can recruit endothelial progenitor cells to

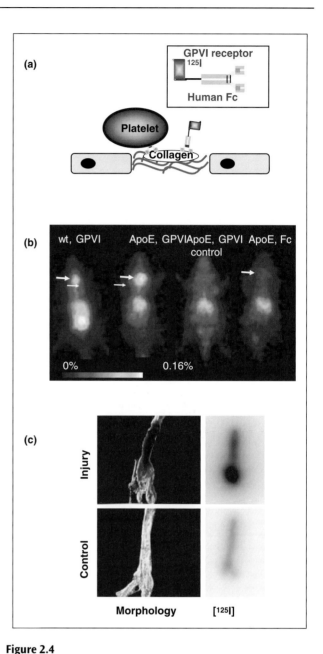

Figure 2.4
Detection of vulnerable plaques by soluble GPVI. (a) A soluble dimeric form of human platelet GPVI conjugated to an Fc fragment, radiolabeled with iodine-125 (^{125}I) was used. GPVI is essential to establish the first interaction of platelets with an exposed collagen surface. Therefore, we made use of this natural mechanism to detect thrombogenic, and thus vulnerable, plaques. (b) Gamma-camera images of wild-type (wt) and *ApoE$^{-/-}$* mice with and without (control animals) experimental carotid injury. Images were aquired 24 hours after administration of 7.4 MBq [^{125}I]GPVI or [^{125}I]Fc-fragment (control compound). The imaging time was 20 minutes. The arrow indicates the area of carotid injury. (c) Representative photomicrographs of injured and control carotid arteries of wild-type mice and the corresponding ex vivo autoradiographs. (see color plate)

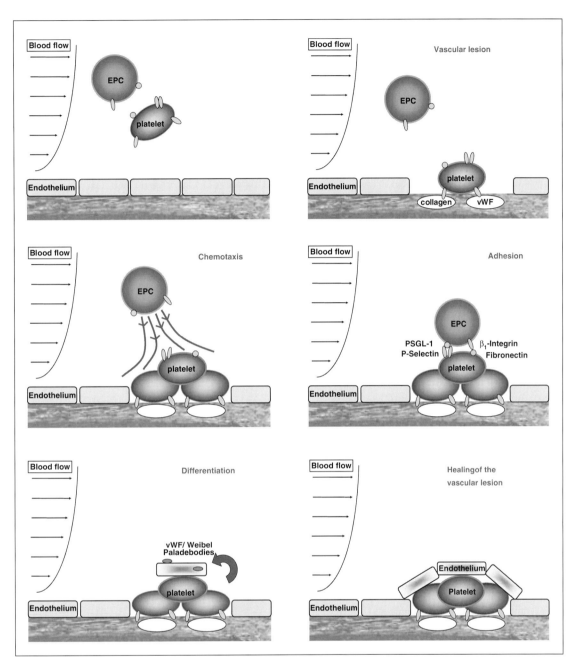

Figure 2.5
Schematic overview of the processes involved in platelet-mediated endothelial progenitor cell (EPC) recruitment to vascular lesions with exposed subendothelial matrix, finally resulting in differentiation to endothelial cells – a process that could initiate and sustain healing of vascular lesions. (see color plate)

exposed collagen at sites of vascular lesions in vitro[35] and in vivo.[36] This mechanisms involves platelet receptors, platelet-derived chemokines, and other mediators, including P-selectin, platelet-derived growth factor (PDGF)-AB, and stromal cell derived factor 1 (SDF-1). Making use of this mechanism, new strategies for the enrichment of progenitor cells at sites of vascular lesions could be developed to improve vascularization and ventricular function in ischemic myocardium (Figure 2.5).

References

1. Lindemann S, Tolley ND, Dixon DA et al. Activated platelets mediate inflammatory signaling by regulated interleukin 1β synthesis. J Cell Biol 2001;154:485–90.

2. Gawaz M, Langer H, May AE. Platelets in inflammation and atherogenesis. J Clin Invest 2005;115:3378–84.

3. Hilf N, Singh-Jasuja H, Schwarzmaier P et al. Human platelets express heat shock protein receptors and regulate dendritic cell maturation. Blood 2002;99:3676–82.

4. Gasic GJ, Gasic TB, Stewart CC. Antimetastatic effects associated with platelet reduction. Proc Natl Acad Sci USA 1968;61:46–52.

5. Hynes RO. Integrins: versatility, modulation, and signaling in cell adhesion. Cell 1992;69:11–25.

6. Massberg S, Gawaz M, Gruner S et al. A crucial role of glycoprotein VI for platelet recruitment to the injured arterial wall in vivo. J Exp Med 2003;197:41–9.

7. Nieswandt B, Watson SP. Platelet–collagen interaction: Is GPVI the central receptor? Blood 2003;102:449–61.

8. Gachet C. Regulation of platelet functions by P2 receptors. Annu Rev Pharmacol Toxicol 2006;46:277–300.

9. Ross R. Atherosclerosis – an inflammatory disease. N Engl J Med 1999;340:115–26.

10. Gawaz M. Do platelets trigger atherosclerosis? Thromb Haemost 2003;90:971–2.

11. Bombeli T, Schwartz BR, Harlan JM. Adhesion of activated platelets to endothelial cells: evidence for a GPIIbIIIa-dependent bridging mechanism and novel roles for endothelial intercellular adhesion molecule 1 (ICAM-1), $\alpha_v\beta_3$ integrin, and GPIbα. J Exp Med 1998;187:329–39.

12. Gawaz M, Neumann FJ, Ott I, Schiessler A, Schomig A. Platelet function in acute myocardial infarction treated with direct angioplasty. Circulation 1996;93: 229–37.

13. Gawaz M, Neumann FJ, Dickfeld T et al. Vitronectin receptor ($\alpha_v\beta_3$) mediates platelet adhesion to the luminal aspect of endothelial cells: implications for reperfusion in acute myocardial infarction. Circulation 1997;96:1809–18.

14. Frenette PS, Johnson RC, Hynes RO, Wagner DD. Platelets roll on stimulated endothelium in vivo: an interaction mediated by endothelial P-selectin. Proc Natl Acad Sci USA 1995;92:7450–4.

15. Massberg S, Enders G, Leiderer R et al. Platelet–endothelial cell interactions during ischemia/reperfusion: the role of P-selectin. Blood 1998;92:507–15.

16. Frenette PS, Moyna C, Hartwell DW et al. Platelet-endothelial interactions in inflamed mesenteric venules. Blood 1998;91:1318–24.

17. Frenette PS, Denis CV, Weiss L et al. P-selectin glycoprotein ligand 1 (PSGL-1) is expressed on platelets and can mediate platelet-endothelial interactions in vivo. J Exp Med 2000;191:1413–22.

18. Johnson RC, Mayadas TN, Frenette PS et al. Blood cell dynamics in P-selectin-deficient mice. Blood 1995;86:1106–14.

19. Subramaniam M, Frenette PS, Saffaripour S et al. Defects in hemostasis in P-selectin-deficient mice. Blood 1996;87:1238–42.

20. Gawaz MP, Loftus JC, Bajt ML et al. Ligand bridging mediates integrin $\alpha_{IIb}\beta_3$ (platelet GPIIb–IIIA) dependent homotypic and heterotypic cell–cell interactions. J Clin Invest 1991;88:1128–34.

21. Massberg S, Enders G, Matos FC et al. Fibrinogen deposition at the postischemic vessel wall promotes platelet adhesion during ischemia–reperfusion in vivo. Blood 1999;94:3829–38.

22. Langer H, May AE, Bultmann A, Gawaz M. ADAM 15 is an adhesion receptor for platelet GPIIb–IIIa and induces platelet activation. Thromb Haemost 2005;94:555–61.

23. Gawaz M, Brand K, Dickfeld T et al. Platelets induce alterations of chemotactic and adhesive properties of endothelial cells mediated through an interleukin-1-dependent mechanism. Implications for atherogenesis. Atherosclerosis 2000;148:75–85.

24. Massberg S, Brand K, Gruner S et al. A critical role of platelet adhesion in the initiation of atherosclerotic lesion formation. J Exp Med 2002;196:887–96.

25. Gawaz M. Role of platelets in coronary thrombosis and reperfusion of ischemic myocardium. Cardiovasc Res 2004;61:498–511.

26. Massberg S, Konrad I, Bultmann A et al. Soluble glycoprotein VI dimer inhibits platelet adhesion and aggregation to the injured vessel wall in vivo. FASEB J 2004;18:397–9.

27. Langer H, Gawaz M. The role of platelets for the pathophysiology of acute coronary syndromes. Hamostaseologie 2006;26:114–18.

28. Gawaz M, Konrad I, Hauser AI et al. Non-invasive imaging of glycoprotein VI binding to injured arterial lesions. Thromb Haemost 2005;93:910–13.

29. Bultmann A, Herdeg C, Li Z et al. Local delivery of soluble platelet collagen receptor glycoprotein VI inhibits thrombus formation in vivo. Thromb Haemost 2006;95:763–6.

30. Griese DP, Ehsan A, Melo LG et al. Isolation and transplantation of autologous circulating endothelial cells into denuded vessels and prosthetic grafts: implications for cell-based vascular therapy. Circulation 2003;108:2710–15.

31. Walter DH, Rittig K, Bahlmann FH et al. Statin therapy accelerates reendothelialization: a novel effect involving mobilization and incorporation of bone marrow-derived endothelial progenitor cells. Circulation 2002;105:3017–24.

32. Fujiyama S, Amano K, Uehira K et al. Bone marrow monocyte lineage cells adhere on injured endothelium in a monocyte chemoattractant protein-1-dependent manner and accelerate reendothelialization as endothelial progenitor cells. Circ Res 2003; 93:980–9.

33. Fernandez-Aviles F, San Roman JA, Garcia-Frade J et al. Experimental and clinical regenerative capability of human bone marrow cells after myocardial infarction. Circ Res 2004;95:742–8.

34. Wollert KC, Meyer GP, Lotz J et al. Intracoronary autologous bone-marrow cell transfer after myocardial infarction: the BOOST randomised controlled clinical trial. Lancet 2004;364:141–8.

35. Langer H, May AE, Daub K et al. Adherent platelets recruit and induce differentiation of murine embryonic endothelial progenitor cells to mature endothelial cells in vitro. Circ Res 2006;98:e2–10.

36. Massberg S, Konrad I, Schurzinger K et al. Platelets secrete stromal cell-derived factor 1α and recruit bone marrow-derived progenitor cells to arterial thrombi in vivo. J Exp Med 2006;203:1221–33.

3

Laboratory assessment of platelet function and coagulation

Alan D Michelson, Andrew L Frelinger III, and Jeffrey I Weitz

Introduction

Platelet function and coagulation can be assessed in the laboratory by numerous tests. Consistent with the focus of this book, this chapter will focus specifically on tests that can be used to guide the clinical use of antithrombotic drugs in coronary artery disease.

Laboratory assessment of platelet function

Introduction

Platelets have a well-defined, critical role in coronary artery thrombosis and in other common cardiovascular diseases, including stroke, peripheral vascular disease, and diabetes mellitus.[1,2] Accordingly, antiplatelet therapy has been demonstrated to be beneficial in these clinical settings.[3] However, there is variability between patients in the response of their platelets to antiplatelet therapy.[4] There is therefore increasing interest in the use of platelet function tests to monitor the effects of antiplatelet drugs in cardiovascular diseases, with the goal of guiding antiplatelet therapy to the optimal dose for prevention or treatment of thrombosis while minimizing hemorrhagic side-effects.[4] In the setting of cardiovascular disease, these tests are frequently used for the measurement of 'aspirin resistance' or 'clopidogrel resistance'.[4-6] The clinical relevance of 'resistance', also referred to as response variability, is discussed in subsequent chapters in this book. This chapter will review the current options for platelet function testing, with a particular focus on point-of-care tests. Tables 3.1 and 3.2 summarize laboratory methods that can potentially be used to guide the clinical use of antiplatelet drugs in coronary artery disease.

The bleeding time

The bleeding time, the first test of platelet function, was developed in the early 1900s.[7] The basis of the test is the timed, platelet-dependent cessation of bleeding from a standardized in vivo wound. Although the bleeding time is therefore a physiologically relevant test, it has many disadvantages: non-specificity (e.g., affected by von Willebrand factor), insensitivity, high interoperator variability, and frequent scar formation.[7] The bleeding time is therefore no longer recommended as a clinical test of platelet function.

Platelet aggregometry

Although a number of other platelet function tests were developed subsequent to the bleeding time, platelet aggregometry, as described in 1962 by Born, became the de facto 'gold standard'.[8] In this test, platelet-to-platelet aggregation in response to an agonist is measured in platelet-rich plasma by turbidometry or, as described subsequently, in whole blood by electrical impedance. The fundamental advantage of platelet aggregometry is that it measures, albeit in an ex vivo system, the most important function of platelets – their aggregation with each other in a glycoprotein (GP) IIb/IIIa (integrin $\alpha_{IIb}\beta_3$)-dependent manner.

Turbidometric platelet aggregation has been the platelet function test most often used in clinical trials. Several studies have reported that platelet aggregometry can predict major adverse cardiac events (MACE), although the number of MACE in all these studies was low.[9-11]

Nevertheless, there are major disadvantages to platelet aggregometry as a clinical test of platelet function, including poor reproducibility, high sample volume, requirement for sample preparation, length of assay time, requirement of a skilled technician, and expense.[8]

Table 3.1 *Methods for the laboratory assessment of platelet function*

Test	Basis	Advantages	Disadvantages
Turbidometric aggregometry	Platelet aggregation	Historical gold standard	High sample volume Sample preparation Time-consuming
Impedance aggregometry	Platelet aggregation	Whole blood assay	High sample volume Sample preparation Time-consuming
VerifyNow	Platelet aggregation	Simple, rapid Point-of-care (no pipetting required) Low sample volume Whole blood assay	Limited hematocrit and platelet count range
Plateletworks	Platelet aggregation	Minimal sample preparation Whole blood assay	Not well studied
Platelet surface P-selectin, activated GPIIb/IIIa, leukocyte–platelet aggregates (flow cytometry)	Activation-dependent changes in platelet surface	Low sample volume Whole blood assays Fixed samples can be mailed to core laboratory	Sample preparation Requires flow cytometer and experienced technician
TEG PlateletMapping system	Platelet contribution to clot strength	Whole blood assay Clot information	Not commercially available Limited studies
Impact cone and plate(let) analyzer	Shear-induced platelet adhesion	Simple, rapid Point-of-care Low sample volume No sample preparation Whole blood assay	Requires pipeting Instrument not widely available Requires pipetting
PFA-100	In vitro cessation of high-shear blood flow by platelet plug	Simple, rapid Point-of-care Low sample volume No sample preparation Whole blood assay	Dependent on von Willebrand factor and hematocrit Requires pipetting Does not correlate well with clopidogrel therapy
VASP phosphorylation state (flow cytometry)	Activation-dependent signaling	Dependent on clopidogrel target, $P2Y_{12}$ Low sample volume Whole blood assay Blood samples can be mailed at RT to core laboratory	Sample preparation Requires flow cytometer and experienced technician
Serum thromboxane B_2 (ELISA)	Activation-dependent release from platelets	Directly dependent on aspirin target, COX-1	Indirect measure Not platelet-specific
Urinary 11-dehydrothromboxane B_2/creatinine ratio	Stable urinary metabolite of thromboxane B_2	Directly dependent on aspirin target, COX-1	Indirect measure Not platelet-specific

Table 3.2 *Platelet function tests for the monitoring of response to aspirin and clopidogrel*

Aspirin

Thromboxane as the endpoint:
- Serum thromboxane B_2
- Urinary 11-dehydrothromboxane B_2

Arachidonic acid as the stimulus:
- VerifyNow aspirin assay
- Platelet aggregation (turbidometric)
- Platelet aggregation (impedance)
- Platelet surface P-selectin, platelet surface-activated GPIIb/IIIa, leukocyte–platelet aggregates (flow cytometry)
- Plateletworks
- Thromboelastogram
- Impact cone and plate(let) analyzer

Other:
- Platelet function analyzer 100 (PFA-100)

Clopidogrel

P2Y$_{12}$ signaling-dependent:
- Vasodilator-stimulated phosphoprotein (VASP) phosphorylation state

ADP as the stimulus:
- VerifyNow (P2Y$_{12}$ assay)
- Platelet aggregation (turbidometric)
- Platelet aggregation (impedance)
- Platelet surface P-selectin, platelet surface-activated GPIIb/IIIa, leukocyte–platelet aggregates (flow cytometry)
- Plateletworks
- Thromboelastogram
- Impact cone and plate(let) analyzer (with ADP)

Reproduced with permission from Michelson AD et al. Eur Heart J 2006;8:G53–8.[25]

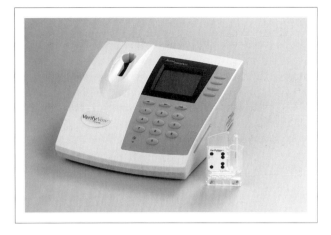

Figure 3.1
VerifyNow point-of-care device for the measurement of platelet function.

VerifyNow

VerifyNow (Accumetrics, San Diego, CA) (Figure 3.1), formerly known as the Ultegra rapid platelet function analyzer (RPFA), is a point-of-care test that is FDA-approved to measure the aspirin- or thienopyridine-induced defects in platelet function. VerifyNow uses the same principle (and therefore has the same fundamental advantage) as platelet aggregometry, i.e., it measures the most important function of platelets – their aggregation with each other in a GPIIb/IIIa-dependent manner. Fibrinogen-coated beads are included in the VerifyNow system to augment the GPIIb/IIIa-dependent signal.[12] There is a direct relationship between the results of testing with the VerifyNow GPIIb/IIIa assay and both platelet aggregometry and GPIIb/IIIa receptor

occupancy. Advantages of the VerifyNow system include point-of-care, simplicity, rapidity (results in 5 minutes), low sample volume, no sample preparation, and a whole blood system.

There are three currently available VerifyNow assays: the GPIIb/IIIa assay (sensitive to GPIIb/IIIa antagonists), the Aspirin Assay (sensitive to aspirin), and the P2Y$_{12}$ Assay (sensitive to thienopyridines).[12] In the VerifyNow Aspirin Assay, arachidonic acid is used as the agonist. This assay is aspirin-specific because arachidonic acid-induced platelet aggregation requires the activity of cyclooxygenase-1 (COX-1) – which is specifically blocked by aspirin. In the VerifyNow P2Y$_{12}$ Assay, adenosine diphosphate (ADP) is used as the agonist. ADP stimulates platelet aggregation via its two receptors: P2Y$_1$ and P2Y$_{12}$. While the agonist utilized in the VerifyNow P2Y$_{12}$ assay is ADP 20 µmol/l, a second agent, prostaglandin E_1 (PGE$_1$) 22 nmol/l is also added in order to suppress intracellular free calcium levels and thereby to reduce the platelet activation contribution from ADP binding to its P2Y$_1$ receptor.

The level of platelet function, as determined by VerifyNow GPIIb/IIIa Assay, predicts the incidence of MACE in patients treated with a GPIIb/IIIa antagonist (abciximab).[13] In aspirin-treated patients pre-percutaneous coronary intervention (PCI) the level of platelet function (or 'aspirin resistance'), as determined by the VerifyNow Aspirin Assay, predicts the incidence of post-PCI myonecrosis.[14]

TEG PlateletMapping system

The thromboelastograph (TEG) was invented more than 50 years ago, but has recently been updated as the TEG PlateletMapping system (Haemoscope, Niles, IL). As blood clots in a rotating sample cup, the cup motion is transmitted by the strengthening clot to a suspended pin. In the PlateletMapping system, a weak clot is generated in heparinized blood by the addition of reptilase and factor XIII. By adding a platelet agonist (arachidonic acid or ADP) the clot strength is greatly enhanced, allowing this test to be sensitive to inhibition of platelet function.[15] Advantages of the TEG PlateletMapping system include that it is a point-of-care (although, unlike the VerifyNow device, pipetting is required), whole blood assay that also provides information on clot formation and clot lysis. Although small studies suggest that the TEG PlateletMapping system can predict MACE, additional studies need to be performed to determine its possible role in monitoring antiplatelet therapy.

Impact cone and plate(let) analyzer

In the Impact cone and plate(let) analyzer (Diamed, Cressier, Switzerland), whole blood is exposed to uniform shear by the spinning of a cone in a standardized cup.[16] After automated staining, platelet adhesion to the cup is evaluated by image analysis software. Advantages of the Impact include point-of-care, simplicity, rapidity, low sample volume, physiologically relevant high shear, and a whole blood system. The assay has been used to monitor GPIIb/IIIa antagonist therapy. The ex vivo addition of arachidonic acid or ADP enable the Impact to be used to monitor aspirin or thienopyridines, respectively.[16] However, additional studies need to be performed to determine its possible role in monitoring antiplatelet therapy.

PFA-100

The Platelet Function Analyzer 100 (PFA-100 assay, Dade Behring, Newark, DE) draws an anticoagulated blood sample under high-shear conditions through a 150 μm diameter, collagen-coated aperture in the presence of ADP or epinephrine (adrenaline).[17] The time taken for a clot to occlude the aperture is reported as the closure time. Advantages of the PFA-100 include simplicity, rapidity, low sample volume, physiologically relevant high shear, no sample preparation (although, unlike the VerifyNow device, pipetting of the blood sample is required), and a whole blood system. Although it is conceptually less specific for aspirin resistance than the other assays listed in Table 3.2 (all of which are directly dependent on the aspirin-sensitive arachidonic acid/COX-1/thromboxane A_2 metabolic pathway), the PFA-100 has been widely used in clinical studies of aspirin resistance.[17] Furthermore, aspirin non-responder status in patients with recurrent cerebral ischemic attacks has been reported to predict MACE.[18] The PFA-100 has also been used to monitor GPIIb/IIIa antagonists, and failure to observe non-closure in the PFA-100 may be associated with an increased incidence of subsequent MACE.[19] However, the PFA-100 is not recommended for monitoring clopidogrel therapy.[17,20]

VASP phosphorylation state

As in the VerifyNow $P2Y_{12}$ assay, the combination of ADP and PGE_1 is used in the flow cytometry-based vasodilator-stimulated phosphoprotein (VASP) assay.[21] Under these conditions, the phosphorylation of VASP (identified by a monoclonal antibody specific for the phosphorylated form of VASP) is directly proportional to the degree of inhibition of the $P2Y_{12}$ receptor.[22] Comparison of the VASP assay with ADP-induced platelet aggregation (turbidometry) demonstrated that the level of thienopyridine-induced inhibition is higher in the VASP assay, presumably because platelet aggregation can still occur via ADP stimulation of $P2Y_1$ in the presence of a thienopyridine.[21] Patients with a poorer platelet response to clopidogrel, as determined by the VASP assay, have been reported to have a higher incidence of subacute stent thrombosis.[23] The advantages of the VASP assay include direct dependence on the target of clopidogrel ($P2Y_{12}$), low sample volume, and a whole blood system. Disadvantages of the VASP assay include the expense and the need for sample preparation, a flow cytometer, and an experienced technician.

Summary

Because of the variability between patients in the response of their platelets to antiplatelet therapy, there is increasing interest in the use of platelet function tests to monitor the effects of antiplatelet drugs, with the ultimate goal of guiding antiplatelet therapy to the optimal dose for prevention or treatment of thrombosis while minimizing side-effects. Aspirin 'resistance' or response variability can be assessed by assays that use thromboxane as the end point or arachidonic acid as the stimulus (Table 3.2). Clopidogrel 'resistance' or response variability can be assessed by a $P2Y_{12}$ signaling-dependent assay (VASP phosphorylation state) or by using ADP as the stimulus (although ADP activates platelets via two receptors, $P2Y_1$ and $P2Y_{12}$, only the latter of which is blocked by thienopyridines[24]) (Table 3.2).

Turbidometric platelet aggregation remains the gold standard platelet function test, in part because most large clinical trials of antiplatelet agents have used this endpoint. However, turbidometric platelet aggregation has many disadvantages, e.g., expense and the requirements for a high sample volume, a skilled technician, and sample preparation. True point-of-care assays, e.g., VerifyNow, overcome these problems and therefore show great promise for clinical utility in patients with coronary artery disease who are treated with antiplatelet agents. In patients treated with antiplatelet drugs, the degree of platelet inhibition, as determined by VerifyNow and several other new platelet function assays, has been shown to predict MACE.[4,25] Nevertheless, no published studies address the clinical effectiveness of altering therapy based on a laboratory finding of aspirin or clopidogrel 'resistance' or hyporesponsiveness.[5,25]

Laboratory assessment of coagulation

Introduction

Anticoagulants are central to the prevention and treatment of venous thromboembolism and are widely used in acute coronary syndromes. For many years, unfractionated heparin was the cornerstone of parenteral anticoagulation therapy. Although low-molecular-weight heparin (LMWH) and fondaparinux have challenged heparin for treatment of acute coronary syndromes, heparin is still used in patients undergoing PCI. The anticoagulant response to heparin is unpredictable, and when given in conjunction with other antithrombotic drugs, there is a risk of bleeding with heparin. Consequently, coagulation monitoring is recommended to optimize efficacy while maintaining safety.

Bivalirudin has emerged as an alternative to heparin in PCI patients. Although there may be less of a need to monitor bivalirudin than there is for heparin, coagulation monitoring is often performed. LMWH and fondaparinux are not routinely monitored. However, there are circumstances in which coagulation monitoring is helpful. For example, quantification of LMWH or fondaparinux levels at the time of PCI would better inform decisions about supplemental heparin. Likewise, assessment of drug levels in patients with renal impairment is important, because both LMWH and fondaparinux are renally excreted. Therefore, adjusted doses may be needed to avoid drug accumulation.

For chronic anticoagulation, oral agents are preferred over parental drugs. Currently, the vitamin K antagonists are the only available oral anticoagulants. These drugs, the prototype of which is warfarin, require coagulation monitoring because they have a narrow therapeutic window. In addition, their metabolism is influenced by common genetic polymorphisms, they interact with numerous other drugs and the anticoagulant response is dependent on dietary intake of vitamin K. Several new oral anticoagulants are under development. In contrast to warfarin, which inhibits the synthesis of factors II (prothrombin), VII, IX, and X, these novel agents target specific clotting enzymes. Drugs that block thrombin or factor Xa are in the most advanced stages of development. Although designed to be administered in fixed doses without coagulation monitoring, there are likely to be circumstances in which monitoring will be needed. For example, some of these drugs are renally excreted and they may accumulate in patients with renal impairment. In addition, assessment of drug levels is important in patients who require urgent surgery or to inform management decisions in those with major hemorrhagic complications.

Overview of coagulation assays

Several techniques, including clot-based tests, chromogenic or color assays, and enzyme immunoassays (EIA), are used for coagulation testing. Of these, clot-based and chromogenic assays are used most often. Whereas clot-based tests provide a more global assessment of coagulation function, chromogenic assays are designed to measure the level of function of specific clotting factors.

Clot-based assays

Clot-based assays are often used for evaluation of patients with suspected bleeding abnormalities and to monitor anticoagulation therapy (Table 3.3).[26] Most of these tests are performed in citrated plasma, and the endpoint for all of them is fibrin clot formation. Some of the technical and analytic variables that can influence assay results are listed in Table 3.4.

Prothrombin time (PT)

This test is performed by adding a thromboplastin reagent that contains tissue factor (which can be recombinant in origin or derived from an extract of brain, lung, or placenta) and calcium to plasma and measuring the clotting time (Figure 3.2a). The PT varies with reagent and coagulometer, but typically ranges between 10 and 14 s. The PT is prolonged with deficiencies of factors VII, X, and V, of prothrombin, or of fibrinogen, and by antibodies directed against these factors.[27] This test also is abnormal in patients with inhibitors of the fibrinogen-to-fibrin conversion reaction, including high doses of heparin and the presence of fibrin degradation products. Typically, PT reagents contain excess phospholipid so that non-specific inhibitors (i.e., lupus anticoagulants), which react with anionic phospholipids, do not prolong the clotting time.[28] The PT is most frequently used to monitor warfarin therapy.

Commercially available thromboplastins vary in their tissue factor source and method of preparation, leading to differing sensitivities to factor deficiencies;[29] therefore, PT results reported using different reagents are not interchangeable.[30] The International Normalized Ratio (INR) corrects for differences in thromboplastin potency. The World Health Organization has established a reference thromboplastin against which commercially available reagents are compared. The International Sensitivity Index (ISI) describes the responsiveness of each thromboplastin reagent to reductions in the vitamin K-dependent clotting factors compared with a sensitive standard, which is assigned an ISI of 1.0. Commercial thromboplastins derived from animal sources are less sensitive than the reference standard and commonly have ISI values of 1.2–2.8.[31] Using the ISI, we can convert PT to an INR with the formula $INR = (\text{patient PT}/\text{mean normal PT})^{ISI}$. Although the INR has helped to standardize anticoagulant monitoring, problems persist. The precision of INR determination varies, depending on reagent–coagulometer combinations.

Table 3.3 *Causes of clot-based assay prolongation*

Scenario	aPTT	INR	TCT
Factor deficiency • HMWK • Prekallikrein • Factor XII • Factor XI • Factor IX • Factor VIII	Prolonged	Normal	Normal
Factor deficiency • Factor X • Factor V • Prothrombin	Prolonged	Prolonged	Normal
Factor deficiency • Factor VII	Normal	Prolonge	Normal
Factor deficiency • Fibrinogen	Prolonged	Prolonged	Prolonged
Non-specific inhibitor	May be prolonged (depends on reagent)	Usually normal	Normal
Heparin (therapeutic doses)	Prolonged	Less affected than aPTT, may be normal	Prolonged
LMWH	Normal	Normal	Prolonged
Hirudin, bivalirudin, argatroban	Prolonged	Variably prolonged	Prolonged
Warfarin (therapeutic doses)	Less affected than INR, may be normal	Prolonged	Normal
Vitamin K deficiency	Less affected than INR, may be normal	Prolonged	Normal
Liver dysfunction	Less affected than INR, may be normal	Usually prolonged	Prolonged
DIC	Less affected than INR	Usually prolonged	Usually prolonged

aPTT, activated partial thromboplastin time;
INR, International Normalized Ratio;
LMWH, low-molecular-weight heparin;
TCT, thrombin clotting time;
HMWK, high-molecular-weight kininogen;
DIC, disseminated intravascular coagulation.

Unreliable reporting of the ISI by thromboplastin manufacturers also complicates INR determination.[32] Finally, with new batches of thromboplastin reagent, each laboratory must establish a mean normal PT using blood from at least 20 healthy volunteers.[32]

Activated partial thromboplastin time (aPTT)

The aPTT is performed by first adding a surface activator (e.g., kaolin, celite, ellagic acid, or silica) and diluted phospholipid (e.g., cephalin) to citrated plasma (Figure 3.2b). The phospholipid in this assay is called partial thromboplastin because tissue factor is absent. After incubation to allow optimal activation of contact factors (factor XII, factor XI, prekallikrein, and high-molecular-weight kininogen), calcium is then added, and the clotting time is measured.[27]

Although the clotting time varies according to the reagent and coagulometer used, the aPTT typically ranges between 22 and 40 s. The aPTT may be prolonged with deficiencies of contact factors, of factors IX, VIII, X or V, of prothrombin, or of fibrinogen. Specific factor inhibitors, as well as non-specific inhibitors, may also prolong the aPTT. Fibrin degradation products and anticoagulants (e.g., heparin, direct thrombin inhibitors, or warfarin) also prolong the aPTT, although the aPTT is less sensitive to warfarin than is the PT.[33]

Thrombin clotting time (TCT)

The TCT is performed by adding excess thrombin to plasma (Figure 3.2c). The TCT is prolonged in patients with low fibrinogen levels or dysfibrinogenemia and in those with elevated levels of fibrin degradation products.[28] These abnormalities are commonly seen with disseminated

Table 3.4   *Variables that can influence the accuracy of clotting test results*

Assay	Variable	Explanation
Clot-based and chromogenic assays (e.g., activated activated partial thromboplastin time, International Normalized Ratio, thrombin clotting time, and anti-factor Xa assays)	Improper filling of tube	Overfilling or underfilling the tube changes the ratio of blood to anticoagulant. Consequently, overfilling may cause falsely low results, whereas underfilling may cause falsely high results
	Abnormal hematocrit	A hematocrit >60% can produce falsely elevated results, whereas a hematocrit <20% can cause inappropriately low results
	Clotted specimen	Poor blood collection technique can induce clotting that results in consumption of coagulation factors (especially fibrinogen) and a falsely prolonged result
	Delay in performing assay	Failure to separate plasma from cells and the subsequent neutralization of heparin by platelet factor 4 released from platelets may result in falsely low values in heparinized samples
	Anticoagulant contamination	If the sample is drawn from an indwelling line used for anticoagulant infusion, it can easily be contaminated, even if the initial volume drawn is discarded. Samples are best drawn from peripheral veins
Whole blood assays (e.g., activated clotting time)	Platelet count and function	Decreased platelet count or function may result in a falsely prolonged ACT
	Hemodilution	Decreased concentration of clotting factors may result in falsely prolonged results
	Anticoagulant contamination	If the sample is drawn from an indwelling line used for anticoagulant administration, it can easily be contaminated. Samples are best drawn from peripheral veins

intravascular coagulation. The TCT is also prolonged by heparin and direct thrombin inhibitors.[28]

Activated clotting time (ACT)

The ACT (Figure 3.2d) is a point-of-care whole blood clotting test used to monitor high-dose heparin therapy or treatment with bivalirudin.[28] The dose of heparin or bivalirudin required in these settings is beyond the range that can be measured with the aPTT.[34] Typically, whole blood is collected into a tube or cartridge containing a coagulation activator (e.g., celite, kaolin, or glass particles) and a magnetic stir bar, and the time taken for the blood to clot is then measured.[28] The reference value for the ACT ranges between 70 and 180 s. The desirable range for anticoagulation depends on the indication and the test method used. During cardiopulmonary bypass surgery, the desired ACT range with heparin may exceed 400–500 s.[35] In contrast, in patients undergoing PCI, a target ACT of 200 s is advocated when heparin is administered in conjunction with a GPIIb/IIIa antagonist, whereas an ACT between 250 and 350 s is targeted in the absence of such adjunctive therapy.[36] The ACT does not correlate well with other coagulation tests.

Ecarin clotting time (ECT)

For the ECT, venom from the *Echis carinatus* snake is used to convert prothrombin to meizothrombin, a prothrombin intermediate that is sensitive to inhibition by direct thrombin inhibitors.[37] The ECT cannot be used to detect states of disturbed coagulation and is useful only for therapeutic drug monitoring. This assay is insensitive to heparin because steric hindrance prevents the heparin–antithrombin complex from inhibiting meizothrombin.[37] Because ecarin also activates the non-carboxylated prothrombin found in plasma of warfarin-treated patients, levels of direct thrombin

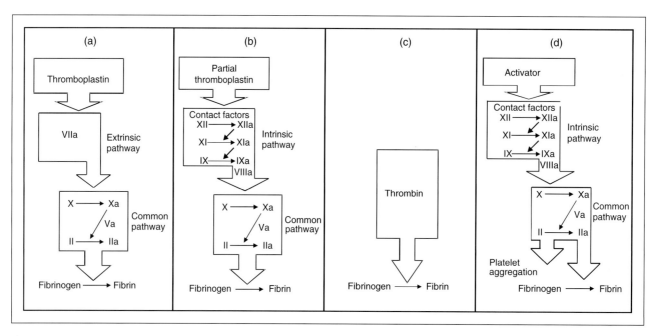

Figure 3.2
(a) Prothrombin time (PT). Thromboplastin reagent containing tissue factor (TF) and calcium is added to citrated plasma. Formation of extrinsic tenase results in rapid fibrin formation via the extrinsic and common pathways. (b) Activated partial thromboplastin time (aPTT). A partial thromboplastin reagent consisting of a surface activator and dilute phospholipid is added to citrated plasma. After incubation to allow activation of the contact factors and generation of factor IXa, calcium is added to induce clotting via the intrinsic and common pathways. (c) Thrombin clotting time (TCT). Thrombin is added to citrated plasma and directly converts fibrinogen to fibrin. (d) Activated clotting time (ACT). In contrast to the PT, aPTT, and TCT, which are done in citrated plasma, the ACT is performed in whole blood. Clotting is initiated by adding an activator of the intrinsic pathway, such as celite, kaolin, or glass beads. Once thrombin (factor IIa) is generated, it induces both platelet aggregation and fibrin formation.

inhibitors can be assayed even with concomitant warfarin treatment.[37] Although the ECT has been used in preclinical research, the test has yet to be standardized and is not widely available. A chromogenic variant of this assay has also been developed in which ecarin is added to a plasma sample and meizothrombin generation is measured with a chromogenic substrate.[38]

Chromogenic assays

Anti-factor Xa assays are used to measure levels of heparin and LMWH. These are chromogenic assays that use a factor Xa substrate onto which a chromophore has been linked (Figure 3.3). Factor Xa cleaves the chromogenic substrate, releasing a colored compound that can be detected with a spectrophotometer and is directly proportional to the amount of factor Xa present.[39] When a known amount of factor Xa is added to plasma containing heparin (or LMWH), the heparin enhances factor Xa inhibition by antithrombin, rendering less factor Xa available to cleave the substrate.[28] By correlating this result with a standard curve produced with known amounts of heparin, it is possible to calculate the heparin concentration in the plasma.

Use of anticoagulant assays to monitor therapy

Anticoagulant drugs in clinical use include vitamin K antagonists (such as warfarin), heparins (unfractionated heparin, LMWH, and fondaparinux) and thrombin inhibitors (bivalirudin, hirudin, and argatroban).

Vitamin K antagonists (VKAs)

VKAs are effective for primary and secondary prevention of venous thromboembolic events in patients with atrial fibrillation or prosthetic heart valves, for prevention of stroke, recurrent infarction, or cardiovascular death in patients with acute myocardial infarction, and for the primary prevention of acute myocardial infarction in high-risk men.[32] The VKA dosage is usually adjusted to attain a desired INR (Table 3.5). Because of the variability in the anticoagulant response to VKA,[40] which reflects genetic variations in metabolism and environmental factors such as medications, diet, and concomitant illness,[40] regular coagulation monitoring and dosage adjustment are required to maintain the INR within the therapeutic range.[40]

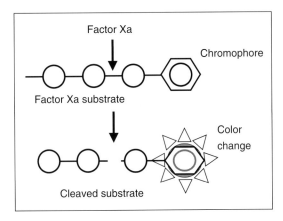

Figure 3.3
Factor Xa heparin assay. Factor Xa is added to plasma containing a synthetic factor Xa substrate that has a chromophore attached to one end. When the substrate is cleaved by factor Xa, the chomophore undergoes a color change, which can be quantified. The extent of color change is directly proportional to the enzyme activity. If heparin or low-molecular-weight heparin (LMWH) is present in the plasma sample, it will promote factor Xa inhibition by antithrombin, rendering less factor Xa available to cleave the substrate. By comparing the result with the extent of substrate hydrolysis in samples containing known amounts of heparin, the heparin concentration in the plasma can be calculated.

Table 3.5 *Optimal therapeutic range for the INR in various indications*

Indication for warfarin therapy	Therapeutic INR range
Venous thromboembolism (prevention and treatment)	2.0–3.0
Atrial fibrillation	2.0–3.0
Valvular heart disease	2.0–3.0
Heart valves:	
• Tissue valves	2.0–3.0
• Mechanical valves	
– Bileaflet aortic position	2.0–3.0
– High-risk valve	2.5–3.5
Acute myocardial infarction:	
• Prevention of embolism	2.0–3.0
• Prevention of reinfarction	3.5–4.5

Heparins

Heparins are indirect anticoagulants that activate antithrombin and promote its capacity to inactivate thrombin and factor Xa.[41,42] To catalyze thrombin inhibition, heparin binds both to antithrombin via a high-affinity pentasaccharide sequence and to thrombin. In contrast, to promote factor Xa inhibition, heparin needs only to bind to antithrombin via its pentasaccharide sequence. Heparin molecules containing < 18 saccharide units are too short to bind to both

thrombin and antithrombin, and therefore cannot catalyze thrombin inhibition. However, these shorter heparin fragments can catalyze factor Xa inhibition, provided that they contain the pentasaccharide sequence.[43] Because almost all of the chains of unfractionated heparin are of sufficient length to bridge antithrombin to thrombin, heparin promotes thrombin and factor Xa inhibition equally well and is assigned a ratio of anti-Xa to anti-IIa of 1.[44]

The anticoagulant response to heparin is unpredictable because of variable non-specific binding to endothelial cells, monocytes, and plasma proteins.[44] Because of this variable anticoagulant response, coagulation monitoring is routinely performed when heparin is given in greater than prophylactic doses. The aPTT is the test most often used to monitor heparin.[35] Unfortunately, aPTT reagents vary in their responsiveness to heparin, and the aPTT therapeutic range differs, depending on the sensitivity of the reagent and the coagulometer used for the test.[45,46] The aPTT has proved more difficult to standardize than the PT, and the commonly quoted therapeutic range of 1.5–2.5 times the control value often leads to systematic administration of subtherapeutic heparin doses.[35] Consequently, it is recommended that the therapeutic aPTT for heparin correspond to that which results in a heparin concentration of 0.35–0.7 anti-factor Xa units/ml.[35] However, evidence supporting the concept of an aPTT therapeutic range that predicts efficacy and safety (with respect to bleeding) is tenuous.[47]

Approximately 25% of patients require doses of heparin of >35 000 U/day to obtain a therapeutic aPTT and are called heparin-resistant.[48] Most of these patients have therapeutic heparin levels when measured with the anti-factor Xa assay, and the discrepancy between the two tests is the result of high concentrations of procoagulants such as fibrinogen and factor VIII, which shorten the aPTT.[49] Heparin therapy in these patients can be managed safely with heparin levels.[49] Less often, patients with a subtherapeutic aPTT also have a subtherapeutic heparin level despite large doses of heparin. This scenario usually reflects a combination of increased levels of heparin-binding proteins and increased heparin clearance.[50] Rarely, this form of heparin resistance is caused by low levels of antithrombin.

Although the aPTT response is linear with heparin levels within the therapeutic range, the aPTT becomes immeasurable with higher heparin doses.[28] Thus, a less sensitive test of global anticoagulation such as the ACT is used to monitor the level of anticoagulation in patients undergoing PCI or aortocoronary bypass surgery.[34] Although several retrospective studies have defined an inverse relationship between the likelihood of a thrombotic event and the ACT after heparin administration for PCI,[51,52] more recent data suggest that ischemic endpoints do not increase with decreasing ACT values, provided that the ACT is ≥ 200 s.[53]

LMWH is derived from unfractionated heparin by chemical or enzymatic depolymerization. With a mean molecular weight about one-third that of unfractionated heparin, only

25–50% of LMWH molecules contain ≥18 saccharides.[35] Consequently, these agents have ratios of anti-factor Xa to anti-factor IIa that range from 2:1 to 4:1.

LMWH has gradually replaced heparin for most indications. LMWH is typically administered in fixed doses when given for prophylactic purposes or in weight-adjusted doses when given for treatment. LMWH has advantages over heparin that enable once- or twice-daily subcutaneous administration without coagulation monitoring (Table 3.6). Exceptions include patients with renal dysfunction (shorter LMWH chains are cleared via the kidneys), those at extremes of weight, and perhaps infants and pregnant women who are receiving full treatment doses.[35,54–56] LMWH has little effect on the aPTT. Consequently, when monitoring is required, anti-factor Xa levels are measured with an LMWH standard.[48,57]

Pitfalls in the monitoring of LMWH by anti-factor Xa levels include poor comparability between commercially available anti-factor Xa chromogenic assays,[54] differences in ratios of anti-factor Xa to anti-factor IIa among the various LMWH preparations,[54] and the importance of timing of blood sampling in relation to dosing.[54] In general, it is recommended that blood samples for LMWH monitoring be obtained 4 hours after a subcutaneous injection. Although the relationship between anti-factor Xa levels and clinical outcomes is unclear,[54,58] typically recommended therapeutic anti-factor Xa levels for twice-daily LMWH therapy range from 0.5 to 1.0 U/ml and for once-daily treatment between 1.0 and 2.0 U/ml.[28]

Although the aPTT may be prolonged with high doses of LMWH, this assay is not used for monitoring. Because LMWH has less effect on the ACT than heparin does,[59–61] empiric LMWH dosing algorithms have been developed in the PCI setting.[36,62]

The most recent heparin derivative is fondaparinux. A synthetic analog of the antithrombin-binding pentasaccharide found in heparin and LMWH, fondaparinux binds antithrombin with high affinity. Fondaparinux increases the rate of factor Xa inhibition by antithrombin by about two orders of magnitude. Because it is too short to bridge antithrombin to thrombin, fondaparinux has no effect on the rate of thrombin inhibition by antithrombin.

Fondaparinux has almost no effect on clot-based tests of coagulation. Routine coagulation monitoring is not recommended with fondaparinux. If monitoring is required, however, anti-factor Xa levels can be measured using fondaparinux as the reference standard. This test will allow assessment of drug levels in μg/ml. With a specific activity of about 700 anti-factor Xa U/mg, drug levels of fondaparinux in μg/ml can be converted to U/ml. However, the relationship between anti-Xa levels and clinical outcomes is uncertain.

Direct thrombin inhibitors

Direct thrombin inhibitors bind directly to thrombin and block the interaction of thrombin with its substrates. Three parenteral direct thrombin inhibitors have been licensed for limited indications in North America. Hirudin and argatroban are approved for treatment of patients with heparin-induced thrombocytopenia, whereas bivalirudin is licensed as an alternative to heparin in patients undergoing PCI, as is argatroban.

Hirudin and argatroban require routine monitoring. The TCT is too sensitive to small amounts of hirudin and argatroban to be used for this purpose.[28] Although the ACT has been used to monitor the higher doses of direct thrombin inhibitors required in interventional settings, it does not provide an optimal linear response at high concentrations.[39] The aPTT is recommended for therapeutic monitoring; however, each direct thrombin inhibitor has its own dose response, and the sensitivity of the test to drug levels varies between aPTT reagents. When hirudin therapy is monitored with the aPTT, the dose is adjusted to maintain an aPTT that is 1.5–2.5 times the control, whereas for argatroban, the target aPTT is 1.5–3 times the control (but not to exceed 100 s). The aPTT appears less useful in patients requiring higher doses of direct thrombin inhibitor in cardiopulmonary bypass procedures, because this test becomes less responsive at increasing drug concentrations.[63] The ECT appears to be useful for both low and high concentrations of direct thrombin inhibitors and is less affected by interfering substances than the aPTT.[39] However, as stated above, it is not routinely available.

The responsiveness of the INR to different drug concentrations differs with assay reagent and with the type of direct thrombin inhibitor.[39] Although all direct thrombin inhibitors prolong the INR, argatroban has the greatest effect on this test. This feature complicates the transitioning of patients with heparin-induced thrombocytopenia from argatroban to VKA.[64] In general, with doses of argatroban up to 2 μg kg^{-1} min^{-1}, argatroban can be discontinued when

Table 3.6 *Advantages of LMWH over heparin and their consequences*

Advantage	Mechanism
Better bioavailability after subcutaneous injection	Can be given subcutaneously for prevention or treatment of thrombosis
Longer half-life	Can be given once- or twice-daily
More predictable anticoagulant response	Routine coagulation monitoring is not necessary
Less platelet activation and binding to platelet factor 4	Reduced risk of heparin-induced thrombocytopenia

Table 3.7 *Examples of point-of-care anticoagulant monitoring devices*

Device	Tests	Deflection method
Hemochron tube	ACT, PT, aPTT	Rotating magnet
Hemochron cuvette	ACT, PT, aPTT	Forced flow through narrow channel
Hepcon	ACT, PT, aPTT	Movement of plunger in and out of blood
i-STAT	ACT	Cleavage of thrombin substrate detected electrochemically
Coumatrak	ACT, PT, aPTT	Blood flow through capillary channel
CoaguChek		
CoaguChek S	PT	Movement of iron particles in blood

the INR is >4.[65] After argatroban is discontinued, the INR is repeated in 4–6 hours. If the repeat INR is below the therapeutic range, the argatroban infusion is resumed, and the procedure is repeated daily until the desired therapeutic INR on VKA alone is reached. For doses >2 $\mu g\,kg^{-1}\,min^{-1}$, the effect of argatroban on the INR is less predictable. It is recommended that the dose of argatroban be temporarily reduced to 2 $\mu g\,kg^{-1}\,min^{-1}$ and the INR checked after 4–6 hours. The procedure outlined previously should then be followed.

Another approach, which avoids discontinuation of the argatroban infusion, is to use factor X levels to monitor the VKA. These levels can be determined using a chromogenic assay. Factor X levels <45% are associated with INR values >2 when the effect of argatroban has been eliminated.[66]

Point-of-care monitoring

Most coagulation assays are performed in centralized laboratories using blood collected from indwelling lines or via venipuncture. This approach introduces problems with respect to turnaround time, venous access requirements, and difficulties associated with sample transport and processing. To circumvent these problems, several point-of-care coagulation tests have been introduced. These devices use various methods for clot detection in venous or capillary blood (Table 3.7). Of these, the ACT remains the most commonly used, reflecting, at least in part, the lack of rapid, readily available, inexpensive alternatives.

Point-of-care INR monitoring is both feasible and practical[67] and is used by many specialized coagulation clinics to streamline care. Although there are concerns about discrepancies between INR results obtained by near-patient testing and those measured in hospital laboratories, several investigators have reported that self-management with point-of-care INR devices is safe for selected patients and results in the same quality of care provided by specialized anticoagulation clinics.[68–71] Although point-of-care aPTT results appear to be clinically reliable and reproducible, there is less experience with these techniques.[72] The varying responsive-

ness of aPTT reagents and the need for calibration with heparin levels to establish an appropriate aPTT range limit the utility of these tests. There is a point-of-care device that can be used to monitor anti-Xa levels. This clot-based test detects LMWH levels above or below 1.0 U/ml. Warfarin, liver disease, and coagulation factor deficiencies can produce falsely high readings with this system.[39] A point-of-care test based on the ECT has also been developed for monitoring direct thrombin inhibitors, but the test has yet to be fully validated.[73,74]

Point-of-care tests are more expensive than centralized assays.[72] Therefore, cost–effectiveness analyses are needed to justify their widespread use.

Conclusions and future directions

With heparin and warfarin still firmly entrenched in our armamentarium of anticoagulants, coagulation monitoring remains an integral part of optimal patient management. The evolution to new heparin derivatives and oral anticoagulants that require little or no monitoring is likely to reduce the need for coagulation testing. However, even with these new agents, monitoring will still be necessary – at least in certain circumstances. This need will be challenging, because the correlation between drug levels and clinical outcomes for these new agents is largely unknown. Furthermore, many of the new drugs have little effect on clot-based tests of coagulation, and their effects on chromogenic assays are variable among members of the same drug class. Therefore, drug-specific monitoring assays may be needed, which will be a challenge for treating physicians, patients, and laboratory management. How these challenges will play out is likely to become clearer as development of these new drugs progresses.

References

1. Michelson AD, ed. Platelets, 2nd edn. San Diego: Elsevier Academic Press, 2007.
2. Ruggeri ZM. Platelets in atherothrombosis. Nat Med 2002;8:1227–34.

3. Antithrombotic Trialists' Collaboration. Collaborative meta-analysis of randomised trials of antiplatelet therapy for prevention of death, myocardial infarction, and stroke in high risk patients. BMJ 2002;324:71–86.

4. Michelson AD. Platelet function testing in cardiovascular diseases. Circulation 2004;110:e489–93.

5. Michelson AD, Cattaneo M, Eikelboom JW et al. Aspirin resistance: position paper of the Working Group on Aspirin Resistance. J Thromb Haemost 2005;3:1309–11.

6. Cattaneo M. Aspirin and clopidogrel: efficacy, safety and the issue of drug resistance. Arterioscler Thromb Vasc Biol 2004;24:1980–7.

7. Lind SE, Kurkjian CD. The bleeding time. In: Michelson AD, ed. Platelets, 2nd edn. San Diego: Elsevier Academic Press, 2007:485–94.

8. Jennings LK, White MM. Platelet aggregation. In: Michelson AD, ed. Platelets, 2nd edn. San Diego: Elsevier Academic Press, 2007: 495–508.

9. Gum PA, Kottke-Marchant K, Welsh PA, While J, Topol EJ. A prospective, blinded determination of the natural history of aspirin resistance among stable patients with cardiovascular disease. J Am Coll Cardiol 2003;41:961–5.

10. Mueller MR, Salat A, Stangl P et al. Variable platelet response to low-dose ASA and the risk of limb deterioration in patients submitted to peripheral arterial angioplasty. Thromb Haemost 1997;78:1003–7.

11. Matetzky S, Shenkman B, Guetta V et al. Clopidogrel resistance is associated with increased risk of recurrent atherothrombotic events in patients with acute myocardial infarction. Circulation 2004;109:3171–5.

12. Steinhubl SR. The VerifyNow system. In: Michelson AD, ed. Platelets, 2nd edn. San Diego: Elsevier Academic Press, 2007:509–18.

13. Steinhubl SR, Talley JD, Braden GA et al. Point-of-care measured platelet inhibition correlates with a reduced risk of an adverse cardiac event after percutaneous coronary intervention: results of the GOLD (AU-Assessing Ultegra) multicenter study. Circulation 2001;103:2572–8.

14. Chen WH, Lee PY, Ng W, Tse HF, Lau CP. Aspirin resistance is associated with a high incidence of myonecrosis after non-urgent percutaneous coronary intervention despite clopidogrel pretreatment. J Am Coll Cardiol 2004;43:1122–6.

15. Harrison P, Keeling D. Clinical tests of platelet function. In: Michelson AD, ed. Platelets, 2nd edn. San Diego: Elsevier Academic Press, 2007:445–74.

16. Varon D, Savion N. Impact cone and plate(let) analyzer. In: Michelson AD, ed. Platelets, 2nd edn. San Diego: Elsevier Academic Press, 2007:535–44.

17. Francis JL. The platelet function analyzer (PFA)-100. In: Michelson AD, ed. Platelets, 2nd edn. San Diego: Elsevier Academic Press, 2007:519–34.

18. Grundmann K, Jaschonek K, Kleine B et al. Aspirin non-responder status in patients with recurrent cerebral ischemic attacks. J Neurol 2003;250:63–6.

19. Madan M, Berkowitz SD, Christie DJ et al. Determination of platelet aggregation inhibition during percutaneous coronary intervention with the platelet function analyzer PFA-100. Am Heart J 2002;144:151–8.

20. Hayward CP, Harrison P, Cattaneo M et al. Platelet function analyzer (PFA)-100 closure time in the evaluation of platelet disorders and platelet function. J Thromb Haemost 2006;4:312–19.

21. Aleil B, Ravanat C, Cazenave JP et al. Flow cytometric analysis of intraplatelet VASP phosphorylation for the detection of clopidogrel resistance in patients with ischemic cardiovascular diseases. J Thromb Haemost 2005;3:85–92.

22. Schwarz UR, Geiger J, Walter U, Eigenthaler M. Flow cytometry analysis of intracellular VASP phosphorylation for the assessment of activating and inhibitory signal transduction pathways in human platelets – definition and detection of ticlopidine/clopidogrel effects. Thromb Haemost 1999;82:1145–52.

23. Gurbel PA, Bliden KP, Samara W et al. Clopidogrel effect on platelet reactivity in patients with stent thrombosis. Results of the CREST study. J Am Coll Cardiol 2005;46:1827–32.

24. Cattaneo M. ADP receptor antagonists. In: Michelson AD, ed. Platelets, 2nd edn. San Diego: Elsevier Academic Press, 2007:1127–44.

25. Michelson AD, Frelinger AL, Furman MI. Resistance to antiplatelet drugs. Eur Heart J 2006;8:G53–8.

26. Suchman AL, Griner PF. Diagnostic uses of the activated partial thromboplastin time and prothrombin time. Ann Intern Med 1986;104: 810–16.

27. White GC II, Marder VJ, Colman RW et al. Approach to the bleeding patient. In: Colman RW, Hirsh J, Marder VJ, Salzman EW, eds. Hemostasis and Thrombosis: Basic Principles and Clinical Practice, 3rd edn. Philadelphia: JB Lippincott, 1994:1134–47.

28. Van Cott EM, Laposata M. Coagulation. In: Jacobs DS, Oxley DK, DeMott WR, eds. The Laboratory Test Handbook, 5th edn. Cleveland: Lexi-Comp, 2001:327–58.

29. Kirkwood TBL. Calibration of reference thromboplastins and standardization of the prothrombin time ratio. Thromb Haemost 1983;49:238–44.

30. Zucker S, Cathey MH, Sox PJ, Hallec EC. Standardization of laboratory tests for controlling anticoagulant therapy. Am J Clin Pathol 1970;53:348–54.

31. Bussey HI, Force RW, Bianco TM, Leonard AD. Reliance on prothrombin time ratios causes significant errors in anticoagulation therapy. Arch Intern Med 1992;152:278–82.

32. Hirsh J. Oral anticoagulant drugs. N Engl J Med 1991;324:1865–75.

33. Hauser VM, Rozek SL. Effect of warfarin on the activated partial thromboplastin time. Drug Intell Clin Pharm 1986;2:964–6.

34. Dougherty K, Gaos C, Bush IL et al. Activated clotting times and activated partial thromboplastin times in patients undergoing coronary angioplasty who receive bolus doses of heparin. Cathet Cardiovasc Diagn 1992;26:260–3.

35. Hirsh J, Raschke R. Heparin and low-molecular-weight heparin: the Seventh ACCP Conference on Antithrombotic and Thrombolytic Therapy. Chest 2004;126:188S–203S.

36. Popma JJ, Berger P, Ohman EM et al. Antithrombotic therapy during percutaneous coronary intervention: the Seventh ACCP Conference on Antithrombotic and Thrombolytic Therapy. Chest 2004;126:576S–99S.

37. Nowak G. The ecarin clotting time, a universal method to quantify direct thrombin inhibitors. Pathophysiol Haemost Thromb 2003/4;33:173–83.

38. Lange U, Nowak G, Bucha E. Ecarin chromogenic assay – a new method for quantitative determination of direct thrombin inhibitors like hirudin. Pathophysiol Haemost Thromb 2003/4;33:184–91.

39. Walenga JM, Hoppensteadt DA. Monitoring the new antithrombotic drugs. Semin Thromb Hemostast 2004;30:683–95.

40. Ansell J, Hirsh J, Poller L et al. The pharmacology and management of the vitamin K antagonists. Chest 2004;126:204S–33S.

41. Rosenberg RD, Bauer KA. The heparin–antithrombin system: a natural anticoagulant mechanism. In: Colman RW, Hirsh J, Marder VJ, Salzman EW, eds. Hemostasis and Thrombosis: Basic Principles and Clinical Practice, 3rd edn. Philadelphia: JB Lippincott, 1994:837–60.

42. Jesty J, Lorenz A, Rodriguez J, Wan TC. Initiation of the tissue factor pathway of coagulation in the presence of heparin: control by antithrombin III and tissue factor pathway inhibitor. Blood 1996;87:2301–17.

43. Casu B, Oreste P, Torri G et al. The structure of heparin oligosaccharide fragments with high anti-(factor Xa) activity containing the minimal antithrombin III-binding sequence. Biochem J 1981;97:599–609.

44. Hirsh J. Heparin. N Engl J Med 1991;324:1565–74.

45. Brill-Edwards P, Ginsberg JS, Johnston M, Hirsh J. Establishing a therapeutic range for heparin therapy. Ann Intern Med 1993;119:104–9.

46. Bates SM, Weitz JI, Johnston M et al. Use of a fixed activated partial thromboplastin time ratio to establish a therapeutic range for unfractionated heparin. Arch Intern Med 2001;161:385–91.

47. Hirsh J, Bates S. The multiple faces of the partial thromboplastin time APTT. J Thromb Haemost 2004;2:2254–6.

48. Hirsh J, Salzman EW, Marder VJ. Treatment of venous thromboembolism. In: Colman RW, Hirsh J, Marder VJ, Salzman EW, eds. Hemostasis and Thrombosis: Basic Principles and Clinical Practice, 3rd edn. Philadelphia: JB Lippincott, 1994:1346–66.

49. Levine MN, Hirsh J, Gent M et al. A randomized trial comparing the activated partial thromboplastin time with heparin assay in patients with acute venous thromboembolism requiring large daily doses of heparin. Arch Intern Med 1994;154:49–56.

50. Young E, Prins M, Levine MN, Hirsh J. Heparin binding to plasma proteins, an important mechanism for heparin resistance. Thromb Haemost 1992;67:639–43.

51. Topol EJ, Bonan R, Jewitt D et al. Use of a direct antithrombin, hirulog, in place of heparin during coronary angioplasty. Circulation 1993;87:1622–9.

52. Narins CR, Hillegass WB, Nelson CL et al. Relationship between activated clotting time during angioplasty and abrupt closure. Circulation 1996;93:667–71.

53. Brener SJ, Moliterno DJ, Lincoff M et al. Relationship between activated clotting time and ischemic or hemorrhage complications. Analysis of 4 recent randomized clinical trials of percutaneous coronary intervention. Circulation 2004;110:994–8.

54. Bounameaux H, de Moerloose P. Is laboratory monitoring of low-molecular-weight heparin therapy necessary? No. J Thromb Haemost 2004;2:551–4.

55. Sutor A, Masticate P, Leaker M, Andrew M. Heparin therapy in pediatric patients. Semin Thromb Hemost 1997;23:303–19.

56. Massicotte P, Julian JA, Gent M et al, and the REVIVE Study Group. An open-label randomized trial of low-molecular-weight heparin compared to heparin and Coumadin for the treatment of venous thromboembolic events in children: the REVIVE trial. Thromb Res 2003;109:85–92.

57. Kitchen S, Lampietro R, Wooley AM, Preston FE. Anti-factor Xa monitoring during treatment of LMWH or danaparoid: inter-assay variability. Thromb Haemost 1999;82:1289–93.

58. Alhenc-Gelas M, Jestin-Le Guernic C, Vitoux JF et al. Adjusted versus fixed-doses of the low-molecular-weight heparin Fragmin in the treatment of deep vein thrombosis. Thromb Haemost 1994;71:698–702.

59. Greiber S, Weber U, Galle J et al. Activated clotting time is not a sensitive parameter to monitor anticoagulation with low molecular-weight heparin in hemodialysis. Nephron 1997;76:15–9.

60. Rabah MM, Premmereur J, Graham M et al. Usefulness of intravenous enoxaparin for percutaneous coronary intervention in stable angina pectoris. Am J Cardiol 1999;84:1391–5.

61. Linkins L-A, Julian JA, Rischke J et al. In vitro comparison of the effect of heparin, enoxaparin and fondaparinux on tests of coagulation. Thromb Res 2002;107:241–4.

62. The SYNERGY Trial Investigators. Enoxaparin vs. unfractionated heparin in high-risk patients with non-ST segment elevation acute coronary syndromes managed with an intended early invasive strategy. Primary results of the SYNERGY randomized trial. JAMA 2004;292:45–54.

63. Nowak G. Clinical monitoring of hirudin and direct thrombin inhibitors. Semin Thromb Haemost 2001;27:537–41.

64. Sheth SB, DiCicco RA, Hursting MJ et al. Interpreting the International Normalized Ratio (INR) in individuals receiving argatroban and warfarin. Thromb Haemost 2001;85:435–40.

65. Harder S, Graff J, Klinkhardt U et al. Transition from argatroban to oral anticoagulation with phenprocoumon or acenocoumarol: effects on prothrombin time, activated partial thromboplastin time, and ecarin clotting time. Thromb Haemost 2004;91:1137–45.

66. Arpino PA, Demirjian Z, Van Cott EM. Use of the chromogenic factor X assay to predict the international normalized ratio in patients transitioning from argatroban to warfarin. Pharmacotherapy 2005;25:157–64.

67. McCurdy SA, White RH. Accuracy and precision of a portable anti-coagulation monitor in a clinical setting. Arch Intern Med 1992;152:589–92.

68. Cromheecke ME, Levi M, Colly LP et al. Oral anticoagulation self-management and management by a specialist anticoagulation clinic: a randomized cross-over comparison. Lancet 2000;356:97–102.

69. Taborski U, Muller-Berghaus G. State of the art patient self-management for control of oral anticoagulation. Semin Thromb Hemost 1999;25:43–7.

70. Gadisseur APA, Breukink-Engbers WGM, van der Meer FJM et al. Comparison of the quality of oral anticoagulation therapy through patient self-management and management by specialized anticoagulation clinics in the Netherlands. A randomized clinical trial. Arch Intern Med 2003;163:2639–46.

71. Menedez-Jandula B, Souto JC, Oliver A et al. Comparing self-management of oral anticoagulant therapy with clinic management. A randomized trial. Ann Intern Med 2005;142:1–10.

72. Zimmerman CR. The role of point-of-care anticoagulation monitoring in arterial and venous thromboembolic disorders. J Thromb Thrombolysis 2000;9:187–2000.

73. Cho L, Kottke-Marchant K, Lincoff AM et al. Correlation of point-of-care ecarin clotting time versus activated clotting time with bivalirudin concentrations. Am J Cardiol 2003;91:1110–13.

74. Casserly IP, Kereiakes DJ, Gray WA et al. Point-of-care ecarin clotting time versus activated clotting time in correlation with bivalirudin concentration. Thromb Res 2004;113:115–21.

Section II.A

Antithrombotic drugs: oral antiplatelet drugs

4

Cyclooxygenase inhibition in atherothrombotic disease

Orina Belton, Sarah McClelland, and Des Fitzgerald

Introduction

Cyclooxygenases are rate-limiting enzymes in the generation of products that exert a broad spectrum of effects in human systems. The enzymes have been the target for the development of inhibitors in the treatment of inflammation and pain, most recently the 'coxibs' or cyclooxygenase-2 selective inhibitors. Cyclooxygenases also have potent effects in the cardiovascular system, and their inhibition has both therapeutic and harmful effects in patients with atherothrombosis, heart failure, and other forms of cardio-vascular disease.

Overview of cyclooxygenase and prostaglandin generation

The prostanoids, which include the prostaglandins (PGI$_2$ (prostacyclin), PGE$_2$, PGD$_2$, and PGF$_2$) and thromboxane (TXA$_2$), are a group of biologically active lipids that play a critical role in several physiological and pathological processes such as gastric cytoprotection, renal haemodynamics, modulation of vascular tone, and the regulation of inflammation and thrombosis.

PGs mediate their effects in part through transmembrane G-protein-coupled receptors, several of which exist for each prostaglandin.[1] For example, there are at least four different PGE-type (EP) receptors and two TXA$_2$ receptors (TP), the latter being alternatively spliced variants derived from a single gene.[2] As these are cell surface receptors, PGs act in a paracrine or autocrine fashion. PGs also activate peroxisomal proliferator-activated receptors (PPARs), nuclear membrane proteins that dimerize with other proteins to form transcription factors.[3] In this way, PGs may act as intracellular signaling molecules and regulate gene expression.[4]

PGs and TXA$_2$ are derived from arachidonic acid by cyclooxygenases (COX), also referred to as prostaglandin H synthases (PGHS). Two isoforms of COX exist: COX-1 and COX-2 (although a COX-3 has been described, this is an alternatively spliced variant of COX-1). The COX enzymes are homodimers; however heterodimerization has been described. COX-1 and COX-2 are bifunctional enzymes that carry out two sequential reactions in spatially distinct but mechanistically coupled active sites: a cyclooxygenase reaction, in which arachidonic acid is converted to PGG$_2$, an unstable intermediate; and a peroxidase reaction, where PGG$_2$ undergoes a two-electron reduction to PGH$_2$.[5] PGH$_2$ serves as a substrate for cell-specific isomerases and synthases to produce the PGs and TXA$_2$. Cells tend to express a predominant isomerase (PGI$_2$ synthase, TXA$_2$ synthase, PGE$_2$ synthase, and PGD synthase) closely coupled with COX that largely determines which product is generated. However, cyclooxygenases can couple to different isomerases in the same cell[6] and cells can express more than one isomerase.[7] A summary of the action of the COX enzymes is shown in Figure 4.1.

Although COX-1 and COX-2 catalysis are indistinguishable, the differences in gene and promoter structure, in protein sequence, and in subcellular localization explain the differential regulation of COX-1 and COX-2 in tissues. The primary structures of COX-1 and COX-2 from numerous species are known.[5] Both isoforms contain signal peptides of varying lengths. Mature, processed COX-1 and COX-2 contain 576 and 587 amino acids, respectively. There is a 60–65% sequence identity between COX-1 and COX-2 from the same species and 85–90% identity among individual isoforms from different species. X-ray crystallographic studies have shown that the overall topology of the enzymes is not affected by the variations in amino acid residues and that the structures of human and murine COX-1 are virtually superimposable on those of COX-2.[8,9] The major sequence differences between COX isoforms occur in

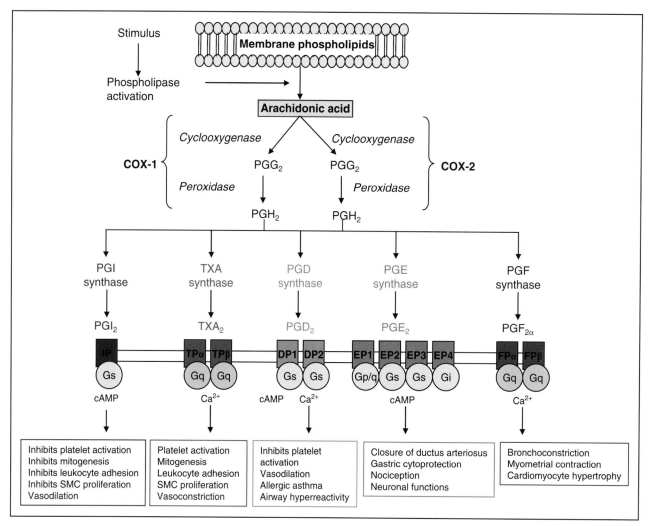

Figure 4.1

Overview of eicosanoid biosynthesis and their biological effects. Cyclooxygenase COX-1 and -2 catalyse identical reactions. The cyclooxygenase reaction results in the formation of prostaglandin G_2 (PGG_2) from arachidonic acid. In a subsequent peroxidase reaction, PGG_2 undergoes a two-electron reduction to PGH_2. PGH_2 serves as a substrate for cell-specific isomerases and synthases, producing the individual PGs and thromboxane A_2 (TXA_2). The eicosanoids exert their effects via a panel of cell-specific G-protein coupled receptors to mediate a broad range of biological effects. cAMP, cyclic adenosine monophosphate; SMC, smooth muscle cell.

the membrane binding domains[10] and in the active site – the latter resulting in important differences in substrate and inhibitor selectivity (discussed below).

The gene structure of *COX-1* facilitates continuous transcription of a stable message, and therefore, traditionally, it has been believed that COX-1 is constitutively expressed under physiological conditions and that COX-1-derived PGs play an important role in cellular housekeeping functions. However, there is now increasing evidence to suggest that COX-1 is induced at sites of inflammation[11] and in atherosclerosis.[12] Conversely COX-2, which is constitutively expressed in some tissues, such as kidney and brain,[13] under normal conditions is a highly inducible enzyme. The structure of *COX-2* is similar to that of immediate early genes such as intercellular cell adhesion molecule 1 (ICAM-1),

and its expression is rapidly induced in response to cytokines,[14] growth factors,[15] free radicals,[16] and oxidized lipids[17] – factors known to play a role in atherothrombotic disease. While COX-2 potentiates early inflammation, recent evidence suggests a role for COX-2 in the resolution phase.[18] Furthermore, while COX-2 was initially believed to function only in pathophysiological responses, it is now clear that it also plays a physiological role in the brain, kidney, and cardiovascular systems.

Cyclooxygenase inhibitors

Both COX isoforms are targets of non-steroidal anti-inflammatory drugs (NSAIDs). NSAIDs, including aspirin are a structurally diverse group of agents with proven anti-inflammatory, analgesic, and antithrombotic properties. The NSAIDs share a common mechanism of action in that they are competitive or non-competitive inhibitors of the COX enzyme(s). Most of the traditional NSAIDs, such as indomethacin and ibuprofen, are reversible competitive inhibitors of COX. Aspirin differs from other NSAIDs in that it covalently modifies the enzyme and consequently is an irreversible inhibitor. Aspirin inhibits both COX-1 and COX-2 by acetylation of Ser530 and Ser516, respectively, in the substrate-binding site. This modifies the positioning of arachidonic acid relative to Tyr385, which initiates the oxidation of the substrate.[19] In the case of COX-1, this abolishes the enzymatic activity, and in the case of COX-2, it converts the enzyme to a lipoxygenase.

NSAIDs show some level of isoform selectivity. Various experimental models have been used to test the selectivity of NSAIDs in vitro, including purified enzymes, intact cell systems, and cells transfected with recombinant enzymes. The selectivity of the compound is evaluated by calculating a ratio of the IC_{50} values for COX-2 and COX-1. However, depending on the model used, the absolute IC_{50} value and values for the IC_{50} ratio of COX-2 to COX-1 vary, although the order of selectivity stays constant from one model to another. Aspirin is 10 to 100 times more potent against COX-1 than COX-2, as the acetylserine side-chain can rotate in the slightly larger site of COX-2, allowing limited access of substrate to the active site.[20] Naproxen and diclofenac are equipotent in inhibiting COX-1 and COX-2, whereas indomethacin, piroxicam, sulindac, and tolmetin are more active against COX-1 than COX-2.[21]

The available evidence suggests that the anti-inflammatory and analgesic properties of traditional NSAIDs are a consequence of COX-2 inhibition, whereas the gastrointestinal (GI) toxicity associated with chronic administration of these compounds is due to inhibition of COX-1 (although it has been suggested that inhibition of both isoforms is necessary for gastric damage to occur). Because of the difference in expression profiles between COX-1 and COX-2, it was believed that selective inhibitors of COX-2 would have the beneficial effects of traditional NSAIDs while sparing the GI tract. As discussed above, although COX-1 and COX-2 are similar in structure and catalytic activity, a single amino acid change in the substrate pocket (from isoleucine in COX-1 to valine in COX-2 at residue 523), creates a side-pocket or channel accessed by selective COX-2. This side-channel is blocked off by the larger isoleucine in COX-1.

COX-1 and COX-2 in atherothrombotic disease

Thrombosis is the late complication of atherosclerosis, a progressive inflammatory disease characterized by mononuclear infiltration, macrophage and foam cell formation, smooth muscle cell proliferation, and lipid accumulation. Platelet and leukocyte recruitment on endothelial cells occurs early in the course of vascular inflammation. As seen at sites of inflammation in general, there is increased expression of COX-1 and COX-2[22] and disordered PG generation.[23] The main products generated are TXA_2, a potent platelet activator and vasoconstrictor, largely derived from COX-1 in platelets; PGI_2, a potent platelet inhibitor and vasodilator, largely generated via COX-2 in vascular endothelium; and PGE_2, which has both pro- and anti-inflammatory activity.[24]

COX-1 and TXA_2 generation

COX-1 plays a key role in atherothrombosis. It is the only COX isoform expressed in the platelet, where it is responsible for the generation of its principal product, TXA_2.[25,26] Studies have shown enhanced TXA_2 biosynthesis (measured as increased urinary excretion of its stable metabolite 11-dehydro-TXB_2) in patients with atherosclerosis and coronary artery thrombosis,[27] and several studies have shown increased TXA_2 generation in murine models of atherosclerosis.[12,28]

Platelets adhere to injured vascular endothelium early in the course of atherosclerosis and are activated. Activated platelets in turn release mitogenic factors such as platelet-derived growth factor (PDGF) and epidermal growth factor (EGF), which promote the development of atherothrombotic lesions by stimulating the proliferation and migration of vascular smooth muscle cells (VSMCs) through a distinct TXA_2/PGH_2 receptor,[29] leading to atherosclerotic plaque formation. TXA_2 also promotes platelet activation and so contributes to the development of arterial thrombosis and the complications of atherosclerosis, such as myocardial infarction and stroke. Antagonism of the TP receptor has been shown to retard plaque formation in hypercholesterolaemic rabbits,[30] prevent arterial thrombosis in rats,[31] and decrease atherosclerosis in the apoE$^{-/-}$[32] and LDLR$^{-/-}$[33] mouse models. This is supported by other studies, which show that deletion of the TP receptor gene retards murine atherogenesis.[34]

Similarly, several studies have implicated COX-1 in the development of atherothrombotic disease. Selective inhibition of COX-1, at a dose that suppressed the increase in TXA_2, markedly attenuated lesion development in the ApoE$^{-/-}$ mouse.[12] Likewise, inhibition of COX-1 and COX-2 (but not of COX-2 alone),[35] and low-dose aspirin[36] inhibit the development of atherosclerotic lesion formation in the LDLR knockout model. In experimental models, disruption of the *COX-1* gene abolishes TXA_2 formation. However, in human disease, COX-1 may not be the sole source of the increased TXA_2 generation seen in atherosclerosis. Continued TXA_2 formation is seen in patients on doses of aspirin that abolish platelet COX-1 activity.[37,38] These reports further show that continued TXA_2 formation in patients on aspirin is associated with carotid intima–medial thickness and subsequent risk of serious cardiovascular events. In one study, the persistent TXA_2 formation in patients with unstable angina treated with aspirin was abolished by the addition of a non-selective COX inhibitor, which, together with other studies, suggests an extraplatelet source for the increased TXA_2.

This is supported by two recent studies. In the first, selective disruption of COX-1 in bone marrow-derived cells failed to suppress atherosclerosis in apoE$^{-/-}$ or LDLR$^{-/-}$ mouse models despite elimination of platelet TXA_2 production. In contrast, COX-1$^{-/-}$ disruption abolishes atherosclerosis in the apoE$^{-/-}$ mouse.[39] Similarly, selective disruption of the TP receptor in bone marrow-derived cells fails to prevent atherosclerosis, suggesting that TP expression in cells other than platelets (and macrophages) contributes to the protective effect.[40]

COX-2 and PGI$_2$ generation

PGI$_2$ is generated by large-vessel endothelium and VSMCs, and its biosynthesis is increased in vascular disease. PGI$_2$ inhibits platelet activity and the release of mitogens such as PDGF and EGF from platelets, endothelial cells, and macrophages, and thus, when synthesized by endothelial cells, will suppress VSMC proliferation in atherosclerotic plaques.[41] PGI$_2$ also inhibits leukocyte adhesion and activation, platelet aggregation, and VSMC migration.

PGI$_2$ mediates its actions largely through the IP receptor, a transmembrane G-protein coupled receptor, predominantly coupled to Gs. Genetic disruption of the IP receptor leads to increased vascular deposition of platelets in the mouse following arterial injury, reinforcing the importance of PGI$_2$ in maintaining vascular homeostasis. The IP receptor also mediates the vascular effects of PGI$_2$ in the carageenan-induced paw injury model of inflammation, with IP receptor-deficient mice displaying reduced inflammatory swelling.[42]

PGI$_2$ is generated through COX-1 and COX-2, although COX-2 is the major source of PGI$_2$ in patients with atherosclerosis, based on studies of metabolite excretion.[23] COX-2 expression is increased in atherosclerotic plaque, which is not surprising given the role of cytokines and growth factors in the pathogenesis of this disease. The increase in COX-2 expression is evident in endothelial cells, VSMCs, monocytes, and macrophages.[22,43] COX-2 expression in macrophages and VSMCs generates eicosanoids that might be expected to have proinflammatory effects such as increased vascular permeability, chemotaxis, and cell proliferation. COX-2 limits cell death (a feature of

atherosclerotic plaques) in several tissues, including cardiomyocytes,[16] and so could promote VSMC growth indirectly.

Several studies have examined a role for COX-2 and PGI$_2$ generation in atherothrombotic disease. The majority of these studies have employed selective inhibitors in the apoE$^{-/-}$ and LDLR$^{-/-}$ murine atherosclerotic models. The results to date have been conflicting and variable in concluding that COX-2 promotes, inhibits, or has no effect on the development of atherosclerosis. A summary of the outcomes of in vivo studies is shown in Table 4.1. Most evidence suggests that COX-2 promotes atherosclerotic plaque formation in that selective COX-2 inhibition in the apoE$^{-/-}$ and LDLR$^{-/-}$ knockout models decreases atherosclerosis. This is further supported by a study that showed that genetic deletion of macrophage COX-2 reduces lesion formation – consistent with the strong evidence of macrophage involvement in lesion formation. However, a recent study has shown that selective inhibition increases the rate of atherosclerotic lesion formation in mice,[44] while accelerated atherosclerotic plaque formation has been reported in mice deficient in both apoE and the IP receptor.[34] Interestingly, it has also been shown that PGI$_2$ mediates the atheroprotective effects of estrogen in female mice, in that deletion of the IP receptor abrogates the effect of estrogen.[45]

One possible explanation for these disparate findings is that COX-2 is involved in both the initiation and resolution phases of inflammation. COX-2 expression in the early phase of the inflammatory reaction is associated with infiltration of polymorphonuclear neutrophils whereas at later time points it is associated with the egression of inflammatory cells and resolution.[18] A possible explanation is that the PGs generated by COX-2 differ during the phases of inflammation and resolution. Thus, PGE$_2$ increases during the acute inflammatory response, whereas cyclopentenone PGs form as the inflammation resolves.[46] Therefore, it is possible that COX-2 plays a differential role in early and later atherosclerosis.

Cardiovascular effects of COX inhibition

Aspirin and atherothrombosis

Given their often opposing roles in the production of the pro- and antithrombotic prostanoids, it is unsurprising that inhibition of the COX isoforms has variable effects depending on which isoform is inhibited and on the balance of inhibition. Platelets express only COX-1, producing TXA_2, which, acting on the TP receptors on the platelet surface, activates the platelet, or enhances its activation. Hence, the product of COX-1 in the platelet is prothrombotic. The vascular endothelium expresses both COX-1 and COX-2.

Table 4.1 *Summary of the effect of COX-2 inhibition on the development of atherosclerosis in murine models of the disease*

Ref	Model	Intervention	Duration	Outcome
35	LDLR$^{-/-}$	Nimesulide	18 weeks	No change in lesion size
60	LDLR$^{-/-}$	Rofecoxib	6 weeks	>30% reduction
61	apoE$^{-/-}$	MF-tricyclic	16 weeks	No change in lesion size
12	apoE$^{-/-}$	SC-236	8 and 16 weeks	No change in lesion size
62	apoE$^{-/-}$	Celecoxib	15 weeks	No change in lesion size
63	apoE$^{-/-}$	MF-tricyclic	3 weeks	84% increase
64	C57Bl/6	COX-2$^{-/-}$ bone marrow	8 weeks	>50% reduction
65	apoE$^{-/-}$	Indomethicin phenethylamide	9 weeks	>50% reduction
66	apoE$^{-/-}$ LDLR$^{-/-}$	COX-1$^{-/-}$ bone marrow	8 weeks	Increased atherosclerosis
44	apoE$^{-/-}$	Rofecoxib Celecoxib	16 weeks	Increased atherosclerosis on normal chow
67	COX-2$^{-/-}$ C57Bl/6	Chow /1% cholesterol Rofecoxib	3 weeks 10 days	Increased aortic lipid Pro-inflammatory high-density lipoprotein

The major product of COX-2 in this setting is PGI_2, which suppresses platelet activation and causes vasorelaxation. The balance between the pro- and antithrombotic effects of COX in the vasculature was proposed in 1976 to be a critical factor in regulating hemostasis in vivo,[47] and this balance is altered by inhibition of the COX isozymes. Inhibition of COX-1 and COX-2 results in the balanced inhibition of platelet TXA_2 generation and endothelial PGI_2 generation.

Aspirin, the only known irreversible COX inhibitor, inhibits COX-1 preferentially for several reasons.[21] As aspirin irreversibly inhibits COX, new COX protein must synthesized de novo to overcome the effect of aspirin on platelets. However, endothelial cells can quickly synthesize new COX-2 protein, and thus vascular PGI_2 production is restored. Hence, COX blockade by aspirin is intrinsically antithrombotic, as it tips the balance between platelet COX-1-derived TXA_2, and endothelium-derived PGI_2, towards the antithrombotic effects of PGI_2.

Low-dose aspirin (75 mg/day) is routinely prescribed for the secondary prevention of myocardial infarction and stroke, due to its aforementioned antithrombotic properties. A meta-analysis concluded that aspirin therapy reduces the combined endpoint of serious vascular events by one-quarter and vascular mortality by one-sixth in high-risk patients with vascular disease.[48] Interestingly, aspirin does not prevent the majority of primary cardiovascular events.[49] In atherosclerotic vascular disease, especially in unstable coronary syndromes, TXA_2 synthesis is only partly suppressed by aspirin. This is evidenced by relatively large amounts of thromboxane metabolites in urine despite inhibition of platelet TXA_2 production.[50] Therefore, the

benefit of aspirin in patients with atherothrombosis may exceed that which is explained by platelet TXB_2 inhibition alone. It has been proposed that aspirin inhibits platelets independently of COX acetylation, has anticoagulant properties, suppresses vascular inflammation, and enhances fibrinolysis.[51] However, very low doses of aspirin are effective, and prevention of clinical events appears to be dose-independent. This supports the theory that platelet COX suppression is the primary mechanism by which benefit is derived. However, some aspirin benefit may occur downstream from platelet inhibition. For example, proteins secreted by activated platelets adhere to the vessel wall and promote atherosclerosis and thrombosis.[52] Low-dose aspirin downregulates soluble CD40 ligand, a platelet inflammatory mediator the expression of which closely correlates with urinary 11-dehydro-TXB_2, a marker of in vivo platelet activation and hence is mediated in part by the platelet.[53] Furthermore, aspirin indirectly suppresses the peroxidase function of the COX enzyme, thereby inhibiting hydroperoxide generation and vascular nitric oxide inactivation.[54]

Chronic administration of aspirin, however, is associated with serious side-effects, most notably in the GI tract. COX-1 in the gut wall is responsible for the production of cytoprotective PGs, in particular PGE_2. Inhibition of these PGs leads to the development of severe gastric pathologies. Since the adverse effects of aspirin and indeed traditional NSAIDs were attributed to COX-1 inhibition and the beneficial inflammatory effects to COX-2 inhibition, it was postulated that selective COX-2 inhibition would provide anti-inflammatory and analgesic effects without the GI side-effects.

COX-2 inhibitors and atherothrombosis

Heralded as a major breakthrough in the management of chronic inflammatory conditions, the coxibs showed at least equal clinical efficacy in terms of pain relief and resolution of inflammation as the traditionas NSAIDs, with significantly fewer gastric side-effects.[55,56] In clinical trials, etoricoxib was shown to be effective in the treatment of rheumatoid arthritis,[57] while lumiracoxib was found to be superior to the traditional NSAIDs diclofenac and naproxen in patients with osteoarthritis.[58]

However, despite their beneficial GI profile, concerns were soon raised regarding the cardiovascular safety of selective COX-2 inhibitors. It was feared that ongoing platelet TXA_2 generation (platelets express only COX-1), combined with inhibition of endothelial COX-2, with the resultant suppression of antiplatelet PGI_2 generation, would tip the balance of pro versus antithrombotic prostanoid formation in the vasculature, resulting in thrombosis.

Despite these early safety concerns, no clinical trials were designed to address the cardiovascular effects of COX-2 inhibition directly. Data came initially from studies to address the efficacy and GI effects of the coxibs, and later from studies addressing the potential role of COX-2 inhibition in colon cancer chemoprevention. The outccomes of trials investigating the efficacy of selective COX-2 inhibitors are summarized in Table 4.2.

The results of two large-scale clinical trials published in 2000 pointed towards a potential increase in cardiovascular events in coxib-treated patients; however, the data generated in these trials were difficult to interpret and compare. The CLASS (Celecoxib Long-term Arthritis Safety Study) trial reported no increase in cardiovascular events;[55] however, the VIGOR (Vioxx Gastrointestinal Outcomes Research) trial reported a twofold increase in cardiovascular events in the rofecoxib (Vioxx)-treated group.[56] Patient populations differed significantly between the two trials, however, with osteoarthritis patients being examined in CLASS and rheumatoid arthritis patients, who may have been at increased risk for cardiovascular events, in VIGOR. Placebos used also differed, with ibuprofen and diclofenac being used in CLASS, and naproxen in VIGOR. It was suggested that, since naproxen has significant antiplatelet effects, it may have lowered the cardiovascular event rate in the placebo group, thereby artificially inflating the event rate in the rofecoxib-treated group.

Definitive evidence for an increased risk of cardiovascular events in patients receiving selective COX-2 inhibitors came in 2005, when two long-term studies designed to examine the cancer chemoprotective effects of rofecoxib (APPROVE: Adenomatous Polyp Prevention on Vioxx)[68] or celecoxib (APC: Adenoma Prevention with Celecoxib),[70] were halted prematurely due to increased cardiovascular events in the coxib-treated groups. The APPROVe trial found that patients receiving 25 mg/day rofecoxib were almost four times as likely to experience a cardiovascular event as those receiving placebo, while the APC trial found that the risk of cardiovascular events was increased 2.3-fold in patients receiving 200 mg/day celecoxib and 3.4-fold in

Table 4.2	*Summary of cardiovascular outcomes in clinical trials investigating the effects of selective COX-2 inhibitors*				
Trial	Drug	Duration	Control	Cardiovascular (CV) outcome	
CLASS ($n=8059$)[55]	Celecoxib 800 mg/day	1 year	Ibuprofen 2400 mg/day and diclofenac	No change in CV risk reported	
VIGOR ($n=8076$)[56]	Rofecoxib 50 mg/day	9 months	Naproxen 500 mg/day	Increased CV risk in rofecoxib group	
TARGET ($n=18000$)[58]	Lumiracoxib	1 year	Naproxen or ibuprofen	Trend towards increased CV events (0.86 vs 0.75 per 100 patient-years)	
APPROVe[68] ($n=2600$)	Rofecoxib 50 mg/day	3 years	Placebo	Increased incidence of CV events (3-fold) with rofecoxib. Trial halted after 18 months	
CRESCENT ($n=404$)[69]	Rofecoxib 25 mg/day	12 weeks	Celecoxib or naproxen	Increase in 24-hour systolic blood pressure with celecoxib	
APC study ($n=2035$)[70]	Celecoxib 200 mg or 400 mg twice daily	2.8–3.1 years	Placebo	Dose-related increase in CV events with celecoxib. Trial halted after 18 months	
CABG surgery study ($n=1671$)[71]	Parecoxib (40 mg/day intravenously) and valdecoxib (20 mg/day)	30 days	Placebo	Increased CV events with parecoxib and valdecoxib vs placebo	

those receiving 400 mg/day celecoxib. Rofecoxib was subsequently voluntarily withdrawn from the market by its manufacturer. A third trial published in 2005, designed to assess the suitability of use of the selective COX-2 inhibitor valdecoxib and its intravenous prodrug parecoxib for pain relief following coronary artery bypass graft (CABG) surgery also uncovered an increased risk of thrombotic cardiovascular events, this time over a short term (10 days). The incidence of adverse cardiovascular events was increased fourfold in the paracoxib/valdecoxib treatment group.[59]

Interestingly, the increased cardiovascular event rate found in the APPROVe and APC trials was seen only after 18 months of daily coxib administration. Therefore, it seems unlikely that the increase in thrombotic events is a direct result of an imbalance between platelet TXA$_2$ and endothelial PGI$_2$ generation, and is suggestive of additional and as yet unidentified pathological mechanisms. This is an ongoing area of intensive research, with recent studies suggesting a possible link between chronic COX-2. inhibition and atherosclerotic plaque destabilization,[33] and also providing evidence that atherosclerotic risk factors are increased in

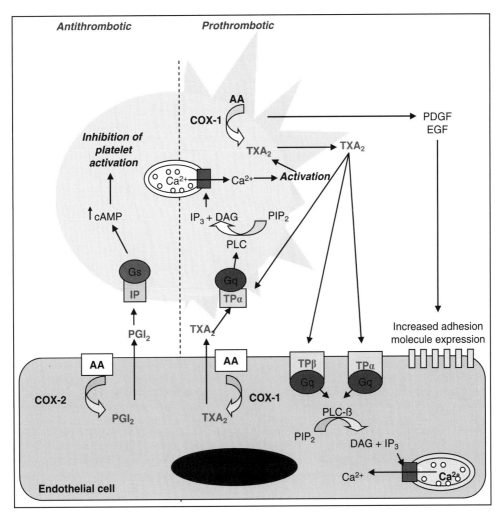

Figure 4.2
Schematic representation of the role of COX-1 and COX-2 on the vasculature. Endothelial cells express both COX-1 and COX-2, resulting in the generation of PGI$_2$ and TXA$_2$, respectively. Conversely, platelets express only COX-1. PGI$_2$ and TXA$_2$ mediate opposing effects on the platelet. TXA$_2$ is a potent platelet activator, whereas PGI$_2$ is a platelet inhibitor. In atherosclerosis, PGI$_2$ generation inhibits TXA$_2$-induced platelet activation and aggregation. Administration of a non-selective non-steroidal anti-inflammatory drug (NSAID) decreases generation of both TXA$_2$ and PGI$_2$, leading to reduced platelet aggregation. However, selective inhibition of COX-2 decreases PGI$_2$ without a concomitant inhibition of TXA$_2$, and hence increases platelet aggregation. AA, arachidonic acid; PDGF, platelet-derived growth factor; EGF, epidermal growth factor; cAMP, cyclic adenosine monophosphate; IP$_3$, inositol trisphosphate; DAG, diacylglycerol; PIP$_2$ phosphatidylinositol biphosphate; PhC, phospholipase C. (see color plate)

murine models genetically deficient in COX-2 A complete understanding of the role of the COX isoforms in the vasculature, in particular in the pathogenesis of atherosclerosis and thrombosis, is as yet elusive.

Conclusions

COX-1 and COX-2 are expressed widely throughout the vasculature, and are responsible for the production of prostanoid products that have pro- and anti-thrombotic, -inflammatory, and -atherosclerotic actions. Pharmacological inhibitors of the COX enzymes are widely used both for resolution of inflammation and pain, in the case of the non-selective NSAIDs, and for secondary prevention of thrombotic cardiovascular events, in the case of aspirin. Indeed, important insights into the complex vascular roles of the COX isoforms have been gleaned from the use of selective COX inhibitors. The disparity in the cardiovascular effects of COX-1 and COX-2 inhibition highlights the importance of, and critical differences between, the roles of the COX isoforms in the vasculature (shown schematically in Figure 4.2). While the beneficial effects of platelet COX-1 inhibition have been successfully harnessed for thrombosis prophylaxis, the pathological prothrombotic effects of selective COX-2 inhibitors have underlined the importance of establishing the precise roles of the COX isozymes in the vasculature.

References

1. Grosser T, Fries S, FitzGerald GA. Biological basis for the cardiovascular consequences of COX-2 inhibition: therapeutic challenges and opportunities. J Clin Invest 2006;116:4–15.
2. Raychowdhury MK, Yukawa M, Collins LJ et al. Alternative splicing produces a divergent cytoplasmic tail in the human endothelial thromboxane A2 receptor. J Biol Chem 1994;269:19256–61 [Erratum 1995;270:7011].
3. Forman BM, Chen J, Evans RM. Hypolipidemic drugs, polyunsaturated fatty acids, and eicosanoids are ligands for peroxisome proliferator-activated receptors alpha and delta. Proc Natl Acad Sci U S A 1997;94:4312–17.
4. Gupta RA, Brockman JA, Sarraf P et al. Target genes of peroxisome proliferator-activated receptor gamma in colorectal cancer cells. J Biol Chem 2001;276:29681–7.
5. Smith WL, Garavito RM, DeWitt DL. Prostaglandin endoperoxide H synthases (cyclooxygenases)-1 and -2. J Biol Chem 1996; 271: 33157–6.
6. Caughey GE, Cleland LG, Penglis PS et al. Roles of cyclooxygenase (COX)-1 and COX-2 in prostanoid production by human endothelial cells: selective up-regulation of prostacyclin synthesis by COX-2. J Immunol 2001;167:2831–8.
7. Brock TG, McNish RW, Peters-Golden M. Arachidonic acid is preferentially metabolized by cyclooxygenase-2 to prostacyclin and prostaglandin E2. J Biol Chem 1999;274:11660–6.
8. Picot D, Garavito RM. Prostaglandin H synthase: implications for membrane structure. FEBS Lett 1994;346:21–5.
9. Kurumbail RG, Stevens AM, Gierse JK et al. Structural basis for selective inhibition of cyclooxygenase-2 by anti-inflammatory agents. Nature 1996;384:644–8.
10. Spencer AG, Thuresson E, Otto JC et al. The membrane binding domains of prostaglandin endoperoxide H synthases 1 and 2. Peptide mapping and mutational analysis. J Biol Chem 1999;274:32936–42.
11. McAdam BF, Mardini IA, Habib A et al. Effect of regulated expression of human cyclooxygenase isoforms on eicosanoid and isoeicosanoid production in inflammation. J Clin Invest 2000;105:1473–82.
12. Belton OA, Duffy A, Toomey S, Fitzgerald DJ. Cyclooxygenase isoforms and platelet vessel wall interactions in the apolipoprotein E knockout mouse model of atherosclerosis. Circulation 2003;108: 3017–23.
13. Hetu PO, Riendeau D. Cyclo-oxygenase-2 contributes to constitutive prostanoid production in rat kidney and brain. Biochem J 2005;391:561–6.
14. Jones DA, Carlton DP, McIntyre TM et al. Molecular cloning of human peroxide synthase type II and demonstration in response to cytokines. J Biol Chem 1993;268:9049–54.
15. Xie W, Herschman HR. Transcriptional regulation of prostaglandin synthase 2 gene expression by platelet-derived growth factor and serum. J Biol Chem 1996;271:31742–8.
16. Adderley SR, Fitzgerald DJ. Oxidative damage of cardiomyocytes is limited by extracellular regulated kinases 1/2-mediated induction of cyclooxygenase-2. J Biol Chem 1999;274:5038–46.
17. Smith LH, Boutaud O, Breyer M et al. Cyclooxygenase-2-dependent prostacyclin formation is regulated by low density lipoprotein cholesterol in vitro. Arterioscler Thromb Vasc Biol 2002;22:983–8.
18. Gilroy DW, Colville-Nash PR, Willis D et al. Inducible cyclooxygenase may have anti-inflammatory properties. Nat Med 1999;5: 698–701.
19. Loll PJ, Picot D, Garavito RM. The structural basis of aspirin activity inferred from the crystal structure of inactivated prostaglandin H2 synthase. Nat Struct Biol 1995;2:637–43.
20. Lecomte M, Laneuville O, Ji C et al. Acetylation of human prostaglandin endoperoxide synthase-2 (cyclooxygenase-2) by aspirin. J Biol Chem 1994;269:13207–15.
21. Mitchell JA, Akarasereenont P, Thiemermann C et al. Selectivity of nonsteroidal antiinflammatory drugs as inhibitors of constitutive and inducible cyclooxygenase. Proc Natl Acad Sci U S A 1993;90: 11693–7.
22. Schonbeck U, Sukhova GK, Graber P et al. Augmented expression of cyclooxygenase-2 in human atherosclerotic lesions. Am J Pathol 1999;155:1281–91.
23. Belton O, Byrne D, Kearney D et al. Cyclooxygenase-1 and -2-dependent prostacyclin formation in patients with atherosclerosis. Circulation 2000;102:840–5.
24. Libby P. Inflammation in atherosclerosis. Nature 2002;420:868–74.
25. Sciulli MG, Renda G, Capone ML et al. Heterogeneity in the suppression of platelet cyclooxygenase-1 activity by aspirin in coronary heart disease. Clin Pharmacol Ther 2006;80:115–25.
26. Evangelista V, Manarini S, Di Santo A et al. De novo synthesis of cyclooxygenase-1 counteracts the suppression of platelet thromboxane biosynthesis by aspirin. Circ Res 2006;98:593–5.
27. Fitzgerald DJ, Doran J, Jackson E, FitzGerald GA. Coronary vascular occlusion mediated via thromboxane A2-prostaglandin endoperoxide receptor activation in vivo. J Clin Invest 1986;77:496–502.
28. Pratico D, Cyrus T, Li H, FitzGerald GA. Endogenous biosynthesis of thromboxane and prostacyclin in 2 distinct murine models of atherosclerosis. Blood 2000;96:3823–6.
29. Karanian JW, Salem N Jr. Hydroxylated 22-carbon fatty acids in platelet and vascular smooth muscle function: interference with TXA2/PGH2 receptors. Agents Actions Suppl 1995;45:39–45.
30. Osborne JA, Lefer AM. Cardioprotective actions of thromboxane receptor antagonism in ischemic atherosclerotic rabbits. Am J Physiol 1988;255:H318–24.

31. Tanaka T, Sato R, Kurimoto T. Z-335, a new thromboxane A_2 receptor antagonist, prevents arterial thrombosis induced by ferric chloride in rats. Eur J Pharmacol 2000;401:413–18.

32. Cayatte AJ, Du Y, Oliver-Krasinski J et al. The thromboxane receptor antagonist S18886 but not aspirin inhibits atherogenesis in apo E-deficient mice: evidence that eicosanoids other than thromboxane contribute to atherosclerosis. Arterioscler Thromb Vasc Biol 2000;20:1724–8.

33. Egan KM, Wang M, Fries S et al. Cyclooxygenases, thromboxane, and atherosclerosis: plaque destabilization by cyclooxygenase-2 inhibition combined with thromboxane receptor antagonism. Circulation 2005;111:334–42.

34. Kobayashi T, Tahara Y, Matsumoto M et al. Roles of thromboxane A_2 and prostacyclin in the development of atherosclerosis in apoE-deficient mice. J Clin Invest 2004;114:784–94.

35. Pratico D, Tillmann C, Zhang ZB et al. Acceleration of atherogenesis by COX-1-dependent prostanoid formation in low density lipoprotein receptor knockout mice. Proc Natl Acad Sci U S A 2001;98: 3358–63.

36. Cyrus T, Sung S, Zhao L et al. Effect of low-dose aspirin on vascular inflammation, plaque stability, and atherogenesis in low-density lipoprotein receptor-deficient mice. Circulation 2002; 106:1282–7.

37. Ho E, Rooney C, Harhen B et al. Atherosclerosis and oxidative stress contribute to aspirin nonresponse in hypertensive subjects. Circulation 2004;110:608.

38. Pulcinelli FM, Riondino S, Celestini A et al. Persistent production of platelet thromboxane A_2 in patients chronically treated with aspirin. J Thromb Haemost 2005;3:2784–9.

39. McClelland S, Toomey S, Hahren B et al. Cyclooxygenase-1 gene deletion inhibits atherosclerosis in the ApoE$^{-/-}$ mouse model. Arterioscler Thromb Vasc Biol 2004;24:e73 (abst).

40. Zhuge X, Arai H, Xu Y et al. Protection of atherogenesis in thromboxane A_2 receptor-deficient mice is not associated with thromboxane A_2 receptor in bone marrow-derived cells. Biochem Biophys Res Commun 2006;351:865–71.

41. Libby P, Warner SJ, Salomon RN, Birinyi LK. Production of platelet-derived growth factor-like mitogen by smooth-muscle cells from human atheroma. N Engl J Med 1988;318:1493–8.

42. Murata T, Ushikubi F, Matsuoka T et al. Altered pain perception and inflammatory response in mice lacking prostacyclin receptor. Nature 1997;388:678–82.

43. Cipollone F, Prontera C, Pini B et al. Overexpression of functionally coupled cyclooxygenase-2 and prostaglandin E synthase in symptomatic atherosclerotic plaques as a basis of prostaglandin E_2-dependent plaque instability. Circulation 2001;104:921–7.

44. Metzner J, Popp L, Marian C et al. The effects of COX-2 selective and non-selective NSAIDs on the initiation and progression of atherosclerosis in ApoE$^{-/-}$ mice. J Mol Med 2007;85:623–33.

45. Egan KM, Lawson JA, Fries S et al. COX-2-derived prostacyclin confers atheroprotection on female mice. Science 2004;306:1954–7.

46. Colville-Nash PR, Gilroy DW, Willis D et al. Prostaglandin F2α produced by inducible cyclooxygenase may contribute to the resolution of inflammation. Inflammopharmacology 2005;12:473–6.

47. Moncada S, Gryglewski R, Bunting S, Vane JR. An enzyme isolated from arteries transforms prostaglandin endoperoxides to an unstable substance that inhibits platelet aggregation. Nature 1976;263:663–5.

48. Antithrombotic Trialists' Collaboration. Collaborative meta-analysis of randomized trials of antiplatelet therapy for prevention of death, myocardial infarction, and stroke in high risk patients. BMJ 2002;324:71–86.

49. Antiplatelet Trialists' Collaboration. Collaborative overview of randomized trial os anti-platelet therapy-I: prevention of death, myocardial infarction and stroke by prolonged antiplatelet therapy in various categories of patients. BMJ 1994;308:81–106.

50. Eikelboom JW, Hirsh J, Weitz JI. Aspirin-resistant thromboxane biosynthesis and the risk of myocardial infarction, stroke, or cardiovascular death in patients at high risk for cardiovascular events. Circulation 2002;105:1650–5.

51. Ratnatunga CP, Edmondson SF, Rees GM, Kovacs IB. High-dose aspirin inhibits shear-induced platelet reaction involving thrombin generation. Circulation 1992;85:1077–82.

52. Coppinger JA, Cagney G, Toomey S et al. Characterization of the proteins released from activated platelets leads to localization of novel platelet proteins in human atherosclerotic lesions. Blood 2004;103:2096–104.

53. Santilli F, Davi G, Consoli A et al. Thromboxane-dependent CD40 ligand release in type 2 diabetes mellitus. J Am Coll Cardiol 2006;47:391–7.

54. Husain S, Andrews NP, Mulcahy D et al. Aspirin improves endothelial dysfunction in atherosclerosis. Circulation 1998;97: 716–20.

55. Silverstein FE, Faich G, Goldstein JL et al. Gastrointestinal toxicity with celecoxib vs nonsteroidal antiinflammatory drugs for osteoarthritis and rheumatoid arthritis: the CLASS study: a randomized controlled trial. Celecoxib Long-term Arthritis Safety Study. JAMA 2000;284:1247–55.

56. Bombardier C, Laine L, Reicin A et al; VIGOR Study Group. Comparison of upper gastrointestinal toxicity of rofecoxib and naproxen in patients with rheumatoid arthritis. VIGOR Study Group. N Engl J Med 2000;343:1520–8.

57. Collantes E, Curtis SP, Lee KW et al; Etoricoxib Rheumatoid Arthritis Study Group. A multinational randomized, controlled, clinical trial of etoricoxib in the treatment of rheumatoid arthritis [ISRCTN25142273]. BMC Fam Pract 2002;3:10.

58. Schnitzer TJ, Burmester GR, Mysler E et al; TARGET Study Group. Comparison of lumiracoxib with naproxen and ibuprofen in the Therapeutic Arthritis Research and Gastrointestinal Event Trial (TARGET), reduction in ulcer complications: randomised controlled trial. Lancet 2004;364:665–74.

59. Nussmeier NA, Whelton AA, Brown MT et al. Complications of the COX-2 inhibitors parecoxib and valdecoxib after cardiac surgery. N Engl J Med 2005;352:1081–91.

60. Burleigh ME, Babaev VR, Oates JA et al. Cyclooxygenase-2 promotes early atherosclerotic lesion formation in LDL receptor-deficient mice. Circulation 2002;105:1816–23.

61. Olesen M, Kwong E, Meztli A et al. No effect of cyclooxygenase inhibition on plaque size in atherosclerosisprone mice. Scand Cardiovasc J 2002;36:362–7.

62. Bea F, Blessing E, Bennett BJ et al. Chronic inhibition of cyclooxygenase-2 does not alter plaque composition in a mouse model of advanced unstable atherosclerosis. Cardiovasc Res 2003;60: 198–204.

63. Rott D, Zhu J, Burnett MS et al. Effects of MF-tricyclic, a selective cyclooxygenase-2 inhibitor, on atherosclerosis progression and susceptibility to cytomegalovirus replication in apolipoprotein-E knockout mice. J Am Coll Cardiol 2003;41:1812–19.

64. Burleigh ME, Babaev VR, Yancey PG et al. Cyclooxygenase-2 promotes early atherosclerotic lesion formation in ApoE-deficient and C57BL/6 mice. J Mol Cell Cardiol 2005;39:443–52.

65. Burleigh ME, Babaev VR, Patel MB et al. Inhibition of cyclooxygenase with indomethacin phenethylamide reduces atherosclerosis in apoE-null mice. Biochem Pharmacol 2005;70:334–42.

66. Babaev VR, Ding L, Reese J et al. Cyclooxygenase-1 deficiency in bone marrow cells increases early atherosclerosis in apolipoprotein E- and low-density lipoprotein receptor-null mice. Circulation 2006;113:108–17.

67. Narasimha A, Watanabe J, Lin JA et al. A novel anti-atherogenic role for COX-2-potential mechanism for the cardiovascular side effects of COX-2 inhibitors. Prostaglandins Other Lipid Mediat 2007; 84:24–33.

68. Bresalier RS, Sandler RS, Quan H et al. Adenomatous Polyp Prevention on Vioxx (APPROVe) Trial Investigators. Cardiovascular events associated with rofecoxib in a colorectal adenoma chemoprevention trial. N Engl J Med 2005;352:1092–102.

69. Sowers JR, White WB, Pitt B et al. Celecoxib Rofecoxib Efficacy and Safety in Comorbidities Evaluation Trial (CRESCENT) Investigators. The effects of cyclooxygenase-2 inhibitors and nonsteroidal anti-inflammatory therapy on 24-hour blood pressure in patients with hypertension, osteoarthritis, and type 2 diabetes mellitus. Arch Intern Med 2005;165:161–8.

70. Solomon SD, McMurray JJ, Pfeffer MA et al. Adenoma Prevention with Celecoxib (APC) Study Investigators. Cardiovascular risk associated with celecoxib in a clinical trial for colorectal adenoma prevention. N Engl J Med 2005;352:1071–80.

71. Ott E, Nussmeier NA, Duke PC et al. Multicenter Study of Perioperative Ischemia (McSPI) Research Group; Ischemia Research and Education Foundation (IREF) Investigators. Efficacy and safety of the cyclooxygenase 2 inhibitors parecoxib and valdecoxib in patients undergoing coronary artery bypass surgery. J Thorac Cardiovasc Surg 2003;125:1481–92.

5

P2Y$_{12}$ receptor antagonism: from bench to bedside

Dominick J Angiolillo and Esther Bernardo

Introduction

Platelets play a key role in the pathophysiology of acute coronary syndromes (ACS) and complications following percutaneous coronary intervention (PCI). Three classes of platelet-inhibiting drugs – aspirin, thienopyridines, and platelet glycoprotein (GP) IIb/IIIa inhibitors – are most commonly used for the prevention and treatment of disorders of arterial vascular thrombosis.[1] These antiplatelet agents have different mechanisms of action. Aspirin inhibits the cyclooxygenase (COX)-1 enzyme, thereby blocking thromboxane A$_2$ (TXA$_2$) synthesis in platelets.[2] For several decades, aspirin has been the sole option for antiplatelet therapy in the treatment and prevention of the manifestations of cardiovascular disease. Although an incredibly cost-effective therapy, patients at risk continue to experience thrombotic events despite aspirin therapy.[3] Glycoprotein (GP) IIb/IIIa inhibitors are very potent antiplatelet agents, as they inhibit the final common pathway that mediates platelet aggregation. However, although GPIIb/IIIa inhibitors effectively prevent periprocedural thrombotic complications, their short duration of action and parenteral dosing do not allow long-term protection. This has raised interest in developing and testing oral GPIIb/IIIa inhibitors. However, despite the promising rationale behind the use of these agents, clinical trials have failed to show any benefit. In particular, a pooled analysis from oral GPIIb/IIIa antagonist trials have shown increased mortality with these agents.[4] This has led investigators to evaluate the effects obtained with combinations of oral antiplatelet agents inhibiting other platelet-activating pathways, namely aspirin and thienopyridines, which inhibit the adenosine diphosphate (ADP) P2Y$_{12}$ receptor.

Purinergic receptors

ADP is one of the most important mediators of both physiological hemostasis and thrombosis.[5,6] Following platelet activation, ADP is not only released from its intracellular storage granules but also further activates platelets, amplifying this process. There are two main purinergic receptor types in the membrane: the guanosine triphosphate (GTP)-coupled protein receptors known as G-protein-binding sites and the ligand-gated ion channel.[5,6] The latter receptor is designated P2X$_1$ and the former P2Y, and each plays a specific and complementary role in platelet activation and aggregation (Figure 5.1).

P2X$_1$ mediates extracellular calcium influx, utilizes adenosine triphosphate (ATP) as an agonist, and leads to alteration in shape. There are two known P2Y receptors: P2Y$_1$ and P2Y$_{12}$, which utilize ADP as an agonist. Activation of the P2Y$_1$ receptor leads to a series of signaling events that initiate a weak and transient phase of platelet aggregation. In particular, P2Y$_1$ is coupled to a G$_q$ protein, and its intracellular signaling pathways involve activation of phospholipase C (PLC), resulting in diacylglycerol (DAG) and inositol trisphosphate (IP$_3$) production. DAG activates protein kinase C (PKC) leading to phosphorylation of myosin light-chain kinase and granule secretion; IP$_3$ leads to mobilization of intracellular calcium. Activation of the P2Y$_{12}$ receptor results in a complex series of intracellular signaling events that result in activation of the GPIIb/IIIa receptor, granule release, amplification of platelet aggregation, and stabilization of the platelet aggregate. The P2Y$_{12}$ receptor is coupled to a G$_i$ protein, and its intracellular signaling pathways involve activation of

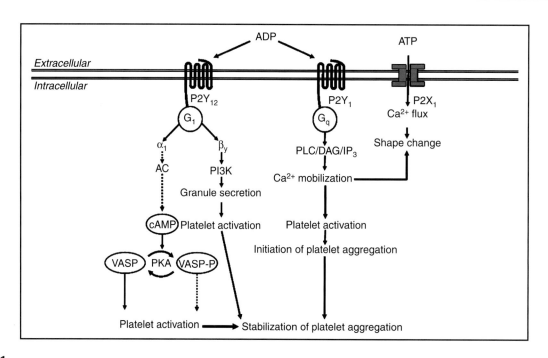

Figure 5.1
Purinergic receptors. Three P2 receptors are present on human platelets: $P2X_1$, $P2Y_1$, and $P2Y_{12}$. $P2X_1$ mediates extracellular calcium influx and utilizes adenosine triphosphate (ATP) as an agonist. $P2Y_1$ and $P2Y_{12}$ are G-coupled proteins that utilize adenosine diphosphate (ADP) as an agonist. The binding of ADP to the G_q-coupled $P2Y_1$ receptor leads to activation of phospholipase C (PLC), which generates diacylglycerol (DAG) and inositol trisphosphate (IP_3), leading to granule secretion and mobilization of intracellular calcium, inducing alteration in shape and initiating by a weak and transient phase of platelet aggregation. The binding of ADP to the G_i-coupled $P2Y_{12}$ receptor liberates the G_i protein subunits α_i and β_γ and leads to stabilization of platelet aggregation. The α_i subunit leads to inhibition of adenylyl cyclase (AC), which reduces cyclic adenosine monophosphate (cAMP) levels. The decrease in cAMP production reduces the activation of specific protein kinases (PKA), which in turn decreases phosphorylation (P) of vasodilator-stimulated phosphoprotein (VASP), leading to increased platelet activation and aggregation; the subunit β_γ activates kinases (PI3K), which induce granule secretion.

phosphatidylinositol 3′-kinase (PI3K) and inhibition of adenylyl cyclase (AC). PI3K activation leads to GPIIb/IIIa activation. Inhibition of AC decreases cyclic adenosine monophosphate (cAMP) levels. Reduction of cAMP levels influences the activity of cAMP-dependent protein kinases, which in turn reduce cAMP-mediated phosphorylation of vasodilator-stimulated phosphoprotein (VASP) and eliminate its protective effect on GPIIb/IIIa receptor activation (Figure 5.1).

$P2Y_{12}$ receptor antagonists: basic principles

Thienopyridines inhibit the ADP $P2Y_{12}$ receptor.[7] Ticlopidine, a first-generation thienopyridine, in combination with aspirin, enhances platelet inhibition.[7,8] This is due to the additive effects on platelet inhibition achieved with blockade of the cyclooxygenase (COX)-1 and $P2Y_{12}$

pathways.[7,8] Dual antiplatelet therapy was first explored in the emerging clinical setting of coronary stenting. In fact, in the initial era of coronary stenting, the antithrombotic regimen of choice for the prevention of stent thrombosis was still not established, and various combinations of antiplatelet agents and anticoagulants were used, with elevated complication rates. The lack of a safe and efficacious antithrombotic drug regimen for patients undergoing coronary stenting significantly limited the growth of coronary interventions. Landmark clinical trials demonstrated that, in patients undergoing coronary stenting, better clinical outcomes were achieved with the combined use of aspirin and ticlopidine than with aspirin alone or aspirin plus warfarin.[9–12] These results, accompanied by a better knowledge of stent deployment techniques,[13] played a pivotal role in the growth of coronary stenting. However, there are two major limitations with the use of ticlopidine: its safety profile (i.e. ticlopidine leads to elevated rates of neutropenia, thrombocytopenia, rash, and adverse gastrointestinal effects) and its inability to induce platelet inhibition rapidly.[14] This led researchers to pursue the development of an antiplatelet agent with the same beneficial properties as ticlopidine, but without its limitations. Thus, clopidogrel, a second-generation thienopyridine, was developed. Today, clopidogrel has largely replaced ticlopidine.

Clopidogrel selectively and irreversibly inhibits the P2Y$_{12}$ receptor.[6] It is an inactive prodrug that requires oxidation by the hepatic cytochrome P450 (CYP) system to generate an active metabolite. In particular, the thiophene ring of clopidogrel is oxidized to form an intermediate metabolite (2-oxoclopidogrel), which is further oxidized, resulting in opening of the thiophene ring and the formation of a carboxyl and a thiol group. The reactive thiol group of the active metabolite of clopidogrel forms a disulfide bridge to one or more cysteine residues of the P2Y$_{12}$ receptor, resulting in its irreversible blockade for the life of the platelet. Thus, P2Y$_{12}$ receptor blockade occurs early in the cascade of events leading to the formation of the platelet thrombus and effectively inhibits platelet activation and aggregation processes.[6] In fact, platelet P2Y$_{12}$ blockade prevents platelet degranulation and the release reaction, which elaborates prothrombotic and inflammatory mediators from the platelet, and also inhibits transformation of the GPIIb/IIIa receptor to the form that binds fibrinogen and links platelets.

The major benefits of clopidogrel over ticlopidine include its better safety profile[14] and its ability to yield antiplatelet effects more rapidly through the administration of a loading dose.[15] The fact that clopidogrel is well tolerated at high doses makes it possible to achieve antiplatelet effects within hours of administration.[15] This has important clinical implications in patients with ACS and PCI, in whom thrombotic occlusions (e.g., reinfarction and stent thrombosis) most commonly occur within the first 24–48 hours. In addition to the better safety and pharmacodynamic profiles, there is also evidence that use of this second-generation thienopyridine leads to better clinical outcomes.[16] In fact, pooled data from more than 10 000 patients undergoing PCI showed lower rates of major adverse cardiac events at 30 days following treatment with clopidogrel than following treatment with ticlopidine.[16] Overall, the safety, pharmacodynamic, and clinical advantages of clopidogrel have led to its widespread adoption over ticlopidine as the antiplatelet agent of choice in patients undergoing PCI.[17]

Clopidogrel: clinical trials

The safety and efficacy of clopidogrel have been tested in a large number of clinical trials. These trials have been performed in patients with different manifestations of atherothrombotic disease, including coronary artery disease, cerebrovascular disease, and peripheral vascular disease. The main results of trials performed over the past decade with clopidogrel are summarized below.

In the CLASSICS trial (CLopidogrel ASpirin Stent International Cooperative Study), the safety/tolerability of clopidogrel versus ticlopidine was assessed.[14] Patients (n=1020) were randomized after successful stent placement and initiated on a 28-day regimen of either (a) 300 mg clopidogrel loading dose and 325 mg/day aspirin on day 1, followed by 75 mg/day clopidogrel and 325 mg/day aspirin; (b) 75 mg/day clopidogrel and 325 mg/day aspirin; or (c) 250 mg twice-daily ticlopidine and 325 mg/day aspirin. The primary endpoint (major peripheral or bleeding complications, neutropenia, thrombocytopenia, or early discontinuation of study drug as the result of noncardiac adverse events) occurred in 9.1% of patients in the ticlopidine group and 4.6% of patients in the combined clopidogrel group (relative risk 0.50; 95% confidence interval (CI) 0.31–0.81; $p = 0.005$).

The CAPRIE (Clopidogrel versus Aspirin in Patients at Risk of Ischemic Events) trial examined the effects of 75 mg clopidogrel once daily versus 325 mg aspirin once daily in a large secondary prevention population consisting of 19 185 patients with recent ischemic stroke, recent myocardial infrction (MI), or established peripheral arterial disease (PAD).[18] Patients were followed up for a mean of 1.9 years. The annual incidence of the primary endpoint (combined incidence of vascular death, MI, or ischemic stroke) was 5.32% with clopidogrel and 5.83% with aspirin, representing an 8.7% reduction in relative risk with clopidogrel above aspirin ($p = 0.043$).

The CURE (Clopidogrel in Unstable Angina to Prevent Recurrent Events) study examined outcomes with clopidogrel plus aspirin versus aspirin alone in patients ($n = 12 562$) with unstable angina or non Q-wave MI.[19] Patients were randomized to receive either clopidogrel (300 mg loading dose and 75 mg thereafter) or placebo in addition to aspirin for up to 1 year. Patients on clopidogrel and aspirin experienced a significant 20% reduction in the first primary outcome (composite vascular death, MI, or stroke) compared with patients receiving aspirin and placebo ($p < 0.001$). Significantly more patients in the clopidogrel plus aspirin group had major bleeding (3.7% vs 2.7%), but there was no increase in life-threatening bleeds. In the PCI–CURE study,[20] which included 2658 patients from the CURE study undergoing PCI, pretreatment with clopidogrel followed by long-term therapy after PCI was shown to be superior to a strategy of no pretreatment and short-term therapy for only 4 weeks after PCI (31% reduction in cardiovascular death or MI; $p = 0.002$).

The CREDO (Clopidogrel for the Reduction of Events During Observation) trial was a randomized, double-blind, placebo-controlled trial conducted among 2116 patients who were to undergo elective PCI or were deemed at high likelihood of undergoing PCI.[21] At 1 year, long-term clopidogrel therapy was associated with a 26.9% relative reduction in the combined risk of death, MI, or stroke (95% CI 3.9–44.4%; $p=0.02$; absolute reduction 3%). Clopidogrel pretreatment (300 mg loading dose) did not significantly reduce the combined risk of death, MI, or urgent target vessel revascularization at 28 days (reduction 18.5%; 95% CI −14.2% to 41.8%; $p=0.23$). However, in a prespecified subgroup analysis, patients who received clopidogrel at least 6 hours before PCI experienced a relative risk reduction of 38.6% (95% CI −1.6% to 62.9%; $p=0.051$) for this endpoint compared with no reduction with treatment less than 6 hours before PCI. In a recent analysis from the CREDO trial, the difference in outcomes between placebo and clopidogrel-pretreated patients was not significant until at least 15 hours of pretreatment, with a 58.8% ($p=0.028$) reduction in the primary endpoint in patients pretreated with clopidogrel for 15 hours or more compared with placebo.[22] The risk of major bleeding at 1 year increased, but not significantly (8.8% with clopidogrel vs 6.7% with placebo; $p=0.07$).

Recently, based on the results of two large-scale clinical trials, the use of clopidogrel has also been approved by the US Food and Drug Administration (FDA) in patients with ST-elevation MI (STEMI).[23,24] The CLARITY (Clopidogrel as Adjunctive Reperfusion Therapy) study and the PCI–CLARITY substudy were designed to address whether a beneficial effect of clopidogrel, including a loading dose, would be attained among STEMI patients who were being treated with thrombolytic therapy and undergoing coronary angiography during the index hospitalization.[25] A total of 3491 patients who presented within 12 hours after the onset of STEMI were randomly assigned to receive clopidogrel (300 mg loading dose followed by 75 mg daily) or placebo. Patients were scheduled to undergo coronary angiography after 48 hours, and those who underwent PCI during the index hospitalization formed the basis of PCI–CLARITY ($n=1863$). Clopidogrel pretreatment significantly reduced the incidence of cardiovascular death or ischemic complications both before and after PCI (at 30 days), without a significant increase in major or minor bleeding. In the COMMIT (ClOpidogrel and Metoprolol in Myocardial Infarction Trial) trial, in which 45 852 patients with acute MI were studied, adding clopidogrel 75 mg daily to aspirin and other standard treatments, including fibrinolytic therapy, safely reduced in-hospital mortality and major vascular events.[24]

In contrast to studies showing a clear benefit of dual antiplatelet therapy across the spectrum of patients with ACS, results of the CHARISMA (Clopidogrel for High Atherothrombotic Risk and Ischemic Stabilization, Management, and Avoidance) trial showed that in high-risk, but non-acute, patients ($n=15603$) with either clinically evident cardiovascular disease or multiple risk factors, clopidogrel plus aspirin was not significantly more effective than aspirin alone in reducing the rate of MI, stroke, or death from cardiovascular causes.[26] This study actually showed dual antiplatelet therapy to be harmful in patients without documented atherothrombotic disease ($n=3284$), as these patients had higher mortality, while in the subgroup of patients with clinically evident atherothrombosis ($n=12153$), there was a 12% relative risk reduction in event rates with clopidogrel ($p=0.046$).[29] Most recently, a subgroup analysis of the CHARISMA trial identified patients who were enrolled with documented prior MI, ischemic stroke, or symptomatic PAD, also known as the CAPRIE-like population ($n=9478$).[27] In this subgroup, there was a 17% relative risk reduction in event rates ($p=0.01$) with clopidogrel. Of note, the greatest benefit was observed in patients with prior MI ($n=3846$), in whom there was a 23% relative risk reduction in event rates ($p=0.031$), whereas no benefits were seen in patients with a history of coronary artery disease (CAD) but without prior MI. The findings of this study suggest that patients with a greater thrombotic burden (e.g., a history of plaque rupture and thrombosis) are most likely to derive benefit from an extended duration of dual antiplatelet therapy. However, studies specifically designed for these patients are warranted to test this hypothesis.

The CARESS (Clopidogrel and Aspirin for Reduction of Emboli in Symptomatic Carotid Stenosis) trail was a randomized, double-blind study in subjects with recently symptomatic ≥50% carotid stenosis.[28] Patients were screened with transcranial Doppler ultrasound, and if asymptomatic microembolic signals (MES) were detected, they were randomized to clopidogrel plus aspirin or aspirin monotherapy. MES, a marker of future stroke and transient ischemic attack (TIA) risk, were detected in 110 of 230 patients by online analysis at baseline, of whom 107 were randomized. In this study, combination therapy with clopidogrel and aspirin was shown to be more effective than aspirin alone in reducing asymptomatic embolization.

ACTIVE W (Atrial Fibrillation Clopidogrel Trial With Irbesartan for Prevention of Vascular Events) was a trial comparing oral anticoagulants (OAC) versus combined antiplatelet therapy with aspirin and clopidogrel for prevention of vascular events (first occurrence of stroke, non-central nervous system (CNS), embolism, MI, or vascular death) in 6706 patients with atrial fibrillation (AF).[29] The incidences of thromboembolic events and major bleeds were compared in patients with paroxysmal AF ($n=1202$) and persistent or permanent AF ($n=5495$). The incidence of stroke and non-CNS embolism was lower for patients treated with OAC, irrespective of the type of AF. There were more bleedings of any type in patients receiving clopidogrel plus aspirin, irrespective of the type of AF. The ACTIVE A arm of this trial will be evaluating, in patients with AF not able or not willing to take OAC, if combined antiplatelet therapy with aspirin and clopidogrel will be superior to aspirin plus placebo for prevention of vascular events. The ACTIVE I arm of this trial will be evaluating if irbesantan is more efficacious than placebo in reducing the composite endpoint in the overall study population.

The MATCH (Management of ATherothrombosis with Clopidogrel in High-risk patients) trial was performed to find out whether aspirin added to clopidogrel would further reduce the risk of recurrent ischemic vascular events in high-risk patients after TIA or ischemic stroke.[30] This was a randomized, double-blind, placebo-controlled trial to compare aspirin (75 mg/day) with placebo in 7599 high-risk patients with recent ischemic stroke or TIA and at least one additional vascular risk factor who were already receiving clopidogrel 75 mg/day. Adding aspirin to clopidogrel in high-risk patients with recent ischemic stroke or TIA was associated with a non-significant difference in reducing major vascular events, and the risk of life-threatening or major bleeding was increased.

P2Y$_{12}$ receptor antagonists: limitations

Despite the clinical benefits achieved with the adjunctive use of clopidogrel in high-risk patients, clinical experience with this drug has led us to appreciate some of its limitations. The major limitations of clopidogrel are attributed to its irreversible antiplatelet effects and to the broad variability of platelet inhibition achieved with this agent.[6] The first limitation, which is inherent to the family of thienopyridines, is a significant increase in bleeding risk in patients requiring surgery who have not withheld clopidogrel treatment for at least 5–7 days (i.e., the life of the platelet). The development of an antiplatelet agent with a reversible mechanism of action, allowing platelet function to return more rapidly to baseline status, would allow patients to undergo surgery more expeditiously without any increase in bleeding risk. The second limitation, platelet inhibition variability, may explain why the antiplatelet effects achieved with a loading dose of clopidogrel are not always rapid and why elevated platelet reactivity may persist in some patients despite the adjunctive use of this antiplatelet drug. Although the mechanisms leading to inadequate clopidogrel-induced antiplatelet effects are not fully elucidated, they may include clinical, cellular, and genetic factors.[6] Furthermore, although the best method of assessing antiplatelet drug response has not been fully established,[6] it is well known that enhanced platelet reactivity plays a key role in atherothrombotic complications. Currently, there is sufficient evidence to support the belief that the persistence of enhanced platelet reactivity, despite the use of clopidogrel, is a clinically relevant entity.

The inefficient conversion of clopidogrel to its active metabolite appears to play a pivotal role in the inadequate clopidogrel-induced antiplatelet effect.[6] In fact, approximately 85% of the prodrug is hydrolyzed by esterases to an inactive carboxylic acid derivative, and only about 15% is metabolized by the CYP system in the liver to generate an active metabolite.[6] One way to increase the generation of the active metabolite of clopidogrel is to raise the dose of the drug, and numerous studies have focused on the impact of high loading doses of clopidogrel. Most of these studies have compared 600 mg with 300 mg loading dose regimens, and have shown that a 600 mg loading dose leads to an earlier, higher, and more sustained (up to 48 hours) inhibition of platelet function, with better response profiles.[31] This may explain why at least 12–15 hours of pretreatment with a 300 mg loading dose are necessary before any clinical benefit can be observed in patients undergoing PCI.[22] Using a 600 mg loading-dose regimen, full antiplatelet effects are achieved after 2 hours.[32] As a result, 600 mg loading doses of clopidogrel have been shown to be equally efficacious if initiated 2–24 hours prior to PCI.[33]

Despite the wide use of high clopidogrel doses in daily clinical practice, studies assessing high-dose regimens are few, and these regimens still have not been approved by the US FDA. To date, the clinical impact of a 600 mg clopidogrel loading dose has been observed in two small studies in patients undergoing PCI, in which pretreatment was shown to be associated with better clinical outcomes – primarily a reduction in periprocedural MI – when compared with pretreatment with a 300 mg loading dose.[34,35] The large ($n \approx 14\,000$) ongoing CURRENT/OASIS-7 (Clopidogrel Optimal Loading Dose Usage to Reduce Recurrent Events/ Optimal Antiplatelet Strategy for Interventions) trial has been designed to determine whether high-dose clopidogrel leads to better clinical outcomes than standard-dose clopidogrel in patients with NSTE–ACS who are undergoing PCI.[6] Patients randomized to the high dose will receive a 600 mg loading dose and then a 150 mg/day maintenance dose from days 2 through 7; patients randomized to the standard dose will receive a 300 mg loading dose and then a 75 mg/day maintenance dose from days 2 through 7. All patients will receive clopidogrel 75 mg/day from days 8 through 30. In addition, all patients will receive aspirin ≥300 mg on day 1, and then be randomized to receive low-dose (75–100 mg) or high-dose (300–325 mg) aspirin.

The impact of increasing the loading dose of clopidogrel to 900 mg has been evaluated recently. Although 600 mg and 900 mg loading doses were associated with greater and faster platelet inhibition than was a 300 mg loading dose, no major differences were observed between the 600 and 900 mg loading-dose regimens.[36,37] Thus, although the clopidogrel response is dose-dependent, there is a threshold (likely attributable to the absorption rate of the drug) that does not allow enhancement of the platelet inhibitory effects beyond a certain dose.[36] Importantly, despite the better degree of platelet inhibition achieved with high loading doses, a wide variability in the effects achieved still persists. A higher maintenance dose of clopidogrel (150 mg/day) has also been evaluated; this resulted in enhanced platelet inhibition compared with the standard 75 mg dose,[38-41] but the antiplatelet effects achieved remain highly variable, and over 50% of patients did not reach the suggested therapeutic targets of $P2Y_{12}$ inhibition.[38,39] The wide variability of antiplatelet effects achieved with clopidogrel points to the need for drugs with more favorable pharmacokinetic and pharmacodynamic profiles.[6] Indeed, the adjunctive use of a GPIIb/IIIa inhibitor in patients with poor clopidogrel response and in whom more potent platelet inhibition is warranted (i.e., high-risk patients) represents a currently available therapeutic option in the acute phase of treatment.[42] Nevertheless, alternative treatment strategies are needed that can yield rapid and potent inhibition in the acute phase of treatment and guarantee sustained platelet inhibition without wide variability in individual response during the maintenance phase of treatment.[6,43] Numerous antiplatelet agents are currently under advanced clinical development, and further studies will address if these agents can be associated with better clinical outcomes without any compromise in safety. These agents include $P2Y_{12}$ receptor antagonists administered orally and intravenously, as well as agents with reversible and irreversible antiplatelet effects. These agents are described in Chapters 9–11 and 14. Other novel antiplatelet agents under advanced clinical testing that block other key platelet receptors and enzymes are described in Chapter 11.

References

1. Duffy B, Bhatt DL. Antiplatelet agents in patients undergoing percutaneous coronary intervention: how many and how much? Am J Cardiovasc Drugs 2005;5:307–18.
2. Patrono C, Garcia Rodriguez LA, Landolfi R, Baigent C. Low-dose aspirin for the prevention of atherothrombosis. N Engl J Med 2005;353:2373–83.
3. Wallentin LC. Aspirin (75 mg/day) after an episode of unstable coronary artery disease: long-term effects on the risk for myocardial infarction, occurrence of severe angina and the need for revascularization. Research Group on Instability in Coronary Artery Disease in Southeast Sweden. J Am Coll Cardiol 1991;18:1587–93.
4. Chew DP, Bhatt DL, Sapp S, Topol EJ. Increased mortality with oral platelet glycoprotein IIb/IIIa antagonists: a meta-analysis of phase III multicenter randomized trials. Circulation 2001;103:201–6.
5. Storey RF, Newby LJ, Heptinstall S. Effects of $P2Y_1$ and $P2Y_{12}$ receptor antagonists on platelet aggregation induced by different agonists in human whole blood. Platelets 2001;12:443–7.
6. Angiolillo DJ, Fernandez-Ortix A, Bernanrdo E et al. Variability in individual responsiveness to clopidogrel: clinical implications, management and future perspectives. J Am Coll Cardiol 2007;49:1505–16.
7. Nagakawa Y, Akedo Y, Orimo H, Yano H. Effect of the combination of antiplatelet agents in man: combination of aspirin, trapidil, ticlopidine and dipyridamole. Thromb Res 1990;60:469–75.
8. Savi P, Herbert JM. Clopidogrel and ticlopidine: P2Y12 adenosine diphosphate-receptor antagonists for the prevention of atherothrombosis. Semin Thromb Hemost 2005;31:174–83.
9. Leon MB, Baim DS, Popma JJ et al. A clinical trial comparing three antithrombotic-drug regimens after coronary-artery stenting. Stent Anticoagulation Restenosis Study Investigators. N Engl J Med 1998;339:1665–71.
10. Urban P, Macaya C, Rupprecht HJ et al. Randomized evaluation of anticoagulation versus antiplatelet therapy after coronary stent implantation in high-risk patients: the Multicenter Aspirin and Ticlopidine Trial after Intracoronary Stenting (MATTIS). Circulation 1998;98:2126–32.
11. Bertrand ME, Legrand V, Boland J et al. Randomized multicenter comparison of conventional anticoagulation versus antiplatelet therapy in unplanned and elective coronary stenting. The Full Anticoagulation versus Aspirin and Ticlopidine (FANTASTIC) study. Circulation 1998;98:1597–603.
12. Schomig A, Neumann FJ, Kastrati A et al. A randomized comparison of antiplatelet and anticoagulant therapy after the placement of coronary-artery stents. N Engl J Med 1996;334:1084–9.
13. Colombo A, Hall P, Nakamura S et al. Intracoronary stenting without anticoagulation accomplished with intravascular ultrasound guidance. Circulation 1995;91:1676–88.
14. Bertrand ME, Rupprecht HJ, Urban P, Gershlick AH. Double-blind study of the safety of clopidogrel with and without a loading dose in combination with aspirin compared with ticlopidine in combination with aspirin after coronary stenting: the Clopidogrel Aspirin Stent International Cooperative Study (CLASSICS). Circulation 2000;102:624–9.
15. Cadroy Y, Bossavy JP, Thalamas C et al. Early potent antithrombotic effect with combined aspirin and a loading dose of clopidogrel on experimental arterial thrombogenesis in humans. Circulation 2000;101:2823–8.
16. Bhatt DL, Bertrand ME, Berger PB et al. Meta-analysis of randomized and registry comparisons of ticlopidine with clopidogrel after stenting. J Am Coll Cardiol 2002;39:9–14.
17. Smith SCJr, Feldman TE, Hirshfeld JW Jr et al. ACC/AHA/SCAI 2005 guideline update for percutaneous coronary intervention: a report of the American College of Cardiology/American Heart Association Task Force on Practice Guidelines (ACC/AHA/SCAI Writing Committee to Update the 2001 Guidelines for Percutaneous Coronary Intervention). J Am Coll Cardiol 2006;47:e1–121.
18. CAPRIE Steering Committee. A randomised, blinded, trial of clopidogrel versus aspirin in patients at risk of ischaemic events (CAPRIE). Lancet 1996;348:1329–39.
19. Yusuf S, Zhao F, Mehta SR et al; Clopidogrel in Unstable Angina to Prevent Recurrent Events Trial Investigators. Effects of clopidogrel in addition to aspirin in patients with acute coronary syndromes without ST-segment elevation. N Engl J Med 2001;345:494–502.
20. Mehta SR, Yusuf S, Peters RJ et al. Clopidogrel in Unstable Angina to Prevent Recurrent Events trial (CURE) Investigators. Effects of pretreatment with clopidogrel and aspirin followed by long-term therapy in patients undergoing percutaneous coronary intervention: the PCI–CURE study. Lancet 2001;358:527–33.
21. Steinhubl SR, Berger PB, Mann JT 3rd et al. CREDO Investigators. Clopidogrel for the Reduction of Events During Observation. Early and sustained dual oral antiplatelet therapy following percutaneous coronary intervention: a randomized controlled trial (CREDO). JAMA 2002;288:2411–20.
22. Steinhubl SR, Berger PB, Brennan DM, Topol EJ for the CREDO Investigators. Optimal timing for the initiation of pre-treatment

with 300 mg clopidogrel before percutaneous coronary intervention. J Am Coll Cardiol 2006;47:939–43.

23. Sabatine MS, Cannon CP, Gibson CM et al. Clopidogrel as Adjunctive Reperfusion Therapy (CLARITY)–Thrombolysis in Myocardial Infarction (TIMI) 28 Investigators. Addition of clopidogrel to aspirin and fibrinolytic therapy for myocardial infarction with ST-segment elevation. CLARITY–TIMI 28 Investigators. N Engl J Med 2005; 352:1179–89.

24. Chen ZM, Jiang LX, Chen YP et al. COMMIT (ClOpidogrel and Metoprolol in Myocardial Infarction Trial) collaborative group. Addition of clopidogrel to aspirin in 45,852 patients with acute myocardial infarction: randomised placebo-controlled trial. Lancet 2005;366:1607–21.

25. Sabatine MS, Cannon CP, Gibson CM et al. Clopidogrel as Adjunctive Reperfusion Therapy (CLARITY)–Thrombolysis in Myocardial Infarction (TIMI) 28 Investigators. Effect of clopidogrel pretreatment before percutaneous coronary intervention in patients with ST-elevation myocardial infarction treated with fibrinolytics: the PCI–CLARITY study. JAMA 2005;294:1224–32.

26. Bhatt DL, Fox KA, Hacke W et al. Clopidogrel for High Atherothrombotic Risk and Ischemic Stabilization, Management, and Avoidance (CHARISMA) Investigators. Clopidogrel and aspirin versus aspirin alone for the prevention of atherothrombotic events. N Engl J Med 2006;354:1706–17.

27. Bhatt DL, Flather MD, Hacke W et al, for the CHARISMA Investigators. Patients with prior myocardial infarction, stroke, or symptomatic peripheral arterial disease in the CHARISMA trial. J Am Coll Cardiol 2007;49:1982–8.

28. Markus HS, Droste DW, Kaps M et al. Dual antiplatelet therapy with clopidogrel and aspirin in symptomatic carotid stenosis evaluated using doppler embolic signal detection: the Clopidogrel and Aspirin for Reduction of Emboli in Symptomatic Carotid Stenosis (CARESS) trial. Circulation 2005;111:2233–40.

29. Hohnloser SH, Pajitnev D, Pogue J et al. Active incidence of stroke in paroxysmal versus sustained atrial fibrillation in patients taking oral anticoagulation or combined antiplatelet therapy: an ACTIVE W substudy. J Am Coll Cardiol 2007;50:2156–61.

30. Diener HC, Bogousslavsky J, Brass LM et al. Aspirin and clopidogrel compared with clopidogrel alone after recent ischaemic stroke or transient ischaemic attack in high-risk patients (MATCH): randomised, double-blind, placebo-controlled trial. Lancet 2004; 364:331–7.

31. Angiolillo DJ, Fernandez-Ortiz A, Bernardo E et al. High clopidogrel loading dose during coronary stenting: effects on drug response and interindividual variability. Eur Heart J 2004;25:1903–10.

32. Hochholzer W, Trenk D, Frundi D et al. Time dependence of platelet inhibition after a 600-mg loading dose of clopidogrel in a large, unselected cohort of candidates for percutaneous coronary intervention. Circulation 2005;111:2560–4.

33. Kandzari DE, Berger PB, Kastrati A et al, for the ISAR–REACT Study Investigators. Influence of treatment duration with a 600-mg dose of clopidogrel before percutaneous coronary revascularization. J Am Coll Cardiol 2004;44:2133–6.

34. Patti G, Colonna G, Pasceri V et al. Randomized trial of high loading dose of clopidogrel for reduction of periprocedural myocardial infarction in patients undergoing coronary intervention: results from the ARMYDA-2 (Antiplatelet therapy for Reduction of MYocardial Damage during Angioplasty) study. Circulation 2005; 111:2099–106.

35. Cuisset T, Frere C, Quilici J et al. Benefit of a 600-mg loading dose of clopidogrel on platelet reactivity and clinical outcomes in patients with non-ST-segment elevation acute coronary syndrome undergoing coronary stenting. J Am Coll Cardiol 2006; 48:1339–45.

36. von Beckerath N, Taubert D, Pogatsa-Murray G et al. Absorption, metabolization, and antiplatelet effects of 300-, 600-, and 900-mg loading doses of clopidogrel: results of the ISAR–CHOICE (Intracoronary Stenting and Antithrombotic Regimen: Choose Between 3 High Oral Doses for Immediate Clopidogrel Effect) trial. Circulation 2005;112:2946–50.

37. Montalescot G, Sideris G, Meuleman C et al. A randomized comparison of high clopidogrel loading-doses in patients with non-ST-elevation acute coronary syndromes: the ALBION trial. J Am Coll Cardiol 2006;48:931–8.

38. Angiolillo DJ, Shoemaker SB, Desai B et al. Randomized comparison of a high clopidogrel maintenance dose in patients with diabetes mellitus and coronary artery disease: results of the Optimizing Antiplatelet Therapy in Diabetes Mellitus (OPTIMUS) study. Circulation. 2007;115:708–16.

39. von Beckerath N, Kastrati A, Wieczorek A et al. A double-blind, randomized study on platelet aggregation in patients treated with a daily dose of 150 or 75 mg of clopidogrel for 30 days. Eur Heart J 2007;28:1814–19.

40. Angiolillo DJ, Costa MA, Shoemaker S et al. Functional effects of high clopidogrel maintenance dosing in patients with inadequate platelet inhibition. Am J Cardiol 2008; in press.

41. Angiolillo DJ, Bernardo E, Palazuelos J et al. Functional impact of high clopidogrel maintenance dosing in patients undergoing elective percutaneous coronary interventions: results of a randomized study. Thromb Haemost 2008; in press.

42. Dalby M, Montalescot G, Bal dit Sollier C et al. Eptifibatide provides additional platelet inhibition in non-ST-elevation myocardial infarction patients already treated with aspirin and clopidogrel. Results of the Platelet Activity Extinction in Non-Q-Wave Myocardial Infarction with Aspirin, Clopidogrel, and Eptifibatide (PEACE) study. J Am Coll Cardiol 2004;43:162–8.

43. Angiolillo DJ. ADP receptor antagonism: What's in the pipeline? Am J Cardiovasc Drugs 2007;7:425–34.

6

Timing, dosing, and length of clopidogrel therapy

Nicolas von Beckerath, and Adnan Kastrati

Timing of clopidogrel therapy

Value of pretreatment

In the initial trials in which dual antiplatelet therapy consisting of aspirin and ticlopidine was compared with aspirin and anticoagulation in patients treated with percutaneous coronary intervention (PCI), ticlopidine pretreatment was not recommended. Despite the lack of pretreatment, dual antiplatelet therapy was clearly more effective than aspirin and anticoagulation in preventing periprocedural thrombotic events.[1] However, soon after long-term post-PCI treatment with thienopyridines became the standard of care for patients receiving stents, reports began to emerge suggesting that pretreatment with these agents might also protect patients from periprocedural thrombotic events.[2,3] Thienopyridine therapy does not achieve its full inhibitory potential before about 7 days unless a loading dose is administered;[4] on the other hand, platelets account for a large proportion of periprocedural ischemic events, including distal embolization of platelet aggregates, thrombotic occlusion of side-branches, and thrombotic occlusion of the treated vessel segment. Steinhubl et al[2] analyzed outcomes in 175 consecutive patients with ticlopidine treatment prior to coronary stenting at the Cleveland Clinic Foundation. Longer duration of ticlopidine pretreatment was strongly associated with a lower incidence of procedure-related non-Q-wave myocardial infarction (MI): the incidence of MI was 29% for a duration of pretreatment <1 day, 14% for 1–2 days, and 5% for ≥3 days; p of the test for trend = 0.002).[2] Results of the early angioplasty trials utilizing aggressive antiplatelet therapy with glycoprotein (GP) IIb/IIIa receptor antagonists suggested that dual antiplatelet therapy without thienopyridine pretreatment does not achieve sufficient platelet inhibition at the time of the procedure. In the EPISTENT (Evaluation of Platelet IIb/IIIa Inhibitor for Stenting) trial, about 1600 patients were randomized to stenting with either placebo or abciximab in addition to aspirin and heparin.[5] Among patients randomized to placebo, ticlopidine pretreatment was associated

with a significant decrease in the incidence of the composite endpoint of death, MI, or target vessel revascularization (TVR) at 1 year (adjusted hazard ratio, 0.73; 95% confidence interval (CI) 0.54–0.98; $p = 0.036$).[3] A similar level of benefit was found in subset analyses of both the PCI-Clarity (PCI-Clopidogrel as Adjunctive Reperfusion Therapy) and PCI-CURE (PCI-Clopidogrel in Unstable Angina to Prevent Recurrent Events) trials.[6,7]

Pretreatment with a 300 mg loading dose

Clopidogrel pretreatment with a 300 mg loading dose given 3–24 hours before the intervention was evaluated in the CREDO (Clopidogrel for the Reduction of Events During Observation) trial.[8] CREDO was a double-blind randomized trial in which clopidogrel pretreatment was compared with placebo pretreatment. The mean duration of pretreatment in this trial was 9.8 hours.[9] Clopidogrel pretreatment did not significantly reduce the combined endpoint of death, MI, or urgent target vessel revascularization at 28 days (reduction 18.5%, 95% CI, −14.2% to 41.8%; $p = 0.23$).[8] Analyses of prespecified subgroups revealed that patients who received clopidogrel at least 6 hours before PCI experience a nearly significant relative risk reduction of 38.6% (95% CI, −1.6% to 62.9%; $p = 0.051$) for the combined endpoint at 28 days compared with no reduction in those patients who were pretreated less than 6 hours before PCI.[8] In a subsequent analysis of the CREDO data in which the duration of clopidogrel pretreatment was entered as a continuous variable, the difference in outcomes between placebo- and clopidogrel-pretreated patients was not significant until at least 15 hours between pretreatment and PCI, with a 58.8% ($p = 0.028$) reduction in the primary endpoint in patients pretreated with clopidogrel (Figure 6.1). In fact, the model in which the time from pretreatment to PCI was entered as a continuous variable suggests that at least 24 hours are needed to achieve the optimal effect of pretreatment when a 300 mg loading dose is used.

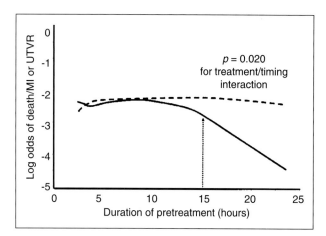

Figure 6.1
Relationship between the duration of study drug treatment before percutaneous coronary intervention and log odds of the primary combined 28-day endpoint of death, myocardial infarction (MI), and urgent target vessel revascularization (UTVR): dashed line, placebo; full line, clopidogrel. (Reprinted with permission from Steinhubl SR et al.[9])

In the light of more recent results on the use of a 600 mg loading dose,[10–12] the authors of this analysis concluded that pretreatment with a 300 mg loading dose should be given at least 15–24 hours before the intervention and, if such long pretreatment period is not possible, pretreatment with 600 mg should be used at least 2 hours before PCI.[9]

Pretreatment with a 600 mg loading dose

Platelet function studies have shown that, in contrast to administration of a 300 mg loading dose of clopidogrel, administration of a 600 mg loading dose results in platelet function inhibition similar to that achieved with chronic therapy within 2 hours.[13,14] In a randomized (albeit small) trial, administration of a 600 mg loading dose significantly reduced the incidence of periprocedural MI in patients treated with PCI as compared with administration of a 300 mg loading dose.[15] Moreover, the results of the ISAR-REACT (Intracoronary Stenting and Antithrombotic Regimen–Rapid Action for Coronary Treatment) trial are highly suggestive for a benefit resulting from pretreatment with a 600 mg loading dose in low- to intermediate-risk patients.[10] In this double-blind randomized trial including 2159 patients, it was tested whether administration of the GPIIb/IIIa antagonist abciximab reduces the incidence of ischemic complications in patients undergoing elective stent placement after pretreatment with a 600 mg loading dose of clopidogrel at least 2 hours before the intervention. The composite endpoint (death, MI, and urgent target-vessel revascularization at 30 days after PCI) was reached in 4%

(45 patients) in the group treated with abciximab and in 4% (43 patients) in the group treated with placebo (relative risk associated with abciximab 1.05; 95% CI 0.69–1.59; $p = 0.82$). The trial could not directly assess the benefits of the 600 mg loading dose, since all patients in the trial received it. However, the event rate was lower than that in low-risk subgroups in the placebo groups of similar controlled trials of a GPIIb/IIIa inhibitor (see, e.g., reference 5). Since other trials have indicated a benefit from a GPIIb/IIIa inhibitor, the data from ISAR-REACT (the lack of such an effect after clopidogrel pretreatment) suggest a favorable effect of the 600 mg loading dose given at least 2 hours before the intervention. In a subsequent analysis of the ISAR-REACT trial, clinical outcomes were examined relative to the duration of pretreatment with the 600 mg loading dose (2–3, 3–6, 6–12, and <12 hours) (Figure 6.2).[16] No significant differences were observed in outcome (the primary endpoint of the trial) between patient groups regarding the duration of pretreatment, irrespective of assignment to abciximab or placebo. In other words, this retrospective analysis of the ISAR-REACT trial suggests that when 600 mg of clopidogrel are given as pretreatment, a pretreatment duration of 2–3 hours is sufficient. Increasing the pretreatment duration above 2–3 hours does not result in an incremental clinical benefit.[16]

It has to be underscored, though, that the results of the ISAR-REACT trial, in which low- to intermediate-risk patients were included, cannot be applied to high-risk patients who present with an acute coronary syndrome. In fact, the ISAR-REACT 2 (Intracoronary Stenting and Antithrombotic Regimen: Rapid Early Action for Coronary Treatment 2) trial has demonstrated that, despite pretreatment with a 600 mg loading dose, adjunctive therapy with the GPIIb/IIIa inhibitor abciximab is beneficial. In this double-blind randomized trial, which included 2022 patients,

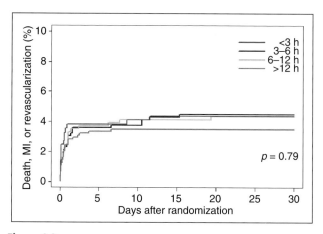

Figure 6.2
Kaplan–Meier event curves for the 30-day occurrence of death, myocardial infarction (MI), or urgent revascularization relative to clopidogrel loading-dose interval. (Adapted from Kandzari DE et al.[16])

abciximab reduced the risk of adverse events in patients with non-ST-segment elevation acute coronary syndromes (ACS) undergoing PCI after pretreatment with a 600 mg loading dose of clopidogrel (relative risk 0.75; 95% CI 0.58–0.97; $p=0.03$).[12] The benefits provided by abciximab, however, were confined to those patients who presented with an elevated plasma level of troponin. Apparently, the higher platelet activity observed in patients with ACS[17,18] requires a more potent inhibition than that provided by clopidogrel alone.

Dosing of clopidogrel therapy

Pharmacology of different loading doses

The effect of clopidogrel on platelet function is most commonly assessed by measuring adenosine diphosphate (ADP)-induced platelet aggregation with optical aggregometry. This method was also used in the initial phase I and II studies on single- and repeated-dose pharmacodynamics.[4,19,20] Single high doses (loading doses) of clopidogrel are being used to achieve a rapid onset of the antiplatelet effect of clopidogrel before PCI. Although other loading doses have also been used, most data are available for 300, 600, and 900 mg loading doses. The effects of single clopidogrel doses ranging from 100 to 600 mg had already been studied in one of the phase I trials.[19] Notably, in this early study, inhibition of ADP-induced platelet aggregation was similar 2 and 24 hours after ingestion of the studied clopidogrel doses (100, 200, 400, and 600 mg), indicating a rapid onset of the effect of single oral doses of clopidogrel. Since similar inhibition of ADP-induced platelet aggregation was observed with the 400 and 600 mg doses, it was assumed that a plateau response is reached in this dosing range.[19] The first study that systematically analyzed the time course of the onset of the antiplatelet effect of a clopidogrel loading dose used a dose of 375 mg.[21] In this study, the bulk of the antiplatelet effect was reached within 2 hours and the maximal effect was reached within 5 hours. Prompted by the need to further optimize peri-interventional thienopyridine therapy and by the failure of the CREDO trial to show a significant reduction of early thrombotic events after PCI by administering a 300 mg dose 6–24 hours before the intervention, more studies followed in which different loading doses were investigated in detail.[13,22,23] At least three studies showed that the administration of a 600 mg loading dose is more effective in suppressing ADP-induced platelet aggregation than a 300 mg dose.[13,22,23] Two randomized studies compared the effects of 300, 600, and 900 mg loading doses.[22,23] The ISAR-CHOICE (Intracoronary Stenting and Antithrombotic Regimen: Choose Between 3 High Oral Doses for Immediate Clopidogrel Effect) trial was a double-blind randomized trial including 60 patients with stable coronary disease prior to cardiac catheterization (20 patients treated with 300, 600, and 900 mg, respectively).[22] In this trial, ADP-induced platelet aggregation was assessed before and 4 hours after administration of clopidogrel. In addition, clopidogrel and its metabolites (the active thiol metabolite and the carboxyl metabolite that lacks any antiplatelet activity) were measured before and serially after administration of clopidogrel. The main results of this trial were that administration of a 600 mg loading dose results in more intense inhibition of platelet aggregation than administration of a 300 mg loading dose and that no further significant inhibition of platelet aggregation can be achieved with administration of a single 900 mg dose (Figure 6.3).

Pharmacokinetic data offer an explanation for both findings. Loading with 600 mg resulted in higher plasma concentrations of unchanged clopidogrel and the active

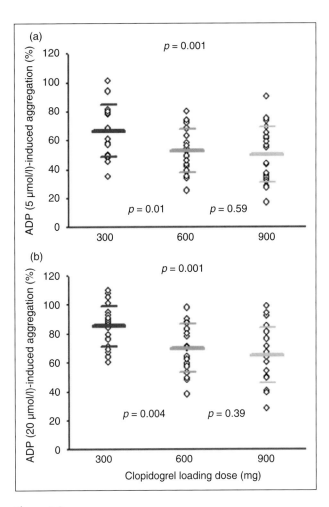

Figure 6.3

Maximal ADP-induced platelet aggregation 4 hours after administration of 300, 600, and 900 mg loading doses of clopidogrel. Platelets were stimulated with a final concentration of 5 μmol/l (a) and 20 μmol/l (b) ADP. Circles represent single measurements and bars denote mean±standard deviation. (Reprinted with permission from von Beckerath N et al.[22])

metabolite compared to loading with 300 mg ($p \leq 0.03$). With administration of 900 mg, no further increases in the plasma concentrations of clopidogrel or its active metabolite ($p \geq 0.38$) were achieved (Figure 6.4). This strongly suggests that intestinal absorption becomes the bottleneck when single doses > 600 mg are administered.

The pharmacokinetic data from ISAR-CHOICE clearly show that by far the largest proportion of clopidogrel is rapidly metabolized to its inactive and more stable carboxyl metabolite. With repeated administration of single high doses of clopidogrel a more intense inhibition of ADP-induced platelet aggregation may be achieved, but the practibility of such an approach is likely to be limited. In the ALBION (Asssessment of the Best Loading Dose of Clopidogrel to Blunt Platelet Activation, Inflammation and Ongoing Necrosis) trial, the antiplatelet effects of 300, 600, and 900 mg loading doses were studied in 103 patients with

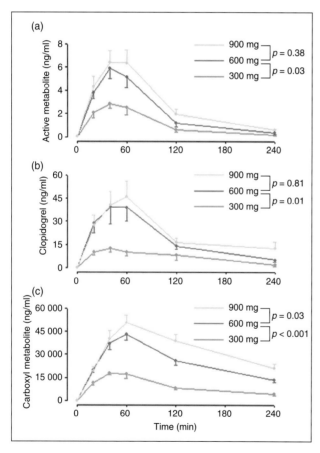

Figure 6.4
Plasma concentrations of the active metabolite (a), unchanged clopidogrel (b), and the carboxyl metabolite (c) before and serially after administration of a 300, 600, and 900 mg doses of clopidogrel. Data are presented as mean±standard error of the mean and analyzed by repeated measures ANOVA with contrasts for the three different clopidogrel doses. (Reprinted with permission from von Beckerath N et al.[22])

non-ST-segment elevation ACS in a randomized manner.[23] The main outcome measure was inhibition of ADP (5 and 20 µmol/l)-induced platelet aggregation (IPA). ADP-induced platelet aggregation was assessed before and 1, 2, 3, 4, 5, 6, and 24 hours after administration of the clopidogrel loading dose. When platelets were stimulated with 5 µmol/l ADP, IPA after administration of 600 and 900 mg was significantly higher than that after administration of 300 mg. No difference was observed between those patients treated with 600 mg and those treated with 900 mg of clopidogrel. When platelets were stimulated with 20 µmol/l ADP, a trend toward higher values for IPA was observed after administration of 900 mg as compared with 600 mg. At no single time point, however, did this difference reach the level of significance. Compared with IPA after 300 mg of clopidogrel, IPA after 900 mg was significantly higher at more time points than IPA after 600 mg. Altogether, the platelet aggregation data from the two studies show that very little (non-significant) extra antiplatelet effect is achieved with single doses exceeding 600 mg.[22,23] Moreover, the data from both trials suggest that the speed of onset of the effect is very similar with all three loading regimens. The difference between the 300 and 600 mg loading doses of clopidogrel is in the degree rather than in the speed of onset of their effect. A large variability in response to clopidogrel loading doses has been observed that (at least partly) results from variable intestinal absorption.[24] In addition, a failure to metabolize clopidogrel to its active thiol metabolite has been observed in individual patients resistant to a high clopidogrel loading dose.[25]

Daily maintenance dose

In the initial studies on repeated-dose pharmacodynamics, the antiaggregatory effects of daily maintenance doses ranging from 10 to 150 mg were studied.[4,20] In these dose-finding studies, with administration of 75 mg once daily the same degree of inhibition of platelet aggregation was achieved as with ticlopidine 250 mg twice daily, which was the target level of inhibition. Based on these results, the currently recommended maintenance dose of clopidogrel (75 mg/day) was chosen for the phase III CAPRIE (Clopidogrel versus Aspirin in Patients at Risk of Ischemic Events) trial and all subsequent clopidogrel trials with clinical endpoints.[26] Thus, all available data showing clinical benefit with clopidogrel therapy stem from the use of a 75 mg daily maintenance dose. This is the only maintenance dose approved by the FDA for the approved indications for this drug. Only recently has restriction to a daily dose of 75 mg as a unique dose for maintenance clopidogrel therapy been questioned.[27] A wide variability in the response to the current maintenance dose regime[28] and an increasing number of reports that show a relationship between the intensity of platelet function inhibition and the incidence of ischemic events after PCI[29] have fueled the discussion on the use of an increased maintenance dose of clopidogrel. Until recently, however, there were only very few data were available on the functional consequences of treatment with an increased (150 mg) daily dose of clopidogrel. The 150 mg daily maintenance dose has only been used in one of the dose-finding studies in healthy male adults.[4] In that study, subjects received either 25 mg ($n=6$), 50 mg ($n=6$), 100 mg ($n=5$), or 150 mg ($n=6$) clopidogrel once daily, and altogether 8 subjects received placebo. The treatment period was 16 days. A direct comparison with the antiplatelet effect of ticlopidine (250 mg twice daily) was missing. A dose-dependent inhibition of ADP-induced platelet aggregation was observed. ADP-induced platelet aggregation before dosing on day 16 was 79%, 55%, 37%, 39%, and 27% for treatment with placebo and daily doses of 25, 50, 100, and 150 mg respectively.[4] In two other dose-finding studies that incorporated a comparison with the antiplatelet effects of ticlopidine (250 mg twice daily) – one in healthy volunteers and one in patients with documented atherosclerotic disease – a similar degree of platelet function inhibition was observed with 75 and 100 mg of clopidogrel daily.[4,20] Therefore, it was assumed that a plateau response is reached with administration of 75 mg once daily. More recent reports, however, clearly show that administration of a higher daily maintenance dose (150 mg) results in a more intense inhibition of platelet aggregation than administration of 75 mg once daily.[30–32] Sixty patients after pretreatment with 600 mg of clopidogrel and within 12 hours after successful PCI were included in the ISAR-CHOICE2 (Intracoronary Stenting and Antithrombotic Regimen: Choose a High Oral maintenance dose for Intensified Clopidogrel Effect 2) trial.[30] They were allocated to receive one of two clopidogrel daily maintenance doses (75 or 150 mg) for 30 days in a double-blind randomized manner. Platelet function was evaluated 30 days after the intervention with optical aggregometry and with a new point-of-care test (VerifyNow P2Y$_{12}$ assay) that has been shown to correlate with the results of optical aggregometry.[33] Maximal ADP (5 μmol/l)-induced platelet aggregation 30 days after PCI in the group treated with 150 mg/day (45.1% ± 20.9%) was significantly lower than in the group treated with 75 mg/day (65.3% ± 12.1%; $p<0.001$).

The VerifyNow P2Y$_{12}$ assay also indicated a higher degree of platelet function inhibition in the group treated with 150 mg/day (60.0 ± 72.0 P2Y$_{12}$ Reaction Units) than in the group treated with 75 mg/day (117.0 ± 64.3 P2Y$_{12}$ Reaction Units; $p=0.004$). In the ExcelsiorACT study, it was shown that in patients with increased ADP-induced platelet aggregation despite pretreatment with a 600 mg loading dose, increasing the daily maintenance dose from 75 to 150 mg results in a significant improvement of platelet inhibition in individual patients.[31] Moreover, in that study, adjustment of the daily maintenance dose after initial testing resulted in

more consistent platelet inhibition of the entire cohort.[31] In the OPTIMUS (Optimizing Antiplatelet Therapy in diabetes MellitUS) trial, it was shown that the 150 mg daily maintenance dose results in more intense inhibition of platelet aggregation in diabetic patients who respond poorly to the 75 mg daily dosing regime.[32] The intensified clopidogrel effect of the 150 mg daily maintenance dose has the potential to further reduce the incidence of ischemic events after PCI. Whether the whole spectrum of patients undergoing PCI or only certain subgroups such as those with an increased thrombotic risk or blunted response to the usual clopidogrel dose would benefit from the daily dose of 150 mg of clopidogrel is still not known This and the optimal duration of such a regime need to be investigated in specifically designed and sufficiently powered clinical trials. These trials will clarify also whether the higher dose carries the risk of increased bleeding complications as compared with the conventional maintenance dose.

Length of therapy after coronary stenting
Bare metal stent implantation

The risk of stent thrombosis after implantation of a bare metal stent is highest during the first few days following the procedure, and disappears almost completely after 4 weeks.[34] Therefore, for a long time, the standard duration of thienopyridine therapy after bare metal stent implantation was 4 weeks. CREDO evaluated not only the possible benefit of clopidogrel loading before PCI but also the possible benefit of long-term (12-month) treatment with clopidogrel after PCI.[8] In the CREDO trial, clopidogrel therapy (loading with 300 mg 3–24 hours before PCI and extended clopidogrel therapy beyond 4 weeks) was associated with a 26.9% relative reduction in the combined risk of death, MI, or stroke (95% confidence interval, 3.9%–44.4%; $p=0.02$; absolute risk reduction, 3%). Although the treatment effect from day 29 until the end of follow-up at 1 year was not a prespecified analysis, continued treatment with clopidogrel beyond 4 weeks was associated with a further relative risk reduction of 37.4% in the combined endpoint (95% CI 1.8–60.1%; $p=0.04$). Thus, clopidogrel therapy beyond 4 weeks was beneficial, at the cost of a non-significant increase in the risk of major bleeding (from 6.7% to 8.8%; $p=0.07$), most cases of which were associated with aortocoronary bypass surgery.[8] Interestingly, prolonged clopidogrel therapy did not result in a reduction in urgent target vessel revascularization (2.0% in the clopidogrel group and 2.2% in the placebo group). Accordingly, the authors suggested that the reduction in the primary endpoint was generated by the reduction in the overall cardiovascular risk of the patients rather than by a reduction of

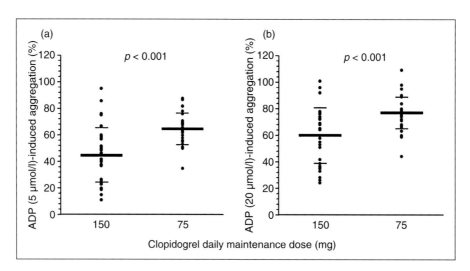

Figure 6.5
Maximal aggregation induced by (a) 5 μmol/l and (b) 20 μmol/l ADP in patients treated with two different clopidogrel daily maintenance doses (150 and 75 mg). Individual data are shown, along with mean (thick lines) and SD (thin lines). (Adapted from von Beckerath N et al. [30])

postprocedural complications.[8] Based on the results of the CREDO trial, the ACC/AHA/SCAI 2005 guideline update for percutaneous coronary intervention recommended at least 4 weeks and ideally up to 12 months of clopidogrel therapy in all patients receiving bare metal stents who are not at a high risk of bleeding.[35]

Drug-eluting stent implantation

Delayed endothelial coverage after drug-eluting stent (DES) implantation prolongs the window of vulnerability to stent thrombosis following the procedure. Instructions for the use in the USA of commercially available DES specify treatment with clopidogrel for at least 3 or 6 months after implantation of sirolimus-eluting or paclitaxel-eluting stents, respectively. These regimens were shown to be safe and effective in the clinical trials for the CYPHER and TAXUS stents when judged by 1-year outcome. European guidelines recommend at least 6 months of clopidogrel therapy after implantation of a drug-eluting stent independent of the drug that is being eluted from the stent.[36] Premature discontinuation of this minimum length of clopidogrel therapy after DES implantation is clearly associated with stent thrombosis.[37,38] Reports about late cases of stent thrombosis[39] and an excess of the combined rate of death and MI occurring after discontinuation of clopidogrel therapy more than 6 months after DES implantation[40] have cast doubt on whether the recommended regimens are sufficient. The prolonged risk of thrombosis after DES implantation has been supported by recent pathological studies.[41] In fact, the process of endothelialization was com-

plete after 6–7 months following bare metal stent implantation, whereas it remained largely incomplete, even after more than 40 months, after DES implantation.[41] A local hypersensitivity reaction to the drug-eluting polymer may also play a role.[41] Moreover, platelet hyperreactivity after cessation of clopidogrel therapy has been hypothesized to contribute to the phenomenon of stent thrombosis soon after scheduled discontinuation of clopidogrel therapy after DES implantation. One-year clopidogrel therapy is the most frequent regimen applied after DES implanation. As more long-term data after DES implantation are being accumulated,[42] the duration of clopidogrel therapy after this procedure is expected to increase, especially in high-risk patients such as those with stenting of the left main coronary artery.

References

1. Rubboli A, Milandri M, Castelvetri C, Cosmi B. Meta-analysis of trials comparing oral anticoagulation and aspirin versus dual antiplatelet therapy after coronary stenting. Clues for the management of patients with an indication for long-term anticoagulation undergoing coronary stenting. Cardiology 2005;104:101–6.
2. Steinhubl SR, Lauer MS, Mukherjee DP et al. The duration of pretreatment with ticlopidine prior to stenting is associated with the risk of procedure-related non-Q-wave myocardial infarctions. J Am Coll Cardiol 1998;32:1366–70.
3. Steinhubl SR, Ellis SG, Wolski K et al. Ticlopidine pretreatment before coronary stenting is associated with sustained decrease in adverse cardiac events: data from the Evaluation of Platelet IIb/IIIa Inhibitor for Stenting (EPISTENT) Trial. Circulation 2001;103:1403–9.

4. Thebault JJ, Kieffer G, Lowe GD et al. Repeated-dose pharmacody-namics of clopidogrel in healthy subjects. Semin Thromb Hemost 1999;25(Suppl 2):9–14.

5. The EPISTENT Investigators. Randomized placebo-controlled and balloon-angioplasty-controlled trial to assess safety of coronary stenting with use of platelet glycoprotein-IIb/IIIa blockade. Lancet 1998;352:87–92.

6. Sabatine MS, Cannon CP, Gibson CM et al. Effect of clopidogrel pre-treatment before percutaneous coronary intervention in patients with ST-elevation myocardial infarction treated with fibrinolytics: the PCI-CLARITY study. JAMA 2005;294:1224–32.

7. Mehta SR, Yusuf S, Peters RJ et al. Effects of pretreatment with clopi-dogrel and aspirin followed by long-term therapy in patients under-going percutaneous coronary intervention: the PCI-CURE study. Lancet 2001;358:527–33.

8. Steinhubl SR, Berger PB, Mann JT 3rd et al. Early and sustained dual oral antiplatelet therapy following percutaneous coronary interven-tion: a randomized controlled trial. JAMA 2002;288:2411–20.

9. Steinhubl SR, Berger PB, Brennan DM, Topol EJ. Optimal timing for the initiation of pre-treatment with 300 mg clopidogrel before percu-taneous coronary intervention. J Am Coll Cardiol 2006;47:939–43.

10. Kastrati A, Mehilli J, Schühlen H et al. A clinical trial of abciximab in elective percutaneous coronary intervention after pretreatment with clopidogrel. N Engl J Med 2004;350:232–8.

11. Mehilli J, Kastrati A, Schühlen H et al. Randomized clinical trial of abciximab in diabetic patients undergoing elective percutaneous coronary interventions after treatment with a high loading dose of clopidogrel. Circulation 2004;110:3627–35.

12. Kastrati A, Mehilli J, Neumann FJ et al. Abciximab in patients with acute coronary syndromes undergoing percutaneous coronary inter-vention after clopidogrel pretreatment: the ISAR-REACT 2 rand-omized trial. JAMA 2006;295:1531–8.

13. Müller I, Seyfarth M, Rüdiger S et al. Effect of a high loading dose of clopidogrel on platelet function in patients undergoing coronary stent placement. Heart 2001;85:92–3.

14. Hochholzer W, Trenk D, Frundi D et al. Time dependence of platelet inhibition after a 600-mg loading dose of clopidogrel in a large, unse-lected cohort of candidates for percutaneous coronary intervention. Circulation 2005;111:2560–4.

15. Patti G, Colonna G, Pasceri V et al. Randomized trial of high loading dose of clopidogrel for reduction of periprocedural myocardial inf-arction in patients undergoing coronary intervention. Results from the ARMYDA-2 (Antiplatelet therapy for Reduction of MYocardial Damage during Angioplasty) study. Circulation 2005;111:2099–106.

16. Kandzari DE, Berger PB, Kastrati A et al. Influence of treatment dura-tion with a 600-mg dose of clopidogrel before percutaneous coro-nary revascularization. J Am Coll Cardiol 2004;44:2133–6.

17. Fitzgerald DJ, Roy L, Catella F, FitzGerald GA. Platelet activation in unstable coronary disease. N Engl J Med 1986;315:983–9.

18. Gawaz M, Neumann FJ, Ott I et al. Platelet function in acute myo-cardial infarction treated with direct angioplasty. Circulation 1996;93:229–37.

19. Thebault JJ, Kieffer G, Cariou R. Single-dose pharmacodynamics of clopidogrel. Semin Thromb Hemost 1999;25(Suppl 2):3–8.

20. Boneu B, Destelle G. Platelet anti-aggregating activity and tolerance of clopidogrel in atherosclerotic patients. Thromb Haemost 1996;76:939–43.

21. Savcic M, Hauert J, Bachmann F et al. Clopidogrel loading dose regi-mens: kinetic profile of pharmacodynamic response in healthy sub-jects. Semin Thromb Hemost 1999;25(Suppl 2):15–19.

22. von Beckerath N, Taubert D, Pogatsa-Murray G et al. Absorption, metabolization, and antiplatelet effects of 300-, 600-, and 900-mg loading doses of clopidogrel: results of the ISAR-CHOICE (Intracoronary Stenting and Antithrombotic Regimen: Choose

Between 3 High Oral Doses for Immediate Clopidogrel Effect) trial. Circulation 2005;112:2946–50.

23. Montalescot G, Sideris G, Meuleman C et al. A randomized comparison of high clopidogrel loading doses in patients with non-ST-segment elevation acute coronary syndromes: the ALBION (Assessment of the Best Loading Dose of Clopidogrel to Blunt Platelet Activation, Inflammation and Ongoing Necrosis) trial. J Am Coll Cardiol 2006;48:931–8.

24. Taubert D, Kastrati A, Harlfinger S et al. Pharmacokinetics of clopi-dogrel after administration of a high loading dose. Thromb Haemost 2004;92:311–16.

25. von Beckerath N, Taubert D, Pogatsa-Murray G et al. A patient with stent thrombosis, clopidogrel-resistance and failure to metabo-lize clopidogrel to its active metabolite. Thromb Haemost 2005;93:789–91.

26. CAPRIE Steering Committee. A randomised, blinded, trial of clopi-dogrel versus aspirin in patients at risk of ischaemic events (CAPRIE). Lancet 1996;348:1329–39.

27. Gurbel PA, Bliden KP, Hayes KM et al. The relation of dosing to clopidogrel responsiveness and the incidence of high post-treatment platelet aggregation in patients undergoing coronary stenting. J Am Coll Cardiol 2005;45:1392–6.

28. Gurbel PA, Bliden KP, Hiatt BL, O'Connor CM. Clopidogrel for coro-nary stenting. Response variability, drug resistance, and the effect of pretreatment platelet reactivity. Circulation 2003;107:2908–13.

29. Hochholzer W, Trenk D, Bestehorn HP et al. Impact of the degree of peri-interventional platelet inhibition after loading with clopidogrel on early clinical outcome of elective coronary stent placement. J Am Coll Cardiol 2006;48:1742–50.

30. von Beckerath N, Kastrati A, Wieczorek A et al. A double-blind rand-omized comparison between two different clopidogrel maintenance doses after percutaneous coronary intervention (ISAR-CHOICE-2 trial). Eur Heart J 2006;27(Abst Suppl):863.

31. Hochholzer W, Trenk D, Müller B et al. Efficacy of adjusted clopidog-rel dosing in patients with insufficient platelet inhibition after elec-tive coronary stenting: the ExcelsiorACT study. Eur Heart J 2006; 27(Abst Suppl):750.

32. Angiolillo DJ, Shoemaker SB, Desai B et al. A randomized compari-son of a high clopidogrel maintenance dose in patients with diabetes mellitus and coronary artery disease: results of the OPTIMUS (Optimizing Antiplatelet Therapy In diabetes MellitUS) study. Circulation 2007;115:708–16.

33. von Beckerath N, Pogatsa-Murray G, Wieczorek A et al. Correlation of a new point-of-care test with conventional optical aggregometry for the assessment of clopidogrel responsiveness. Thromb Haemost 2006;95:910–11.

34. Schühlen H, Kastrati A, Dirschinger J et al. Intracoronary stenting and risk for major adverse cardiac events during the first month. Circulation 1998;98:104–11.

35. Smith SC Jr, Feldman TE, Hirshfeld JW Jr et al. ACC/AHA/SCAI 2005 guideline update for percutaneous coronary intervention – summary article: a report of the American College of Cardiology/ American Heart Association Task Force on Practice Guidelines (ACC/ AHA/SCAI Writing Committee to Update the 2001 Guidelines for Percutaneous Coronary Intervention). Circulation 2006;113:156–75.

36. Silber S, Albertsson P, Aviles FF et al. Guidelines for percutaneous coronary interventions. The Task Force for Percutaneous Coronary Interventions of the European Society of Cardiology. Eur Heart J 2005;26:804–47.

37. Iakovou I, Schmidt T, Bonizzoni E et al. Incidence, predictors, and outcome of thrombosis after successful implantation of drug-eluting stents. JAMA 2005;293:2126–30.

38. Spertus JA, Kettelkamp R, Vance C et al. Prevalence, predictors, and outcomes of premature discontinuation of thienopyridine therapy

after drug-eluting stent placement: results from the PREMIER registry. Circulation 2006;113:2803–9.

39. McFadden EP, Stabile E, Regar E et al. Late thrombosis in drug-eluting coronary stents after discontinuation of antiplatelet therapy. Lancet 2004;364:1519–21.

40. Pfisterer M, Brunner-La Rocca HP, Buser PT et al. Late clinical events after clopidogrel discontinuation may limit the benefit of drug-eluting stents: an observational study of drug-eluting versus bare-metal stents. J Am Coll Cardiol 2006;48:2584–91.

41. Joner M, Finn AV, Farb A et al. Pathology of drug-eluting stents in humans: delayed healing and late thrombotic risk. J Am Coll Cardiol 2006;48:193–202.

42. Eisenstein EL, Anstrom KJ, Kong DF et al. Clopidogrel use and long-term clinical outcomes after drug-eluting stent implantation. JAMA 2007;297:159–68.

7

Resistance to antiplatelet drugs: aspirin

Wai-Hong Chen and Daniel I Simon

Introduction

Platelets play a pivotal role in mediating thrombotic complications of atherosclerotic vascular disease and percutaneous coronary intervention (PCI). Platelets adhere to the subendothelium via interaction with collagen and von Willebrand factor (vVF) at sites of spontaneous or iatrogenic plaque disruption. After adhesion, platelets undergo conformational changes and release agonists with prothrombotic and/or vasoactive properties such as thromboxane A_2 (TXA_2) and adenosine diphosphate (ADP), which result in amplification and propagation of platelet activation and aggregation, eventually leading to thrombus formation in combination with coagulation factors.

Aspirin is the cornerstone of oral antiplatelet therapy for preventing ischemic events of atherothrombotic disease. Aspirin inhibits platelet cyclooxygenase-1 (COX-1) by irreversible acetylation of a serine residue at position 529, which prevents the conversion of arachidonic acid to TXA_2.[1] The antithrombotic effect of aspirin results from the decreased production of TXA_2, a potent vasoconstrictor and platelet agonist. The Antithrombotic Trialists' Collaboration reported that aspirin therapy was associated with 15% reduction in vascular mortality, a 34% reduction in myocardial infarction, and a 25% reduction in stroke among high-risk patients with atherothrombotic disease.[2] Aspirin has also been shown to reduce the acute ischemic complications of coronary angioplasty.[3–5]

While the benefits of aspirin are widely accepted, there are still some patients who suffer 'breakthrough' events despite daily aspirin therapy. It has been estimated that 10–20% of aspirin-treated patients may experience recurrent thrombotic events during long-term follow-up,[6] suggesting that the antiplatelet effects of aspirin may not be equivalent in all patients. In addition to these clinical observations, measurements of platelet aggregation, platelet activation, and bleeding time have indeed confirmed wide variability in patients' responses to aspirin therapy.[7–9] It is on the basis of this constellation of clinical and laboratory evidence of a diminished or absent response to aspirin treatment in some individuals that the concept of 'aspirin resistance' has emerged.

Definition(s) of aspirin resistance

Aspirin resistance may be defined as the inability of aspirin to produce an anticipated effect on one or more in vitro tests of platelet function, mainly platelet aggregation, and has been referred to as laboratory aspirin resistance. A clinical definition of aspirin resistance is the failure of the drug to prevent an atherothrombotic event despite prescription of aspirin. This phenomenon has also been described as aspirin treatment failure. Laboratory definitions of aspirin resistance have involved either detecting the failure of aspirin's pharmacological effect or the failure of aspirin to prevent or inhibit platelet aggregation (Table 7.1). Aspirin resistance, defined by its pharmacological action, is persistent production of TXA_2 despite therapy, measured by the presence of TXA_2 metabolites in serum or urine. In contrast, persistent platelet aggregation despite aspirin treatment defines failure of aspirin-mediated platelet inhibition, and this may occur via non-thromboxane mediated pathways of platelet activation. It has been suggested that aspirin resistance is a misleading term since in some situations, aspirin successfully inhibits thromboxane synthesis, but platelet aggregation persists. The term 'aspirin non-response' encompasses the failure of aspirin to both inhibit thromboxane synthesis and reduce platelet aggregation.[10]

Mechanisms of aspirin resistance

Although much is currently known about the effects of aspirin on platelets, the mechanisms of aspirin resistance have not been fully established. It is likely that clinical, pharmacological, biological, and genetic factors (contribute to the variable platelet response to aspirin (Table 7.2).[11–13] Patient non-compliance with prescribed therapy[14] and reduced gastrointestinal absorption[15] are obvious causes of aspirin resistance/failure. Cigarette smoking has been shown

Table 7.1 *Laboratory assays for measuring antiplatelet effects of aspirin*

	Advantages	Disadvantages
Bleeding time	In vivo test; physiological	Non-specific; operator-dependent; insensitive
Urinary 11-dehydroTXB$_2$	COX-1-dependent; correlation with clinical outcomes	Not platelet-specific; indirect measure; dependent on renal function; uncertain reproducibility
Light transmission aggregometry	Gold standard; correlation with clinical outcomes	Time-consuming; expensive; poor reproducibility
Platelet Function Analyzer-100	Simple; rapid; correlation with clinical outcomes	Dependent on vWF and hematocrit; no instrument adjustment
VerifyNow Aspirin	Simple; rapid; point-of-care; correlation with clinical outcomes	No instrument adjustment

TXB$_2$, thromboxane B$_2$; COX-1, cyclooxygenase-1, vWF, von Willebrand factor.

Table 7.2 *Potential mechanisms of aspirin resistance*

Clinical
- Non-compliance with aspirin prescription
- Reduced aspirin absorption
- Cigarette smoking: accentuation of platelet thrombosis

Pharmacological
- Inadequate dose
- Drug interaction: inhibition of aspirin access to COX-1 binding site by concurrent intake of NSAIDs
- Duration of treatment: reduced antiplatelet response with long-term therapy

Biological
- Increased platelet turnover: newly formed platelets not acetylated by once-daily aspirin dosing
- Alternative pathways of thromboxane biosynthesis: COX-2 in platelets and endothelial cells
- Alternative pathways of platelet activation: erythrocyte-induced platelet activation; increased platelet sensitivity to collagen, ADP, or catecholamine

Genetic
- Polymorphisms of COX-1, COX-2, TXA$_2$ synthase, or other enzymes involved in arachidonic acid metabolism
- Polymorphisms of platelet glycoprotein receptors

COX, cyclooxygenase; NSAIDs, non-steroidal anti-inflammatory drugs; ADP, adenosine diphosphate; TXA$_2$, thromboxane A$_2$.

to increase platelet thrombus formation in aspirin-treated patients with coronary artery disease.[16] Intake of non-steroidal anti-inflammatory drugs (NSAIDs) can interfere with the binding of aspirin to COX-1,[17] but the clinical significance remains controversial.[18,19] The issue of whether a higher aspirin dose is associated with a greater platelet-inhibitory response is also contentious in the literature, and is influenced by the assay used and the platelet agonist

tested.[20–28] Reduction in the platelet-inhibitory effect during long-term treatment has been observed,[29] but the mechanisms remain unknown. Increased platelet turnover as seen after coronary artery bypass graft surgery can lead to inadequate suppression of platelet COX-1 because of increased proportion of non-aspirinated platelets.[30] Alternative pathways of TXA$_2$ production by COX-2 from platelets[31] and endothelial cells[32] have been attributed to aspirin resistance. Persistent platelet activation despite aspirin inhibition of TXA$_2$ may be a reflection of the redundancy of platelet activation pathways from ADP, collagen, and other agonists.[33,34] Genetics plays an important role in determining laboratory response to antiplatelet drugs. Polymorphisms involving COX-1,[35] COX-2,[36] platelet glycoprotein receptors,[37–39] and ADP receptor gene P2Y$_{12}$[40] have all been reported to affect platelet response to aspirin.

Prevalence of aspirin resistance

As the antiplatelet effects of aspirin may not be uniform among all patients and over time, the exact prevalence of aspirin resistance remains uncertain. In the majority of previous studies, it has been reported to range from 5% to 60% of the population. Variability in aspirin-mediated platelet inhibition has been noted not only in patients with cerebrovascular disease, coronary artery disease or presenting for coronary artery bypass surgery, but also in patients with some atherosclerosis-related conditions, and even in normal subjects.[7,8,22,26,41,42] The absence of standardized diagnostic criteria and a single validated method of identifying aspirin-resistant individuals, as well as the lack of precise biological mechanisms for this phenomenon, has led to a wide range of population estimates.

Clinical relevance of aspirin resistance

An emerging number of studies linking laboratory measures of aspirin resistance to adverse clinical outcomes have been reported, and prospective series are summarized in Figure 7.1. Grotemeyer et al[7] determined aspirin responsiveness in 180 stroke patients 12 hours after an oral intake of 500 mg aspirin. Patients with a platelet reactivity index ≤1.25 were categorized as aspirin responders, while those with an index >1.25 were defined as being secondary aspirin non-responders (i.e., aspirin-resistant). All patients were prescribed aspirin 500 mg three times daily and were followed for 24 months. Stroke, myocardial infarction (MI), or vascular death were major outcome measures. The incidence of aspirin resistance was 33%. Complete follow-up was obtained in 174 patients (96%). Major events were noted in 29 patients: 5 (4.4%) in the aspirin-responder group versus 24 (40%) in the aspirin-resistant group ($p <$ 0.0001). More recently, through retrospective Platelet Function Analyzer (PFA)-100 analysis, Grundmann et al[43] reported from a cross-sectional study that, in 53 patients treated with aspirin for secondary prevention of transient

ischemic attack (TIA) or stroke, the rate of aspirin resistance was significantly higher (12/35; 34%) in those with recurrent cerebrovascular events as compared with those without recurrence (0/18; 0%; $p = 0.0006$). Mueller et al[44] studied 100 patients with intermittent claudication undergoing elective percutaneous balloon angioplasty. Aspirin was prescribed at a dose of 100 mg daily. Using corrected whole blood aggregometry, they defined a normal response to aspirin as ≥20% reduction in platelet function with both ADP and collagen as agonists. Fluctuations in aspirin responsiveness among the studied population were noted on serial monitoring. The incidence of aspirin resistance was about 60% at each time point of measurement. At 52-week follow-up, 8 patients in the aspirin resistance group were noted to have reocclusion at the angioplasty site, compared with none of the patients with a normal response to aspirin (87% increase in risk; $p = 0.0093$). Eikelboom et al[10] performed a nested case–control study on 976 aspirin-treated patients, with documented or at high-risk of cardiovascular disease, from the Heart outcomes Prevention Evaluation (HOPE) trial. Aspirin responsiveness was divided into quartiles by urinary 11-dehydrothromboxane B_2 levels, a marker of in vivo thromboxane generation. After

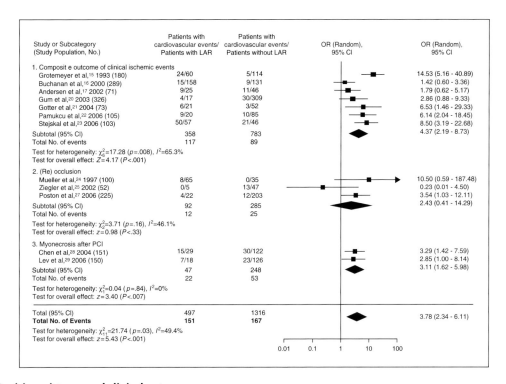

Figure 7.1   Aspirin resistance and clinical outcomes
Odds ratios (ORs) and 95% confidence intervals of the cardiovascular outcome for patients with laboratory-defined aspirin resistance (LAR) vs. those without LAR from eligible studies. Studies are grouped by the outcome parameter used: Group 1 presents a composite outcome of clinical ischemic events, including cardiovascular death, myocardial infarction, stroke, acute coronary syndrome, and revascularization procedure; Group 2, (re)occlusion after bypass grafting or angioplasty; and Group 3, myonecrosis after PCI. The black squares represent ORs for the association between aspirin resistance and cardiovascular outcomes of individual studies. The size of the squares corresponds to the weight of the study in the meta-analysis (Reprinted with permission from Snoep JD et al.[45]).

5 years of follow-up, those patients in the upper quartile had a 1.8-fold increase in risk for the composite of MI, stroke, or cardiovascular death (odds ratio (OR) 1.8; 95% confidence interval (CI) 1.2–2.7; $p = 0.009$) when compared with those in the lower quartile, and the association was independent of traditional risk factors. There was a twofold increase in the risk of MI and a 3.5-fold increase in the risk of cardiovascular death as well. In a 4-year retrospective cohort study among 129 post-MI patients, Andersen et al[46] noted a tendency to a higher incidence of adverse vascular events in aspirin-resistant patients (measured by Platelet Function Analyzer-100) as compared with sensitive patients (36% vs 24%), although the difference did not reach statistical significance ($p = 0.28$). Gum et al[47] enrolled 326 stable patients with cardiovascular disease treated with aspirin 325 mg daily for ≥7 days and defined aspirin resistance as a mean aggregation of ≥70% with 10 μmol/l ADP and a mean aggregation of ≥20% with 0.5 mg/ml arachidonic acid by optical platelet aggregation. Aspirin resistance was noted in 17 patients (5.2%). After a mean follow-up of 1.8 years, major events (death, MI, or stroke) occurred in 4 (24%) patients in the aspirin-resistant group, compared with 30 (10%) patients in the aspirin-sensitive group ($p = 0.03$). The Kaplan–Meier time-to-event curves for event-free survival showed a late divergence of the event curves that remained to be explained. Multivariate analysis demonstrated that, in addition to other risk factors such as increasing age, history of congestive heart failure, and elevated platelet count, aspirin resistance was an independent predictor of adverse outcomes (hazard ratio (HR) 4.14; 95% CI 1.42–12.06; $p = 0.009$). Chen et al[48] examined aspirin responsiveness in patients undergoing elective PCI treated with aspirin at 80–300 mg daily for at least 7 days, clopidogrel pretreatment with a loading dose of 300 mg at least 12 hours before intervention, and procedural anticoagulation using heparin. Using VerifyNow Aspirin, 29 (19.2%) out of the 151 enrolled patients were found to be aspirin-resistant, as defined by an aspirin reaction unit (ARU) ≥550. Patients with aspirin resistance were at increased risk of myocardial necrosis (OR 2.9; 95% CI 1.2–6.9; $p = 0.015$) determined by creatine kinase myocardial band isoenzyme (CK-MB) elevation, when compared with aspirin-sensitive patients. In an elective PCI population ($n = 150$), Lev et al[49] tested for both aspirin and clopidogrel responsiveness in patients receiving aspirin 81–325 mg daily for ≥1 week and clopidogrel at 300 mg loading-dose on completion of the PCI, and 75 mg daily thereafter. Bivalirudin was used for procedural anticoagulation to reduce the confounding effect of heparin on platelet activation. Blood samples were taken at baseline and 20–24 hours after clopidogrel loading. Adopting the criteria of Gum et al[47] and Chen et al,[48] they defined aspirin resistance as the presence of at least two of the following: (i) 0.5 mg/ml arachidonic acid-induced platelet aggregation ≥20%; (ii) 5 μmol/l ADP-induced platelet aggregation ≥70%; (iii) ARU ≥550 by VerifyNow Aspirin.

Clopidogrel resistance was defined as baseline minus post-treatment aggregation ≤10% in response to both 5 and 20 μmol/l ADP. The rates of aspirin and clopidogrel resistance were 12.7% and 24%, respectively. Clopidogrel resistance was noted in 9 (47.4%) of the aspirin-resistant patients and 27 (20.6%) of the aspirin-sensitive patients. Similar to the study results of Chen et al,[48] a significant increase in the incidence of CK-MB elevation was observed in aspirin-resistant patients, when compared with aspirin-sensitive patients (38.9% vs 18.3%; $p = 0.04$). Dual drug-resistant patients were also more likely than dual drug-sensitive patients to have CK-MB elevations (44.4% vs 15.8%; $p = 0.05$). After reporting the predictors and prevalence of aspirin resistance among 468 stable patients with coronary artery disease using VerifyNow Aspirin,[26] Chen et al[50] followed this cohort prospectively, and found that after a mean follow-up of 379 ± 200 days, patients with aspirin resistance ($n = 128$; 27.4%) were at increased risk of the composite outcome of cardiovascular death, MI, unstable angina requiring hospitalization, stroke, and TIA compared with patients who were aspirin-sensitive (15.6% vs 5.3%; HR 3.12; 95% CI 1.65–5.91; $p < 0.001$). Cox proportional hazard regression modeling identified aspirin resistance, diabetes, prior MI, and a low hemoglobin to be independently associated with major adverse long-term outcomes (HR for aspirin resistance 2.46; 95% CI 1.27–4.76; $p = 0.007$).

Conclusions

There is ample evidence to show interindividual variability in platelet responsiveness to aspirin. Analogously to biological responses to other pharmacological agents such as blood pressure and cholesterol-lowering drugs, which display a continuous distribution, similar response to aspirin may exist. Data are accumulating indicating that hypo- or non-responsiveness to aspirin measured in the laboratory (i.e. resistance) is associated with adverse spontaneous (cardiovascular death, acute coronary syndromes, stroke, or peripheral arterial occlusion) or procedure-related (myocardial necrosis after PCI or reocclusion after peripheral angioplasty) clinical events in diverse populations of patients with atherothrombotic disease in stable or unstable phase. Nevertheless, the currently available data are flawed by some major limitations. The sample sizes of these reports are small. Confounding variables are not adequately controlled by the study designs. Different definitions of antiplatelet resistance are used. Variable aspirin dosage, uncertain treatment compliance, and lack of pretreatment platelet activity assessment have been noted in aspirin studies. Clinical application of antiplatelet resistance will require studies on larger populations that define antiplatelet resistance using consistent and reproducible assays, and correlate the measurements with clinical outcomes that can be improved by

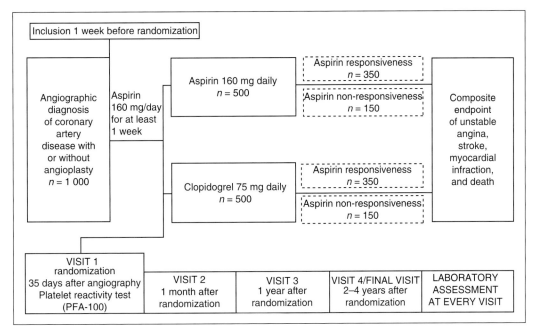

Figure 7.2
Flow chart for the ASCET study. Reproduced from Pettersen AA. Unstable angina, Stroke, Myocardial infarction and death in aspirin non-responders. A prospective, randomized trial. The ASCET (Aspirin non-responsiveness and Clopidogrel Endpoint Trial) design.[53]

alterations in antiplatelet strategy (e.g., increasing the dose of antiplatelet agent, or adding or substituting a second antiplatelet agent). Such prospective randomized trials are currently underway. The CHARISMA (Clopidogrel for High Atherothrombotic Risk and Ischemic Stabilization, Management, and Avoidance) trial compared clopidogrel and aspirin versus placebo and aspirin for high-risk primary or secondary prevention, and has been reported.[51] Urinary 11-dehydrothromboxane B_2 levels have been checked in a substudy, enabling prospective assessment of the addition of clopidogrel to aspirin in reducing adverse events associated aspirin resistance.[52] ASCET (ASpirin non-responsiveness and Clopidogrel Endpoint Trial) is evaluating whether switching to clopidogrel will be superior to continued aspirin therapy in improving clinical outcomes among aspirin-resistant patients with angiographically documented coronary artery disease (Figure 7.2).[53] The practice of antiplatelet therapy tailored to individual response may enter a new era upon validation by these trials.

References

1. Loll PJ, Picot D, Garavito RM. The structural basis of aspirin activity inferred from the crystal structure of inactivated prostaglandin H_2 synthase. Nat Struct Biol 1995;2:637–43.

2. Antithrombotic Trialists' Collaboration. Collaborative meta-analysis of randomised trials of antiplatelet therapy for prevention of death, myocardial infarction, and stroke in high risk patients. BMJ 2002;324:71–86.

3. Barnathan ES, Schwartz JS, Taylor L et al. Aspirin and dipyridamole in the prevention of acute coronary thrombosis complicating coronary angioplasty. Circulation 1987;76:125–34.

4. Schwartz L, Bourassa MG, Lesperance J et al. Aspirin and dipyridamole in the prevention of restenosis after percutaneous transluminal coronary angioplasty. N Engl J Med 1988;318:1714–19.

5. Lembo NJ, Black AJR, Roubin GS et al. Effect of pre-treatment with aspirin versus aspirin plus dipyridamole on frequency and type of acute complications of percutaneous transluminal coronary angioplasty. Am J Cardiol 1990;65:422–26.

6. Patrono C, Coller B, FitzGerald GA et al. Platelet-active drugs: the relationships among dose, effectiveness, and side effects. Chest 2004;126:234S–64S.

7. Grotemeyer KH, Scharafinski HW, Husstedt IW. Two-year follow-up of aspirin responder and aspirin non-responder: a pilot-study including 180 post-stroke patients. Thromb Res 1993;71:397–403.

8. Pappas JM, Westengard JC, Bull BS. Population variability in the effect of aspirin on platelet function. Implications for clinical trials and therapy. Arch Pathol Lab Med 1994;118:801–4.

9. Gum PA, Kottke-Marchant K, Poggio ED et al. Profile and prevalence of aspirin resistance in patients with cardiovascular disease. Am J Cardiol 2001;88:230–5.

10. Eikelboom JW, Hirsh J, Weitz JI et al. Aspirin-resistant thromboxane biosynthesis and the risk of myocardial infarction, stroke, or cardiovascular death in patients at high risk for cardiovascular events. Circulation 2002;105:1650–5.

11. Mason PJ, Jacobs AK, Freedman JF. Aspirin resistance and atherothrombotic disease. J Am Coll Cardiol 2005;46:986–93.

12. Hankey GJ, Eikelboom JW. Aspirin resistance. Lancet 2006;367: 606–17.

13. Wang TH, Bhatt DL, Topol EJ. Aspirin and clopidogrel resistance: an emerging clinical entity. Eur Heart J 2006;27:647–54.

14. Schwartz KA, Schwartz DE, Ghosheh K et al. Compliance as a critical consideration in patients who appear to be resistant to aspirin after healing of myocardial infarction. Am J Cardiol 2005;95:973–5.

15. Gonzalez-Conejero R, Rivera J, Corral J et al. Biological assessment of aspirin efficacy on healthy individuals: heterogeneous response or aspirin failure? Stroke 2005;36:276–80.

16. Hung J, Lam JYT, Lacoste L et al. Cigarette smoking acutely increases platelet thrombus formation in patients with coronary artery disease taking aspirin. Circulation 1995;92:2432–6.

17. Catella-Lawson F, Reilly MP, Kapoor SC et al. Cyclooxygenase inhibitors and the antiplatelet effects of aspirin. N Engl J Med 2001;345:1809–17.

18. MacDonald TM, Wei L. Effect of ibuprofen on cardioprotective effect of aspirin. Lancet 2003;361:573–4.

19. Curtis JP, Krumholz HM. The case for an adverse interaction between aspirin and non-steroidal anti-inflammatory drugs: Is it time to believe the hype? J Am Coll Cardiol 2004;43:991–3.

20. Caterina RD, Giannessi D, Boem A et al. Equal antiplatelet effects of aspirin 50 or 324 mg/day in patients after acute myocardial infarction. Thromb Haemost 1985;54:528–32.

21. Tohgi H, Konno S, Tamura K et al. Effects of low-to-high doses of aspirin on platelet aggregability and metabolites of thromboxane A2 and prostacyclin. Stroke 1992;23:1400–3.

22. Helgason CM, Bolin KM, Hoff JA et al. Development of aspirin resistance in persons with previous ischemic stroke. Stroke 1994;25:2331–6.

23. Dabaghi SF, Kamat SG, Payne J et al. Effects of low-dose aspirin on in vitro platelet aggregation in the early minutes after ingestion in normal subjects. Am J Cardiol 1994;74:720–3.

24. Feng D, McKenna C, Murillo J et al. Effect of aspirin dosage and enteric coating on platelet reactivity. Am J Cardiol 1997;80:189–93.

25. Hart RG, Leonard AD, Talbert RL et al. Aspirin dosage and thromboxane synthesis in patients with vascular disease. Pharmacotherapy 2003;23:579–84.

26. Lee PY, Chen WH, Ng W et al. Low-dose aspirin increases aspirin resistance in patients with coronary artery disease. Am J Med 2005;118:723–7.

27. Mehta SS, Silver RJ, Aaronson A et al. Comparison of aspirin resistance in type 1 versus type 2 diabetes mellitus. Am J Cardiol 2006;97:567–70.

28. Frelinger AL, Furman MI, Linden MD et al. Residual arachidonic acid-induced platelet activation via an adenosine diphosphate-dependent but cyclooxygenase-1- and cyclooxygenase-2-independent pathway: a 700-patient study of aspirin resistance. Circulation 2006;113:2888–96.

29. Pulcinelli FM, Pignatelli P, Celestini A et al. Inhibition of platelet aggregation by aspirin progressively decreases in long-term treated patients. J Am Coll Cardiol 2004;43:979–84.

30. Zimmermann N, Wenk A, Kim U et al. Functional and biochemical evaluation of platelet aspirin resistance after coronary artery bypass surgery. Circulation 2003;108:542–7.

31. Weber AA, Zimmermann KC, Meyer-Kirchrath J, Schror K. Cyclooxygenase-2 in human platelets as a possible factor in aspirin resistance. Lancet 1999;353:900.

32. Karim S, Habib A, Levy-Toledano S, Maclouf J. Cyclooxygenase-1 and -2 of endothelial cells utilize exogenous or endogenous arachidonic acid for transcellular production of thromboxane. J Biol Chem 1996;271:12042–8.

33. Kawasaki T, Ozeki Y, Igawa T, Kambayashi J. Increased platelet sensitivity to collagen in individuals resistant to low-dose aspirin. Stroke 2000;31:591–5.

34. Macchi L, Christiaens L, Brabant S et al. Resistance to aspirin in vitro is associated with increased platelet sensitivity to adenosine diphosphate. Thromb Res 2002;107:45–9.

35. Halushka M, Walker LP, Halushka PV. Genetic variation in cyclooxygenase 1: effects on response to aspirin. Clin Pharmacol Ther 2003;73:122–30.

36. Cipollone F, Toniato E, Martinotti S et al. A polymorphism in the cyclooxygenase 2 gene as an inherited protective factor against myocardial infarction and stroke. JAMA 2004;291:2221–8.

37. Michelson AD, Furman MI, Goldschmidt-Clermont P et al. Platelet GP IIIa Pl(A) polymorphisms display different sensitivities to agonists. Circulation 2000;101:1013–18.

38. Undas A, Brummel K, Musial J et al. Pl(A2) polymorphism of β_3 integrins is associated with enhanced thrombin generation and impaired antithrombotic action of aspirin at the site of microvascular injury. Circulation 2001;104:2666–72.

39. Macchi L, Christiaens L, Brabant S et al. Resistance in vitro to low-dose aspirin is associated with platelet PlA1 (GP IIIa) polymorphism but not with C807T(GP Ia/IIa) and C-5T Kozak (GP Ibα) polymorphisms. J Am Coll Cardiol 2003;42:1115–19.

40. Jefferson BK, Foster JH, McCarthy JJ et al. Aspirin resistance and a single gene. Am J Cardiol 2005;95:805–8.

41. Gum PA, Kottke-Marchant K, Poggio ED et al. Profile and prevalence of aspirin resistance in patients with cardiovascular disease. Am J Cardiol 2001;88:230–5.

42. Wang JC, Aucoin-Barry D, Manuelian D et al. Incidence of aspirin nonresponsiveness using the Ultegra Rapid Platelet Function Assay-ASA. Am J Cardiol 2003;92:1492–4.

43. Grundmann K, Jaschonek K, Kleine B et al. Aspirin non-responder status in patients with recurrent cerebral ischemic attacks. J Neurol 2003;250:63–6.

44. Mueller MR, Salat A, Stangl P et al. Variable platelet response to low-dose ASA and the risk of limb deterioration in patients submitted to peripheral arterial angioplasty. Thromb Haemost 1997;78:1003–7.

45. Snoep JD, Hovens MM, Eikenboom et al. Association of laboratory-defined aspirin resistance with a higher risk of recurrent cardiovascular events. A Systematic Review and Meta-analysis. Arch Intern Med 2007;167:1593–99.

46. Andersen K, Hurlen M, Arnesen H, Seljeflot I. Aspirin non-responsiveness as measured by PFA-100 in patients with coronary artery disease. Thromb Res 2002;108:37–42.

47. Gum PA, Kottke-Marchant K, Welsh PA et al. A prospective, blinded determination of the natural history of aspirin resistance among stable patients with cardiovascular disease. J Am Coll Cardiol 2003;41:961–5.

48. Chen WH, Lee PY, Ng W et al. Aspirin resistance is associated with a high incidence of myonecrosis after non-urgent percutaneous coronary intervention despite clopidogrel pretreatment. J Am Coll Cardiol 2004;43:1122–6.

49. Lev EI, Patel RT, Maresh KJ et al. Aspirin and clopidogrel drug response in patients undergoing percutaneous coronary intervention: the role of dual drug resistance. J Am Coll Cardiol 2006;47:27–33.

50. Chen WH, Cheng X, Lee PY et al. Aspirin resistance and aadverse clinical events in patients with coronary artery Disease. Am J Med 2007;120:631–5.

51. Bhatt DL, Fox KA, Kacke W et al. Clopidogrel and aspirin versus aspirin alone for the prevention of atherothrombotic events. N Engl J Med 2006;354:1706–17.

52. Bhatt DL, Topol EJ. Clopidogrel added to aspirin versus aspirin alone in secondary prevention and high-risk primary prevention: rationale and design of the Clopidogrel for High Atherothrombotic Risk and Ischemic Stabilization, Management, and Avoidance (CHARISMA) trial. Am Heart J 2004;148:263–8.

53. Pettersen AA, Seljeflot I, Abdelnoor M, Arnesen H. Unstable angina, stroke, myocardial infarction and death in aspirin non-responders. A prospective, randomized trial. The ASCET (ASpirin non-responsiveness and Clopidogrel Endpoint Trial) design. Scand Cardiovasc J 2004;38:353–6.

8

Resistance to antiplatelet drugs: clopidogrel

Christian M Valina, Dietmar Trenk, and Franz-Josef Neumann

Introduction

Since the early days of antiplatelet therapy, inadequate or absent platelet inhibition – so-called non-response – has been a matter of concern. The problem of aspirin resistance was identified many years ago. Despite intensive research in this field (see Chapter 7), the impact of non-response to aspirin (i.e., the proportion of patients affected and the clinical consequences) is incompletely understood, thus far.

More recently, several studies have reported non-response after administration of clopidogrel. In these communications, diverse definitions for non-response have been used. These include absolute or relative change in platelet aggregation from baseline <10%, as well as relative reduction of platelet aggregation within the lowest quartile of the cohort analyzed.[1,2] Studies analyzing large populations treated with clopidogrel, however, did not identify a discrete subset of patients with non-response who could be clearly separated from the responders.[3–5] Rather, the observed distribution of platelet responses after treatment with clopidogrel could be adequately modeled by a single normal distribution (Figure 8.1). Nevertheless, the standard deviation of this distribution was very broad, comprising the range from absent platelet responses to adenosine diphosphate (ADP) to near-complete inhibition. Thus, patients identified by the various non-responder definitions published in the literature do not represent a distinct population but rather the lower end of the continuum. In the absence of an evident pharmacological definition of non-response, it is important to arrive at a clinical definition – that is, to define the threshold of on-treatment platelet reactivity above which the risk of atherothrombotic complications increases.

In this chapter, we will first discuss the causes of the wide variability of platelet responses to clopidogrel and address the clinical settings associated with low responses. In the second part, we will present currently available evidence for the clinical relevance of high on-clopidogrel platelet reactivity.

Variability of platelet responses to clopidogrel

Mechanism of action of clopidogrel and receptor binding

ADP-induced platelet aggregation is the result of the interplay between ADP and two distinct G-protein-coupled receptors named $P2Y_1$ and $P2Y_{12}$. Activation of $P2Y_{12}$ receptors causes a cascade of processes that mediate thromboxane A_2 (TXA_2) production, the release of α-granules, and subsequent expression of P-selectin on the surface of activated platelets. ADP-induced platelet aggregation is therefore dependent on stimulation of $P2Y_1$ as well as $P2Y_{12}$ receptors. The $P2Y_{12}$ receptor is the target for the thienopyridine drugs ticlopidine (a first-generation thienopyridine) and clopidogrel (a second-generation thienopyridine) (Figure 8.2).[6] Clopidogrel selectively inhibits the binding of adenosine diphosphate (ADP) to its platelet receptor $P2Y_{12}$ by modifying the platelet ADP receptor (a thiol group within the molecule of a formed metabolite binds via disulfide bonds with a thiol-containing amino acid (cysteine) located on the $P2Y_{12}$ receptor) and the subsequent ADP-mediated activation of the glycoprotein (GP) IIb/IIIa complex, thereby inhibiting platelet aggregation. Because the blockade of the ADP binding by clopidogrel is irreversible, the inhibitory effect lasts the complete lifespan of the platelet. Clopidogrel also inhibits platelet aggregation induced by agonists other than ADP by blocking the amplification of platelet activation by released ADP. It does not inhibit phosphodiesterase activity.

According to the above mechanisms, $P2Y_{12}$ receptor blockade acts early in the cascade of events leading to the formation of the platelet thrombus and effectively inhibits platelet aggregation. Therefore, it was investigated whether polymorphic variations in platelet membrane receptors (e.g., GPIa, GPIIIa, and $P2Y_{12}$), which have been linked to platelet aggregation phenotypes, modulate the individual response to clopidogrel (Table 8.1).[7–22] Fontana et al[23]

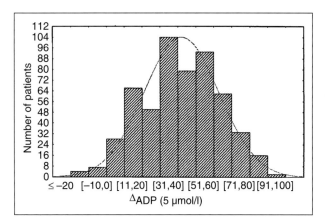

Figure 8.1
Distribution of changes in 5 μmol of adenosine diphosphate (ADP)-induced platelet aggregation, $\Delta_{ADP(5\,\mu mol/l)}$, in 544 patients after receiving clopidogrel therapy, modeled by a single normal distribution. Negative changes in aggregation values represent aggregation values after the administration of clopidogrel that were higher than the baseline readings. (Reproduced with permission from Serebruany VL et al.[5])

examined ADP-induced platelet aggregation responses in 98 healthy volunteers and identified two phenotypic groups of subjects with high and low responsiveness to 2 μmol/l ADP. This was followed by screening of the G_i-coupled ADP receptor gene *P2RY12* for sequence variations. Among the five frequent polymorphisms identified thus far, four were in total linkage disequilibrium, determining haplotypes H1 and H2, with respective allelic frequencies of 0.86 and 0.14. The number of H2 alleles was associated with the maximal aggregation response to ADP in the overall study population ($p = 0.007$). Downregulation of the platelet cyclic adenosine monophosphate (cAMP) concentration by ADP was more marked in 10 H2 carriers than in 10 non-carriers. It was considered that carriers of the H2 haplotype may have an increased risk of atherothrombosis and/or a lesser clinical response to drugs inhibiting platelet function. These findings could not be reproduced by several investigators studying patients with coronary artery disease and treated with clopidogrel (Table 8.1). Angiolillo et al[24] characterized platelet aggregation profiles in patients ($n = 82$) on dual antiplatelet treatment (aspirin plus clopidogrel) for >1 month and assessed whether these may be influenced by the C807T polymorphism of the GPIa gene (carriers: CT + TT genotypes; $n = 51$, non-carriers: CC genotype; $n = 31$). Platelet aggregation varied significantly in patients on long-term dual antiplatelet treatment and was increased in T allele carriers of the 807C/T polymorphism of the GPIa gene. However, this finding could not be replicated by other groups (Table 8.1).

Common sequence variations within the platelet receptor genes do not seem to contribute to a relevant extent to the interpatient variability in clopidogrel efficacy.

Absorption and prehepatic metabolism

Following oral administration of clopidogrel, approximately 50% of the dose is absorbed rapidly from the gastrointestinal tract, as shown by data on urinary excretion of clopidogrel-related metabolites.[25] Peak plasma levels (3 mg/l) of the main circulating metabolite occurring approximately 1 hour after oral dosing of 75 mg clopidogrel (base). The pharmacokinetics of the main circulating metabolite increases linearly with dose in the range of 50–150 mg of clopidogrel. Administration of clopidogrel bisulfate with meals did not significantly modify the bioavailability of clopidogrel as assessed by the pharmacokinetics of the main circulating metabolite. Clopidogrel and the main circulating metabolite bind reversibly in vitro to human plasma proteins (98% and 94%, respectively). The binding is non-saturable in vitro up to a concentration of 100 μg/ml. After absorption, the majority of parent drug is hydrolyzed by esterases to a carboxylic acid derivative that accounts for 85% of clopidogrel-related circulating compounds, which have no effect on platelet aggregation (Figure 8.3). Differences in individual absorption of clopidogrel may lead to clopidogrel response variability.[26]

Hepatic metabolism and drug interaction

Clopidogrel is an inactive prodrug requiring oxidation by hepatic cytochrome P450 to generate an active metabolite (Figure 8.3).[27] Since about 85% of the prodrug is hydrolyzed by esterases in the blood, only about 15% can be metabolized by the cytochrome P450 system in the liver to generate an active metabolite. The active metabolite is generated by hydrolysis of 2-oxoclopidogrel via a cytochrome P450-dependent pathway; in this metabolite, the thiophene ring has been opened to give an unsaturated carboxylic acid side-chain and a highly reactive thiol group, and it is chemically unstable.[27–29] 2-Oxoclopidogrel is considered to be an intermediate metabolite, because it displays no antiplatelet activity in vitro, but marked antiaggregating activity ex vivo when administered to rats.[27,28] This indicates that a further downstream metabolite is responsible for the antiplatelet activity of clopidogrel. The thiol group of the metabolite is responsible for the irreversible binding by formation of a disulfide bridge with the thiol-containing cysteine present in the ADP receptor at the platelet surface.[30,31]

The cytochrome P450 isoenzymes involved in the metabolism of clopidogrel, and especially in the formation of 2-oxoclopidogrel, have been investigated since the early 1990s. Results from studies in patients, from clinical pharmacological investigations, and from in vitro experiments have provided new insights into the metabolic activation of clopidogrel via cytochrome P450 in humans.

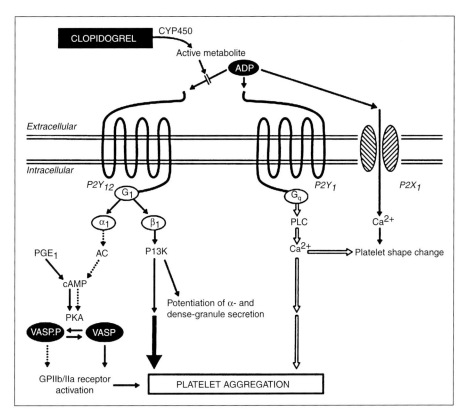

Figure 8.2

Mechanism of action of clopidogrel. Clopidogrel competitively and irreversibly inhibits the adenosine diphosphate (ADP) P2Y$_{12}$ receptor; ADP binds to the P2Y$_1$ receptor to induce change in platelet shape and a weak and transient platelet aggregation. The binding of ADP to its G$_i$-coupled P2Y$_{12}$ receptor liberates the Gi-protein subunits α_{Gi} and β_{γ}. The subunit α_{Gi} leads to the inhibition of adenylyl cyclase (AC), which, in turn, lowers the cyclic adenosine monophosphate (cAMP) level. This inhibits the cAMP-mediated phosphorylation of vasodilator-stimulated phosphoprotein (VASP) (giving VASP-P), which is known to be closely related to the inhibition of glyprotein (GP) IIb/IIIa receptor activation. The subunit β_{γ} activates the phosphatidylinositol 3'-kinase (PI3K), which potentiates dense- and α-granule secretion. Multiple arrows within a given pathway indicate that intermediate steps may be involved. Dotted arrows indicate inhibition and solid arrows indicate activation. CYP450, cytochrome P450; PGE$_1$, prostaglandin E$_1$; PKA, protein kinase activation; PLC, phospholipase C. (Reproduced with permission from Nguyen TA et al.[6])

Evidence supporting the hypothesis that CYP3A4 is one of the cytochrome P450 isoenzymes involved in the metabolic activation of clopidogrel was obtained by Lau et al[32] from pharmacological experiments in healthy subjects. These experiments showed that inhibitors of CYP3A4, such as erythromycin and troleandomycin, attenuated the antiplatelet effects of clopidogrel, while an inducer of CYP3A4 (rifampicin) amplified these effects. In addition, they observed that the inhibition of ADP-induced platelet aggregation was attenuated in a dose-dependent manner in patients treated concomitantly with the CYP3A4-dependent 3-hydroxy-3-methylglutaryl coenzyme A (HMG-CoA)-reductase inhibitor atorvastatin. In contrast, ADP-induced aggregation was not altered in patients treated with pravastatin compared with controls. Because pravastatin, in contrast to atorvastatin, is not a substrate of CYP3A4, it was postulated that CYP3A4 was the key cytochrome P450 isoenzyme responsible for the metabolic activation of clopidogrel and that a drug–drug interaction between atorvasta-

tin and clopidogrel at the level of CYP3A4 is the underlying mechanism for the observed decreased antiplatelet effect of clopidogrel in patients treated with atorvastatin. In contrast to Lau et al,[32] Hochholzer et al[3] and Smith et al[33] found that comedication with CYP3A4-metabolized statins did not appreciably affect platelet aggregation after clopidogrel (Figures 8.4 and 8.5). Ex vivo measurements of the platelet-inhibitory activity of clopidogrel and retrospective analysis of clinical studies enrolling patients with and without concurrent treatment with CYP3A4-metabolized statins failed to confirm any effect on platelet function during treatment with clopidogrel or any impact on clinical outcome measures.[34–42]

The metabolic activity of the CYP3A4 enzyme is under genetic control and varies considerably among individuals.[14,43] Genetic polymorphisms of this and other cytochrome P450 enzymes have been studied, since they may influence the amount of active metabolites of clopidogrel (Table 8.1). Up to now, there have been only two studies suggesting an

at 24 hours ($p = 0.02$), and during the overall study time ($p = 0.025$). The percentage of inhibition of platelet aggregation 24 hours following clopidogrel loading dose was suboptimal (<40%) in 59% and 26% of overweight and normal weight patients, respectively ($p = 0.04$). An elevated body mass index (BMI, 25 kg/m²) was the only independent predictor of suboptimal platelet response, which suggest that overweight patients may need a higher loading dose of clopidogrel and/or an adjunct antithrombotic treatment to adequately inhibit platelet aggregation early after coronary stenting.

Hochholzer et al[47] assessed platelet aggregation of 802 patients immediately before elective PCI in the EXCELSIOR study (for details, see below). Univariable analysis of baseline demographic and clinical characteristics revealed age, diabetes mellitus, BMI, and impaired left ventricular function as predictors for weaker inhibition of platelet aggregation. The multivariable general linear model showed only BMI to be an independent variable for ADP-induced platelet aggregation immediately before PCI.

No significant difference was observed in the plasma levels of the main circulating metabolite between males and females.[25] In the CAPRIE trial, the incidences of clinical outcome events, other adverse clinical events, and abnormal clinical laboratory parameters were similar in men and women.[48] Pharmacokinetic differences due to race have not been studied.

Several comorbidities (e.g., acute coronary syndrome, and rheumatic diseases) have been implicated in heightening platelet reactivity. Therefore, high pretreatment platelet reactivity and thrombotic burden before drug administration may contribute to a reduction in clopidogrel-induced antiplatelet effect.[1,49] Increased platelet aggregation can be found in patients with diabetes mellitus (insulin-dependent diabetes mellitus) or acute coronary syndrome.[50,51]

During maintenance treatment with 75 mg clopidogrel per day, plasma levels of the main circulating metabolite were lower in patients with severe renal impairment (creatinine clearance 5–15 ml/min) compared with subjects with moderate renal impairment (creatinine clearance 30–60 ml/min) or healthy subjects. Although inhibition of ADP-induced platelet aggregation was lower (25%) than that observed in healthy volunteers, the prolongation of bleeding time was similar to that in healthy volunteers receiving 75 mg of clopidogrel per day.

Clinical relevance of high on-clopidogrel platelet reactivity

Much of the recent interest in non-response to clopidogrel is derived from the widespread use of drug-eluting stents for treatment of coronary artery stenosis. Drug-eluting

stents suppress neointima formation after coronary interventions and thus restenosis, but at the same time delay healing. The delayed healing causes an extended need for adequate platelet inhibition by dual antiplatelet therapy with aspirin and clopidogrel. Accordingly, interventional cardiologists have been concerned that inadequate suppression of platelet reactivity may put patients with drug-eluting stents at increased risk for stent thrombosis. This concern has been stimulated a number of studies addressing the impact of the variability of platelet responses to clopidogrel on short- and long-term outcome after placement of drug-eluting stents. These studies will be reviewed below.

Retrospective studies

In an one of the first retrospective studies, Ajzenberg et al[52] reported on platelet function testing in 10 patients with stent thrombosis, and compared these findings with 22 matched control patients without stent thrombosis. They found that shear-induced platelet aggregation was increased on average by more than twofold in patients with stent thrombosis compared with matched controls, a difference that was statistically highly significant ($p = 0.009$) (Figure 8.6). Likewise, Wenaweser et al[53] reported a trend towards increased ADP-induced platelet aggregation in 23 patients with stent thrombosis as compared with 50 matched controls (Figure 8.6). In the CREST study, Gurbel et al[4] took a similar approach and compared 20 patients with stent thrombosis with 100 matched control patients. As shown in Figure 8.7, they found significantly enhanced on-treatment platelet reactivity as assessed by both ADP-induced platelet aggregation, measured by light transmittance aggregometry, and P2Y$_{12}$ reactivity ratio, measured by flow cytometry.

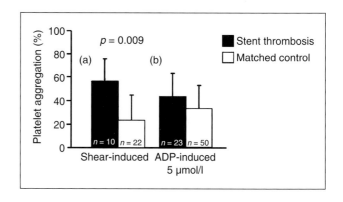

Figure 8.6

(a) Shear-induced platelet aggregation analyzed in patients who had experienced subacute stent thrombosis ($n = 10$) and stented patients without subacute stent thrombosis ($n = 22$).[52] (b) Platelet aggregation (5 μmol ADP in patients with stent thrombosis ($n = 23$) and control patients ($n = 50$).[53]

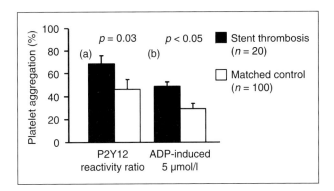

Figure 8.7
P2Y$_{12}$ reactivity ratio (measure of ADP-induced VASP phosphorylation) (a) and platelet aggregation induced by ADP (b) determined in patients who suffered subacute stent thrombosis ($n = 20$) and compared with an age-matched group of patients without stent thrombosis ($n = 100$). (Adapted from Gurbel PA et al.[4])

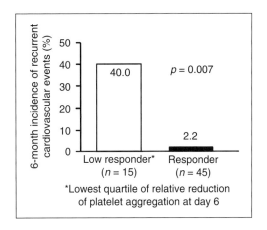

Figure 8.8
Six-month incidence of recurrent events after catheter intervention in acute myocardial infarction depending on responder status to clopidogrel. (Adapted from Matetzky et al.[54])

Prospective observational studies

To the best of our knowledge, Matetzky et al[54] were the first to report a prospective study on the impact of low response to clopidogrel on clinical outcome. Their study included 60 patients with percutaneous coronary intervention (PCI) and stent placement for acute ST-segment elevation myocardial infarction (STEMI). Patients were stratified to quartiles according to the percentage of reduction of ADP-induced platelet aggregation (5 μmol/l). Within the quartile with the lowest response to clopidogrel, 6 of 15 patients incurred a recurrent cardiovascular event (including reinfarction, recurrent acute coronary syndrome, peripheral arterial occlusion, and stroke), whereas only 1 of the 45 remaining patients had an event ($p = 0.007$) (Figure 8.8). Although the findings were suggestive of a relevant impact of low responses to clopidogrel, the data had to be interpreted cautiously because of the low number of patients included in this study.

More recently the STRATEGY trial has addressed myocardial infarction. In this trial, Campo et al[55] investigated the value of platelet reactivity in predicting clinical outcome in patients with STEMI ($n = 70$) undergoing primary PCI assisted by GPIIb/IIIa inhibition. At 1 year, patients with high platelet reactivity at entry showed an adjusted 5- to 11-fold increase in the risk of death, reinfarction, and target vessel revascularization (hazard ratio (HR) 11, 95% confidence interval (CI) 1.5–78 ($p = 0.02$) with Platelet Function Analyzer 100, HR 5.2, 95% CI 1.1–23 ($p = 0.03$) with light transmission aggregometry).

Cuisset et al[56] investigated the platelet response to clopidogrel and aspirin in patients with non-ST-elevation acute coronary syndrome undergoing PCI with stenting ($n = 106$) and found after 1-month follow-up a significant association of clinical events with platelet response to clopidogrel (quartile 4, i.e., 'low-responder', vs quartile 1–3; odds ratio

22.4; 95% CI 4.6–109). In another study, they compared the incidence of periprocedural myocardial infarction in patients with acute coronary syndrome ($n = 190$) between non-responders to dual antiplatelet therapy (high post-treatment platelet reactivity, i.e., ADP (10 μmol/l)-induced platelet aggregation >70%) and 'normo-responders', and showed a significantly higher incidence of periprocedural myocardial infarction in patients with high post-treatment platelet reactivity (43% vs 24%; $p = 0.014$).

The PREPARE POST-STENTING study investigated 192 patients undergoing PCI with stent placement.[58] Most of the patients received a peri-interventional loading dose of clopidogrel (300 mg in 75 patients and 600 mg in 60 patients); 57 patients were on chronic maintenance treatment with 75 mg of clopidogrel. Post-treatment platelet function testing was performed at least 24 hours post procedure and at least 18 hours after cessation of therapy with GPIIb/IIIa inhibitors. Platelet reactivity to ADP was measured by light transmittance aggregometry, and clot strength, a measure of thrombin-induced fibrin and platelet interactions, was measured by thrombelastography. The primary clinical endpoint was the 6-month incidence of cardiovascular death, myocardial infarction, stroke, and unstable angina. The incidence of the primary endpoint was compared between the strata defined by quartiles of platelet function testing. With light transmittance aggregometry, there was a non-significant increase in the incidence of the primary endpoint with increasing quartile of platelet reactivity from 10% in the lowest quartile to 32% in the highest quartile (Figure 8.9). Thrombelastography, however, revealed a strong and statistically highly significant association between quartiles of platelet reactivity assessed by clot strength and outcome, showing an increase from 2% in the lowest quartile of clot strength to 58% in the highest quartile (Figure 8.10).

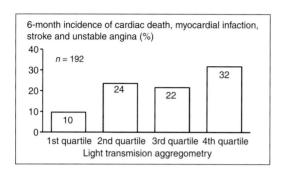

Figure 8.9
Observed incidence of ischemic events according to quartiles of light transmittance aggregometry (LTA) values. (Adapted from Gurbel PA et al. J Am Coll Cardiol 2005;46:1820–6.[58])

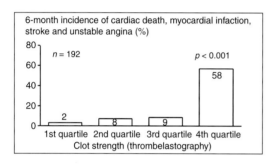

Figure 8.10
Observed incidence of ischemic events according to quartiles of clot strength values. The *p*-value indicates that the proportion of ischemic events in each of the first three quartiles is significantly different from the proportion of ischemic events in the fourth quartile (*p* < 0.001). (Adapted from Gurbel PA et al.[58])

One-hundred patients were also followed for 1 year to assess the incidence of cardiovascular death, stroke, myocardial infarction, and readmission for ischemia. Twenty-three patients incurred one of these events. Platelet reactivity in patients with events was significantly higher than in patients without events (Figure 8.11). Applying thresholds for high on-treatment platelet reactivity derived from the experience in the PREPARE POST-STENTING study, a high on-treatment platelet aggregation was associated with a 1-year incidence of ischemic events of 74%, versus 8% in patients with low platelet reactivity. This difference was statistically highly significant (*p*<0.01) (Figure 8.11).[59]

EXCELSIOR (Impact of Extent of Clopidogrel-Induced Platelet Inhibition During Elective Stent Implantation on Clinical Event Rate) was a prospective observational study in 802 patients undergoing low- to intermediate-risk PCI with stent placement after loading with 600 mg clopidogrel. The primary hypothesis of the study assumed that the 30-day incidence of major adverse cardiovascular events (MACE: death, myocardial infarction, or target vessel revas-

cularization) differed by quartiles of ADP-induced (5 μmol/l) platelet aggregation during PCI. Blood samples were obtained before clopidogrel loading, at the time of catheterization before administration of heparin, and at day 1 after PCI after the first maintenance dose. During a 30-day follow-up, 15 patients (1.9 %) incurred MACE (3 deaths, 8 myocardial infarctions, and 8 target lesion revascularizations). The incidence of 30-day MACE differed significantly (*p*=0.034) between quartiles of platelet aggregation: 0.5% in the first quartile, 0.5% in the second, 1.3% in the third, and 3.5% in the fourth. Platelet aggregation above median incurred a 6.7-fold increase in risk (95% CI 1.25–9.41; *p*=0.03) of 30-day MACE (Figure 8.12). Multivariable logistic regression analysis including pertinent covariables confirmed platelet aggregation as a significant independent predictor of 30-day MACE (adjusted OR 9.6; 95% CI 2.1–44.3; *p*=0.01).[47]

In contrast to the absolute platelet reactivity at the time of intervention, current non-responder definitions based on change in platelet aggregation from baseline were less predictive of events. In patients with an absolute change in platelet aggregation ≤ 10%, the 30-day MACE was 2.2%, as compared with 1.8% in patients not meeting this definition of non-response (*p*=0.56). When patients were stratified according to an alternative non-responder definition (namely, percent inhibition <10 %), there were no significant differences in 30-day MACE either (2.3% vs 1.7%; *p*=0.51). These findings demonstrate that the absolute level of platelet reactivity at the time of intervention is important – irrespective of whether this level is reached by a strong inhibition by clopidogrel or by low baseline platelet reactivity.

Meanwhile, 1-year follow-up data for EXCELSIOR have become available. The EXCELSIOR follow-up study investigated the 1-year incidence of death and myocardial infarction with respect to predischarge ADP-induced (5 μmol/l) residual platelet aggregation (RPA) >14%, which was the threshold for increased risk in the analysis of the 30-day outcome of the EXCELSIOR cohort. Of the 765 patients with predischarge assessment of RPA, 217 had RPA >14%. In these patients, the incidence of the primary endpoint was 6%, whereas it was 2% in patients with RPA ≤14% (*p*=0.004). After adjustment for pertinent baseline variables, the hazard ratio of RPA >14% for the primary endpoint was 3.5 (95% CI 1.5–8.2; *p*=0.004) (Figure 8.13). Even after discontinuation of clopidogrel, a significant difference in the incidence of the primary endpoint between the strata defined by RPA (*p*=0.044) was found. In the 281 patients treated with a drug-eluting stent, the incidence of the primary endpoint was 7.1% when RPA >14%, versus 0.9% in those with RPA ≤14% (HR 7.8; 95% CI 1.5–40.3; *p*=0.004), whereas with a bare-metal stent no significant difference in outcome between the strata defined by residual platelet aggregation was found (HR 2.1; 95% CI 0.8–5.3; *p*=0.13) (Figure 8.13). Thus, the predischarge RPA after administration of clopidogrel was highly predictive for the 1-year incidence of

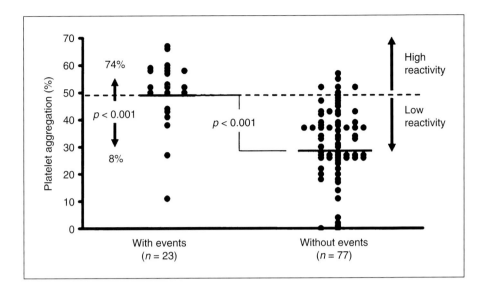

Figure 8.11
Relation of high on-treatment platelet reactivity to ischemic events: graph demonstrating percentage of patients with and without ischemic events displaying high on-treatment platelet reactivity as measured by 5 μmol/l ADP-induced light transmittance aggregometry. The dashed line indicates the cut point for high on-treatment platelet reactivity. (Adapted from Bliden KP et al.[59])

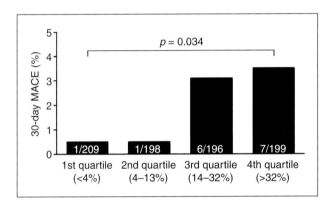

Figure 8.12
Incidence of major adverse cardiac events (MACE) within 30 days after percutaneous coronary intervention by quartiles of ADP-induced platelet aggregation. The *p*-value was determined by a log-rank test.

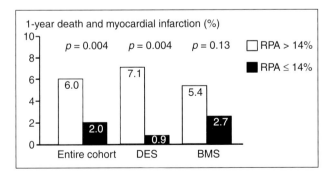

Figure 8.13
One-year incidence of death and myocardial infarction according to strata defined by pre-discharge ADP-induced (5 μmol/l) residual platelet aggregation (RPA) in the entire EXCELSIOR cohort, as well as in the subsets with a drug-eluting stent (DES) or a bare metal stent (BMS).

death and myocardial infarction after coronary stent placement, particularly after placement of a drug-eluting stent.

Whereas the EXCELSIOR study focused on low- to intermediate-risk PCI, the recently published RECLOSE trial investigated higher-risk patients undergoing PCI with placement of a drug-eluting stent.[60] This prospective observational study included 804 patients, more than 50% of whom presented with acute coronary syndromes, 39% with unstable angina, and 27% with acute myocardial infarction. Low responsiveness to clopidogrel was defined by an ADP-induced (10 μmol/l) platelet aggregation >70% on clopidogrel. The primary endpoint of the study – the incidence of definite or probable stent thrombosis during 6-months follow-up – was reached in 2.3% of the patients with an adequate response to clopidogrel and in 8.6% of those with a low response (*p*<0.001). The study also observed a significant difference in cardiac mortality, depending on the response to clopidogrel: cardiac mortality was 8.6% in patients with a low responsiveness, whereas it was 1.4% in those with an adequate response (*p* < 0.01). On multivariable analysis, low responsiveness to clopidogrel was a strong independent predictor of stent thrombosis, with a hazard ratio of 3.08 (95% CI 1.32–7.16; *p*=0.009). The RECLOSE study demonstrates that an inadequate response to clopidogrel is a strong independent predictor of stent thrombosis in high-risk patients receiving sirolimus- and paclitaxel-eluting stents.

In EXCELSIOR and RECLOSE, the stratification according to on-treatment platelet reactivity was based on light transmittance aggregometry. At the 2007 Annual Meeting of the American College of Cardiology, Price and co-workers reported a study with a cartridge-based bedside test of platelet aggregation (VerifyNow). Patients with a platelet reactivity in the upper tertile of the readout of the device were defined as having high post-treatment reactivity.

The study included 380 patients undergoing PCI. At 6 months, the composite incidence of definite, probable, and possible stent thrombosis was 4.0% in patients with high post-treatment reactivity and 0.4% in those with low post-treatment reactivity ($p = 0.02$). The findings of this study confirm the clinical impact of the variability of platelet responses to clopidogrel, and suggest that bedside platelet function tests may be an adequate tool to identify patients with inadequate suppression of platelet function.

Implications

In summary, platelet responses to clopidogrel show a large variability. Clopidogrel is a prodrug with a low bioavailability, and its conversion to the active metabolite depends on absorption, as well as prehepatic metabolism by esterases and hepatic metabolism by the highly polymorphic cytochrome P450 system. Thus, conversion of clopidogrel to its active metabolite is subject to genetically, pharmacologically, and environmentally determined variability in the activity of the cytochrome P450 system. In many patients, the effect of currently approved dosages for clopidogrel is far below the individual maximal plateau. In these patients, increasing the dose of clopidogrel can correct inadequate responses.

Evidence is mounting that the variability of platelet responses to clopidogrel has a major impact on long-term clinical outcome, particularly in patients undergoing placement of a drug-eluting stent. Further studies will be needed to define the optimal platelet function tests as well as the optimal threshold for defining inadequate on-treatment platelet reactivity. Moreover, further studies are needed to test whether correction of inadequate responses to clopidogrel by increasing the dosage or changing to a more potent antiplatelet drug can correct the increased risk associated with low responses to clopidogrel. Until these data are available, it may be prudent to incorporate on-clopidogrel platelet reactivity in clinical decision making with respect to revascularization strategies (surgical vs interventional) and with respect to the choice of stent (bare metal stent vs drug-eluting stent).

References

1. Gurbel PA, Bliden KP, Hiatt BL, O'Connor CM. Clopidogrel for coronary stenting: response variability, drug resistance, and the effect of pretreatment platelet reactivity. Circulation 2003;107:2908–13.
2. Muller I, Besta F, Schulz C et al. Prevalence of clopidogrel non-responders among patients with stable angina pectoris scheduled for elective coronary stent placement. Thromb Haemost 2003;89:783–7.
3. Hochholzer W, Trenk D, Frundi D et al. Time dependence of platelet inhibition after a 600-mg loading dose of clopidogrel in a large, unselected cohort of candidates for percutaneous coronary intervention. Circulation 2005;111:2560–4.
4. Gurbel PA, Bliden KP, Samara W et al. Clopidogrel effect on platelet reactivity in patients with stent thrombosis: results of the CREST study. J Am Coll Cardiol 2005;46:1827–32.
5. Serebruany VL, Steinhubl SR, Berger PB et al. Variability in platelet responsiveness to clopidogrel among 544 individuals. J Am Coll Cardiol 2005;45:246–51.
6. Nguyen TA, Diodati JG, Pharand C. Resistance to clopidogrel: a review of the evidence. J Am Coll Cardiol 2005;45:1157–64.
7. Papp E, Havasi V, Bene J et al. Does glycoprotein IIIa gene (Pl(A)) polymorphism influence clopidogrel resistance? A study in older patients. Drugs Aging 2007;24:345–50.
8. Cuisset T, Frere C, Quilici J et al. Role of the T744C polymorphism of the P2Y12 gene on platelet response to a 600-mg loading dose of clopidogrel in 597 patients with non-ST-segment elevation acute coronary syndrome. Thromb Res 2007; Epub a head of print.
9. Cuisset T, Frere C, Quilici J et al. Lack of association between the 807 C/T polymorphism of glycoprotein Ia gene and post-treatment platelet reactivity after aspirin and clopidogrel in patients with acute coronary syndrome. Thromb Haemost 2007;97:212–17.
10. Sibbing D, von Beckerath O, Schomig A et al. P2Y1 gene A1622G dimorphism is not associated with adenosine diphosphate-induced platelet activation and aggregation after administration of a single high dose of clopidogrel. J Thromb Haemost 2006;4:912–14.
11. Smith SM, Judge HM, Peters G et al. Common sequence variations in the P2Y12 and CYP3A5 genes do not explain the variability in the inhibitory effects of clopidogrel therapy. Platelets 2006;17:250–8.
12. Smith SM, Judge HM, Peters G et al. PAR-1 genotype influences platelet aggregation and procoagulant responses in patients with coronary artery disease prior to and during clopidogrel therapy. Platelets 2005;16:340–5.
13. Suh JW, Koo BK, Zhang SY et al. Increased risk of atherothrombotic events associated with cytochrome P450 3A5 polymorphism in patients taking clopidogrel. CMAJ 2006;174:1715–22.
14. Angiolillo DJ, Fernandez-Ortiz A, Bernardo E et al. Contribution of gene sequence variations of the hepatic cytochrome P450 3A4 enzyme to variability in individual responsiveness to clopidogrel. Arterioscler Thromb Vasc Biol 2006;26:1895–900.
15. Hulot JS, Bura A, Villard E et al. Cytochrome P450 2C19 loss-of-function polymorphism is a major determinant of clopidogrel responsiveness in healthy subjects. Blood 2006;108:2244–7.
16. Lev EI, Patel RT, Guthikonda S et al. Genetic polymorphisms of the platelet receptors P2Y$_{12}$, P2Y$_1$ and GP IIIa and response to aspirin and clopidogrel. Thromb Res 2007;119:355–60.
17. Cooke GE, Liu-Stratton Y, Ferketich AK et al. Effect of platelet antigen polymorphism on platelet inhibition by aspirin, clopidogrel, or their combination. J Am Coll Cardiol 2006;47:541–6.
18. Dropinski J, Musial J, Jakiela B et al. Anti-thrombotic action of clopidogrel and Pl(A1/A2) polymorphism of β_3 integrin in patients with coronary artery disease not being treated with aspirin. Thromb Haemost 2005;94:1300–5.
19. Angiolillo DJ, Fernandez-Ortiz A, Bernardo E et al. Variability in platelet aggregation following sustained aspirin and clopidogrel treatment in patients with coronary heart disease and influence of the 807 C/T polymorphism of the glycoprotein Ia gene. Am J Cardiol 2005;96:1095–9.
20. Angiolillo DJ, Fernandez-Ortiz A, Bernardo E et al. Lack of association between the P2Y12 receptor gene polymorphism and platelet response to clopidogrel in patients with coronary artery disease. Thromb Res 2005;116:491–7.
21. Angiolillo DJ, Fernandez-Ortiz A, Bernardo E et al. 807 C/T polymorphism of the glycoprotein Ia gene and pharmacogenetic modulation of platelet response to dual antiplatelet treatment. Blood Coagul Fibrinolysis 2004;15:427–33.

22. Angiolillo DJ, Fernandez-Ortiz A, Bernardo E et al. PlA polymorphism and platelet reactivity following clopidogrel loading dose in patients undergoing coronary stent implantation. Blood Coagul Fibrinolysis 2004;15:89–93.

23. Fontana P, Dupont A, Gandrille S et al. Adenosine diphosphate-induced platelet aggregation is associated with *P2Y12* gene sequence variations in healthy subjects. Circulation 2003;108: 989–95.

24. Angiolillo DJ, Fernandez-Ortiz A, Bernardo E et al. Variability in platelet aggregation following sustained aspirin and clopidogrel treatment in patients with coronary heart disease and influence of the 807 C/T polymorphism of the glycoprotein Ia gene. Am J Cardiol 2005;96:1095–9.

25. Sanofi-Aventis Canada Inc., West Laval, Quebec, Canada. Product Monograph, February 20, 2007.

26. Taubert D, Kastrati A, Harlfinger S et al. Pharmacokinetics of clopidogrel after administration of a high loading dose. Thromb Haemost 2004;92:311–16.

27. Savi P, Herbert JM, Pflieger AM et al. Importance of hepatic metabolism in the antiaggregating activity of the thienopyridine clopidogrel. Biochem Pharmacol 1992;44:527–32.

28. Savi P, Combalbert J, Gaich C et al. The antiaggregating activity of clopidogrel is due to a metabolic activation by the hepatic cytochrome P450-1A. Thromb Haemost 1994;72:313–17.

29. Humphries RG, Tomlinson W, Ingall AH et al. FPL 66096: a novel, highly potent and selective antagonist at human platelet P2T-purinoceptors. Br J Pharmacol 1994;113:1057–63.

30. Savi P, Pereillo JM, Uzabiaga MF et al. Identification and biological activity of the active metabolite of clopidogrel. Thromb Haemost 2000;84:891–6.

31. Ding Z, Kim S, Dorsam RT et al. Inactivation of the human *P2Y12* receptor by thiol reagents requires interaction with both extracellular cysteine residues, Cys17 and Cys270. Blood 2003;101:3908–14.

32. Lau WC, Gurbel PA, Watkins PB et al. Contribution of hepatic cytochrome P450 3A4 metabolic activity to the phenomenon of clopidogrel resistance. Circulation 2004;109:166–71.

33. Smith SM, Judge HM, Peters G, Storey RF. Multiple antiplatelet effects of clopidogrel are not modulated by statin type in patients undergoing percutaneous coronary intervention. Platelets 2004;15:465–74.

34. Müller I, Besta F, Schulz C et al. Effects of statins on platelet inhibition by a high loading dose of clopidogrel. Circulation 2003;108:2195–7.

35. Neubauer H, Gunesdogan B, Hanefeld C, Spiecker M, Mugge A. Lipophilic statins interfere with the inhibitory effects of clopidogrel on platelet function – a flow cytometry study. Eur Heart J 2003;24:1744–9.

36. Saw J, Steinhubl SR, Berger PB et al. Clopidogrel for the Reduction of Events During Observation Investigators. Lack of adverse clopidogrel–atorvastatin clinical interaction from secondary analysis of a randomized, placebo-controlled clopidogrel trial. Circulation 2003;108:921–4.

37. Wienbergen H, Gitt AK, Schiele R et al. MITRA PLUS Study Group. Comparison of clinical benefits of clopidogrel therapy in patients with acute coronary syndromes taking atorvastatin versus other statin therapies. Am J Cardiol 2003;92:285–8.

38. Gorchakova O, von Beckerath N, Gawaz M et al. Antiplatelet effects of a 600 mg loading dose of clopidogrel are not attenuated in patients receiving atorvastatin or simvastatin for at least 4 weeks prior to coronary artery stenting. Eur Heart J 2004;25:1898–902.

39. Brophy J, Costa V, Babapulle M. A pharmaco–epidemiological study of the interaction between atorvastatin and clopidogrel following percutaneous coronary interventions. J Am Coll Cardiol 2004;43(Suppl A): Abst 1063-55.

40. Hochholzer W, Trenk D, Frundi D et al. Chronic treatment with CYP3A4-metabolized statins has no effect on the antiplatelet activity of a bolus dose of clopidogrel 600 mg. Eur Heart J 2004;25(Suppl):463 (Abst 2778).

41. Mitsios JV, Papathanasiou AI, Rodis FI et al. Atorvastatin does not affect the antiplatelet potency of clopidogrel when it is administered concomitantly for 5 weeks in patients with acute coronary syndromes. Circulation 2004;109:1335–8.

42. Serebruany VL, Midei MG, Malinin AI et al. Absence of interaction between atorvastatin or other statins and clopidogrel. Arch Intern Med 2004;164:2051–7.

43. Beitelshees AL, McLeod HL. Clopidogrel pharmacogenetics: promising steps towards patient care? Arterioscler Thromb Vasc Biol 2006;26:1681–3.

44. Forbes CD, Lowe GD, MacLaren M et al. Clopidogrel compatibility with concomitant cardiac co-medications: a study of its interactions with a beta-blocker and a calcium uptake antagonist. Semin Thromb Hemost 1999;25(Suppl 2):55–60.

45. Peeters PA, Crijns HJ, Tamminga WJ et al. Clopidogrel, a novel antiplatelet agent, and digoxin: absence of harmacodynamic and pharmacokinetic interaction. Semin Thromb Hemost 1999;25(Suppl 2):51–4.

46. Angiolillo DJ, Fernandez-Ortiz A, Bernardo E et al. Platelet aggregation according to body mass index in patients undergoing coronary stenting: Should clopidogrel loading-dose be weight adjusted? J Invasive Cardiol 2004;16:169–74.

47. Hochholzer W, Trenk D, Bestehorn HP et al. Impact of the degree of peri-interventional platelet inhibition after loading with clopidogrel on early clinical outcome of elective coronary stent placement. J Am Coll Cardiol 2006;48:1742–50.

48. CAPRIE Steering Committee. A randomised, blinded, trial of clopidogrel versus aspirin in patients at risk of ischaemic events (CAPRIE). Lancet 1996;348:1329–39.

49. Samara WM, Bliden KP, Tantry US, Gurbel PA. The difference between clopidogrel responsiveness and posttreatment platelet reactivity. Thromb Res 2005;115:89–94.

50. Angiolillo DJ, Fernandez-Ortiz A, Bernardo E et al. Clopidogrel withdrawal is associated with proinflammatory and prothrombotic effects in patients with diabetes and coronary artery disease. Diabetes 2006;55:780–4.

51. Soffer D, Moussa I, Harjai KJ et al. Impact of angina class on inhibition of platelet aggregation following clopidogrel loading in patients undergoing coronary intervention: Do we need more aggressive dosing regimens in unstable angina? Catheter Cardiovasc Interv 2003;59:21–5.

52. Ajzenberg N, Aubry P, Huisse MG et al. Enhanced shear-induced platelet aggregation in patients who experience subacute stent thrombosis: a case–control study. J Am Coll Cardiol 2005;45:1753–6.

53. Wenaweser P, Dorffler-Melly J, Imboden K et al. Stent thrombosis is associated with an impaired response to antiplatelet therapy. J Am Coll Cardiol 2005;45:1748–52.

54. Matetzky S, Shenkman B, Guetta V et al. Clopidogrel resistance is associated with increased risk of recurrent atherothrombotic events in patients with acute myocardial infarction. Circulation 2004;109:3171–5.

55. Campo G, Valgimigli M, Gemmati D et al. Value of platelet reactivity in predicting response to treatment and clinical outcome in patients undergoing primary coronary intervention: insights into the STRATEGY Study. J Am Coll Cardiol 2006;48:2178–85.

56. Cuisset T, Frere C, Quilici J et al. High post-treatment platelet reactivity identified low-responders to dual antiplatelet therapy at increased risk of recurrent cardiovascular events after stenting for acute coronary syndrome. J Thromb Haemost 2006;4:542–9.

57. Cuisset T, Frere C, Quilici J et al. High post-treatment platelet reactivity is associated with a high incidence of myonecrosis after stenting for non-ST elevation acute coronary syndromes. Thromb Haemost 2007;97:282–7.

58. Gurbel PA, Bliden KP, Guyer K et al. Platelet reactivity in patients and recurrent events post-stenting: results of the PREPARE POST-STENTING study. J Am Coll Cardiol 2005;46:1820–6.

59. Bliden KP, DiChiara J, Tantry US et al. Increased risk in patients with high platelet aggregation receiving chronic clopidogrel therapy undergoing percutaneous coronary intervention: Is the current antiplatelet therapy adequate? J Am Coll Cardiol 2007;49:657–66.

60. Buonamici P, Marcucci R, Migliorini A et al. Impact of platelet reactivity after clopidogrel administration on drug-eluting stent thrombosis. J Am Coll Cardiol 2007;49:2312–17.

9

Prasugrel – a third-generation thienopyridine

Stephen D Wiviott and Elliott M Antman

Introduction

Thienopyridine antiplatelet agents represent a major advance in the care of patients with coronary artery disease, particularly those with acute coronary syndromes (ACS) and those undergoing percutaneous coronary intervention (PCI). Clopidogrel has largely replaced ticlopidine because of better tolerability and fewer side-effects. Despite the significant improvement of dual antiplatelet therapy with aspirin and clopidogrel over aspirin alone, significant limitations of this agent exist; relatively modest inhibition of platelet aggregation, delayed onset of antiplatelet activity, and substantial variability of response among individuals.[1] As a result of these limitations, there may be a role for novel antiplatelet agents, including newer-generation thienopyridines. Prasugrel (CS-747, LY 640315) is the first new agent in this class to undergo clinical testing, and is the subject of this chapter.

Chemical structure, metabolism, pharmacokinetics, and preclinical studies

Prasugrel is an investigational member of the thienopyridine class. Its chemical name is (±)-2-[2-acetyloxy-6,7-dihydrothieno[3,2-c]pyridine-5(4H)-yl]-1-cyclopropyl-2-(2-fluorophenyl)ethanone and its structure is shown in Figure 9.1. Compared with clopidogrel, prasugrel has modifications of two side-chains and a substitution of a fluoro for a chloro group. Like clopidogrel, prasugrel is a prodrug requiring metabolism to an active metabolite for its antiplatelet activity (Figure 9.2). Initially prasugrel is rapidly de-esterified to an inactive metabolite R-95913 and subsequently to the active adenosine diphosphate (ADP) receptor antagonist R-13827 by the hepatic cytochrome P450 system, predominantly CYP3A4, but also CYP2B6,

CYP2C9, CYP2C19, and CYP2D6.[2] The predominant difference between the metabolism of prasugrel and clopidogrel is that in the early stages of metabolism of clopidogrel, a significant portion of the prodrug is deactivated, resulting in less potential active metabolite. Absorption and metabolism are rapid with prasugrel, resulting in a median time for maximal concentration (T_{max}) for R-13827 (Payne, ESC 2005) of approximately 30 minutes. Although the active metabolites of the two drugs have similar potency at the level of the platelet, prasugrel achieves 10- to 100-fold higher levels of the concentration of the active metabolite than does clopidogrel.[3] Correspondingly, in animal studies, prasugrel was shown to be rapidly active (within 30 minutes) and approximately 10-fold more potent than clopidogrel on a mg/kg basis when measured by inhibition of platelet aggregation (IPA).[4,5] In summary, prasugrel is a rapid-onset, potent thienopyridine, with the active metabolites of clopidogrel and prasugrel have similar potency of inhibition of platelet aggregation when present in equal concentrations. The differences in pharmacokinetics and dynamics compared with clopidogrel being largely related to more rapid and efficient generation of the active metabolite of prasugrel.

Pharmacodynamics and safety (phase I studies)

A key phase I study of prasugrel was a crossover study in healthy subjects.[3] In this study, 68 healthy subjects not taking aspirin received either a 300 mg loading dose of clopidogrel or a 60 mg loading dose of prasugrel, and after a washout period of 2 weeks, the alternate therapy. Both therapies were well tolerated. Prasugrel was shown to have more rapid onset of antiplatelet action than clopidogrel, with significant inhibition of ADP-induced platelet aggregation evident by 15 minutes and maximal effect within 60 minutes, compared with 4–6 hours for clopidogrel. In addition, the peak IPA was higher for prasugrel

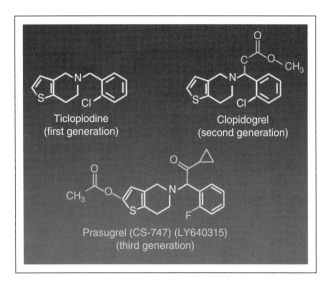

Figure 9.1
Structures of thienopyridine antiplatelet agents. (see color plate)

(mean 78.8% vs 35%; $p < 0.001$) following 20 μmol/l ADP. Strikingly, there was a less interpatient variability among patients receiving prasugrel compared with clopidogrel (Figure 9.4). When thienopyridine resistance was defined as 20% IPA at 24 hours, 42% of subjects were resistant when receiving clopidogrel; however, no subject was resistant when receiving prasugrel. Further, among the clopidogrel-resistant subjects, there was no discernable difference in prasugrel response compared with those subjects who had responded well to clopidogrel. Among subjects responding poorly to clopidogrel, there was less generation of the active metabolite. Taken together, these data suggested that resistance to thienopyridines may be primarily related to levels of active metabolite generation – not to platelet level resistance. This may indicate either limitation at the level of absorption or metabolism to the active metabolite.

In a subsequent three-period crossover study, prasugrel 60 mg loading dose followed by 10 mg daily was compared with clopidogrel 300 mg followed by 75 mg daily or 600 mg followed by 75 mg daily for 7 days with a 14-day washout period between each treatment in 33 subjects.[6] The results of this study are shown in Figure 9.5, and indicated that prasugrel was more rapid in onset and achieved higher levels of inhibition of platelet aggregation than either dose of clopidogrel. Of note, the difference in inhibition of platelet aggregation between prasugrel and 600 mg of clopidogrel was greater than the difference between 600 and 300 mg of clopidogrel. While the differences in aggregation between the two loading doses of clopidogrel had abated by 3 days of follow-up, these differences persisted throughout the study period during maintenance therapy for prasugrel compared to clopidogrel.

The key phase Ib study of prasugrel compared with clopidogrel was performed in patients with stable coronary artery disease receiving aspirin.[7] After an aspirin-only run-in period, subjects were randomized to receive either 300 mg of clopidogrel followed by 75 mg daily (300/75 mg) for 4 weeks or one of four loading and maintenance dosing (LD/MD) regimens of prasugrel (40/5 mg, 40/7.5 mg, 60/10 mg, or 60/15 mg) The primary objective was a comparison of the degree of platelet inhibition achieved between the different groups. The results demonstrated that both prasugrel 40 or 60 mg loading doses achieved more rapid and higher levels of inhibition of platelet aggregation to 20 μmol/l ADP (60.6% and 68.4% vs 30%; $p < 0.001$) and a lower rate of pharmacodynamic non-response (3% vs 52%; $p < 0.0001$). Prasugrel at maintenance doses of 10 and 15 mg per day achieved higher levels of IPA and less non-response (0% vs 45%; $p < 0.0001$) than clopidogrel 75 mg at day 28. Minor bleeding events were numerically, but not statistically, more frequent in the highest-dose prasugrel arm.

An additional evaluation of prasugrel compared to clopidogrel was undertaken in the PRINCIPLE (PRasugrel IN Comparison to Clopidogrel for Inhibition of PLatelet Activation and AggrEgation)–TIMI (Thrombosis In Myocardial Infarction) 44 study.[8] This study was two-phase study of subjects undergoing elective PCI. In the first phase, prasugrel 10 mg will be compared with clopidogrel 600 mg loading dose, with a primary endpoint of ADP-stimulated IPA at 6 hours. In the second phase, subjects received prasugrel 10 mg or clopidogrel 150 mg following the loading dose for 14 days and were then crossed over to the alternate treatment for an additional 14 days. The primary endpoint was IPA following 14 days' treatment. The primary endpoint of the loading phase of the study showed significantly higher levels of IPA for each timepoint with prasugrel compared to clopidogrel (Figure 9.3a). Similarly, IPA was higher following 14 days maintenance therapy with prasugrel compared to high-dose clopidogrel (Figure 9.3b). This study provided important comparative pharmacodynamic information for prasugrel compared with the higher doses of clopidogrel that are used by some practitioners during and following PCI.

Phase II: safety evaluation

The JUMBO (Joint Utilization of Medications to Block Platelets Optimally)–TIMI 26 trial[9] was a phase II, double-blind, double-dummy, dose-ranging study of 904 patients undergoing either elective or urgent PCI with stenting and followed for 30 days. The design is shown in Figure 9.6. Patients were randomized to one of three combinations of loading and maintenance doses of prasugrel – a low- (40/7.5 mg), intermediate- (60/10 mg), or high- (60/15 mg) dose regimen – or to standard-dose clopidogrel (300/75 mg). The loading dose was given at the time of the PCI, and

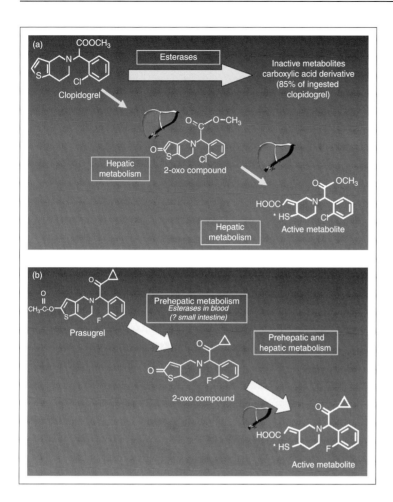

Figure 9.2
Schematics of the metabolism of clopidogrel (a)
and prasugrel (b). (see color plate)

maintenance doses were administered daily for 30 days. As this study was designed to assess the safety of prasugrel in patients undergoing PCI, the primary endpoint was significant non-coronary artery bypass surgery (CABG)-associated hemorrhage at 30 days, defined as the combination of TIMI major plus TIMI minor bleeding. The results showed a higher absolute rate but no significant difference for prasugrel compared with clopidogrel for the primary endpoint of significant bleeding (1.7% vs 1.2%; $p = 0.59$). In addition, rates of bleeding for both groups were similar to or lower than other contemporary studies.[10] TIMI major bleeding was less frequent and similar for prasugrel and clopidogrel (0.5% vs 0.8%; $p = 0.54$). Less severe (TIMI minimal)Nuisance bleeding tended to be higher in the highest-dose prasugrel arm. Although not designed or powered to detect differences in clinical efficacy endpoints, a non-statistically significant but consistently lower rate of ischemic events was observed among the prasugrel treated patients compared with those treated with standard doses of clopidogrel. The primary efficacy endpoint – major adverse cardiovascular events (MACE), consisting of the combination of death, myocardial infarction, stroke, recurrent ischemia requiring rehospitalization, and clinical target vessel thrombosis (urgent revas-

cularization or total target vessel occlusion documented angiographically) – occurred in 7.2% of prasugrel-treated subjects compared with 9.4% of clopidogrel-treated subjects ($p = 0.26$). Myocardial infarction was predominantly periprocedural and also tended to occur less frequently in patients treated with prasugrel (5.7% vs 7.9%; $p = 0.23$). The results of this study suggested that prasugrel had an adequate safety profile to proceed with phase III testing in a trial designed with adequate sample size to detect a clinically meaningful reduction in cardiovascular ischemic events.

Phase III: efficacy evaluation

The efficacy of prasugrel compared with clopidogrel was tested in the registration pathway, phase III study TRITON (TRial to assess Improvement in Therapeutic Outcomes by optimizing platelet inhibitioN with prasugrel) – TIMI 38. This is a randomized, double-blind, parallel-group, multinational clinical trial.[11] The design is shown in Figure 9.7. Approximately 13 600 patients comprise the study population: 10 100 with moderate to high risk unstable angina (TIMI Risk Score ≥3)[12] non-ST-elevation myocardial

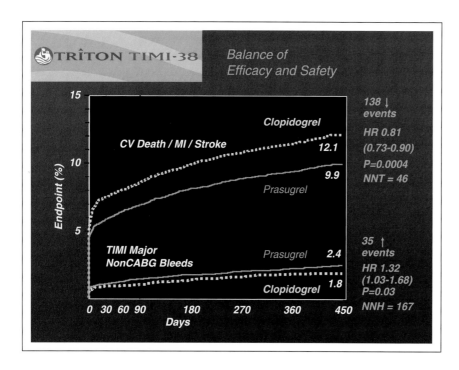

Figure 9.8
(see color plate)

registration pathway trial, testing the efficacy of prasugrel compared with clopidogrel in patients with ACS undergoing PCI. If this drug improves clinical outcomes with acceptable safety, it may be an important addition to the medical antiplatelet options for physicians. In addition to the safety and efficacy of this particular compound, its evaluation will help to determine whether use of an agent or dose of an agent that achieves higher level of ADP-induced platelet aggregation, and less variability in response than current standards, will result in improved clinical outcomes.

References

1. O'Donoghue M, Wiviott SD. Clopidogrel response variability and future therapies: clopidogrel: does one size fit all? Circulation 2006;114:e600–6.

2. Rehmel JL, Eckstein JA, Farid NA et al. Interactions of two major metabolites of prasugrel, a thienopyridine antiplatelet agent, with the cytochromes P450. Drug Metab Dispos 2006;34:600–7.

3. Brandt JT, Payne CD, Wiviott SD et al. A comparison of prasugrel and clopidogrel loading doses on platelet function: magnitude of platelet inhibition is related to active metabolite formation. Am Heart J 2007;153:e69–16.

4. Sugidachi A, Asai F, Ogawa T et al. The in vivo pharmacological profile of CS-747, a novel antiplatelet agent with platelet ADP receptor antagonist properties. Br J Pharmacol 2000;129:1439–46.

5. Niitsu Y, Jakubowski JA, Sugidachi A, Asai F. Pharmacology of CS-747 (prasugrel, LY640315), a novel, potent antiplatelet agent with in vivo P2Y12 receptor antagonist activity. Semin Thromb Hemost 2005;31:184–94.

6. Payne CD, Li YG, Ernets CS et al. A prasugrel 60 mg loading dose achieves faster onset and higher levels of platelet inhibition compared with 300 mg or 600 mg clopidogrel loading doses. Paper presented at Trascatheter Cardiovascular Therapeutics 18th Annual Scientific Symposium, October 2006.

7. Jernberg T, Payne CD, Winters KJ et al. Prasugrel achieves greater inhibition of platelet aggregation and a lower rate of non-responders compared with clopidogrel in aspirin-treated patients with stable coronary artery disease. Eur Heart J 2006;27:1166–73.

8. Wiviott SD, Trenk D, Frelinger AL et al. Prasugrel compared with high loading- and maintenance-dose clopidogrel in patients with planned percutaneous coronary intervention: the Prasugrel in Comparison to Clopidogrel for Inhibition of Platelet Activation and Aggregation-Thrombolysis in Myocardial Infarction 44 trial. Circulation 2007; 116:2923–32.

9. Wiviott SD, Antman EM, Winters KJ et al. Randomized comparison of prasugrel (CS-747, LY640315), a novel thienopyridine P2Y12 antagonist, with clopidogrel in percutaneous coronary intervention: results of the Joint Utilization of Medications to Block Platelets Optimally (JUMBO)-TIMI 26 trial. Circulation 2005; 111:3366–73.

10. Steinhubl SR, Berger PB, Mann JT 3rd et al. Early and sustained dual oral antiplatelet therapy following percutaneous coronary intervention: a randomized controlled trial. JAMA 2002;288:2411–20.

11. Wiviott SD, Antman EM, Gibson CM et al. Evaluation of prasugrel compared with clopidogrel in patients with acute coronary syndromes: design and rationale for the TRial to assess Improvement in Therapeutic Outcomes by optimizing platelet InhibitioN with prasugrel Thrombolysis In Myocardial Infarction 38 (TRITON-TIMI 38). Am Heart J 2006;152:627–35.

12. Antman EM, Cohen M, Bernink PJ et al. The TIMI risk score for unstable angina/non-ST elevation MI: A method for prognostication and therapeutic decision making. JAMA 2000;284:835–42.

13. Wiviott SD, Braunwald E, McCabe CH. Prasugrel versus Clopidogrel in Patients with Acute Coronary Syndromes. NEJM 2007; 357:2001–15.

10

Direct oral P2Y$_{12}$ inhibition: AZD6140 (Ticagrelor)

Steen Husted and Christopher P Cannon

Platelet P2Y receptors

Platelet activation by nucleotides such as adenosine diphosphate (ADP) plays a crucial role in thrombus formation. The nucleotides interact with two large families of purinergic (P) receptors: the ionotropic P2X and the G-protein-coupled P2Y receptors (Figure 10.1). Two types of P2Y and one type of P2X receptors are expressed by human platelets. Among the eight different subtypes of P2Y receptors cloned so far, the P2Y$_1$ and P2Y$_{12}$ types are present on platelets, acting as receptors for ADP. The importance of these receptors in both physiological and pathological platelet function is derived largely from human disorders, mouse models, and pharmacological intervention.

The Gαq-coupled P2Y$_1$ receptor is responsible for inositol triphosphate formation through formation of phospholipase C (PLC), leading to a transient increase in the concentration of intracellular calcium, platelet shape changes, and weak transient platelet aggregation.[1] The P2Y$_1$ receptor plays an essential role in the initiation of platelet ADP-induced activation, thromboxane A$_2$ (TXA$_2$) generation, and platelet activation in response to other agonists.[1]

The negatively coupled G$_i$ P2Y$_{12}$ receptor has extracellular cysteines and is responsible for completion of the platelet aggregation response to ADP[2] with several signalling molecules downstream such as cAMP, vasodilator-stimulated phosphoprotein (VASP), dephosphorylation, phosphatidytinositol 3′-kinase, and Rap1b.

The P2Y$_{12}$ receptor plays a role in dense granule secretion, fibrinogen-receptor activation, P-selectin expression, and thrombus formation, indicating a central role for the hemostatic response.[3,4] The receptor is important not only for ADP-induced aggregation, but also aggregation induced by thrombin, immune complexes, epinephrine (adrenaline), serotonin, TXA$_2$, and the PAR1-selective agonist SFLLRN.[5]

In addition, the P2Y$_{12}$ receptor contributes to phosphatidylserine exposure at the platelet surface, where coagulation factors bind to stimulate thrombin generation[6] and, together with P2Y$_1$, it is involved in the formation of platelet-leucocyte conjugates, which leads to tissue factor exposure.[7]

Oral P2Y$_{12}$ receptor blockers – limitations of clopidogrel

Oral antiplatelet therapy with clopidogrel, a thienopyridine, is central to the treatment of patients with atherothrombotic disease. Clopidogrel is a prodrug requiring hepatic cytochrome P450 metabolism to release its active metabolite, which binds irreversibly to the P2Y$_{12}$ receptor such that recovery of platelet function is precluded.

Numerous studies have documented the efficacy of treatment with the thienopyridines clopidogrel and ticlopidine.[8–11] Clopidogrel has, however, largely superseded ticlopidine due to its better safety and tolerability profile, particularly its lower incidence of neutropenia and thrombotic thrombocytopenic purpura (TTP).

However, evidence suggests that there is a considerable interindividual variability in the response to clopidogrel as measured by platelet aggregation and flow cytometry.[12] The terms clopidogrel 'resistance', 'non-responsiveness', and 'hyporesponsiveness' have been used interchangeably to indicate a less-than-expected inhibition of ADP-induced platelet aggregation/activation following standard clopidogrel therapy.[13] The incidence of resistance to clopidogrel

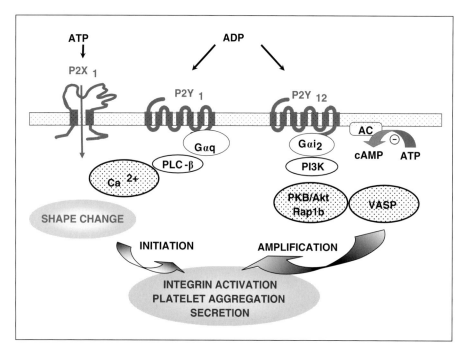

Figure 10.1
The G-protein-coupled platelet P2Y receptors. ATP, adenosine triphosphate; ADP, adenosine diphosphate; cAMP, cyclic adenosine monophosphate; PKB, protein kinase B; PI3K, phosphatidylinositol 3'-kinase; VASP, vasodilator-stimulated phosphoprotein.

varies from 5% to 46%.[13] The mechanisms of clopidogrel resistance are multifactorial, but important factors are patient non-compliance, physician failure to prescribe/inadequate dosing, effects on the cytochrome P450 system such as drug–drug interaction or gene polymorphisms of the CYP3A4 system affecting generation of the active metabolite, and polymorphisms of the $P2Y_{12}$ receptor.[14] Also, a heightened degree of of platelet activation may be an important determinant of low response.[15]

Other limitations of clopidogrel (Table 10.1) include a suboptimal onset of action and a relatively modest inhibition of ex vivo platelet response to ADP both following a loading dose of 300 or 600 mg and at steady state on a daily dose of 75 mg.[16]

Moreover, a few small studies have correlated inadequate platelet inhibition with the occurrence of adverse clinical events, including recurrent ischemia post percutaneous coronary interventing (PCI) and stent thrombosis.[17–19]

Oral $P2Y_{12}$ receptor blockers – direct acting non-thienopyridines: AZD6140 (Ticagrelor)

The non-thienopyridine $P2Y_{12}$ receptor antagonists, such as cangrelor and AZD6140, have chemical structures that

Table 10.1 *Limitations of clopidogrel*

- High interpatient variability in pharmacokinetics and pharmacodynamics (resistance/non-responders)
- Modest inhibition of platelet response ex vivo
- Irreversible $P2Y_{12}$ receptor binding
- Requires metabolic activation
- Onset of action suboptimal

differ substantially from those of the thienopyridines (Figure 10.2). In contrast to the thienopyridines, cangrelor and AZD6140 bind reversibly to the platelet receptor.

AZD6140 (Ticagrelor) is the first member of a class of high-affinity, stable, and selective $P2Y_{12}$ receptor antagonists known as cyclopentyltriazolopyrimidines (Figure 10.2). The drug is a non-phosphate and competitive $P2Y_{12}$ antagonist with high affinity properties resulting from substitution at the 2 position in the adenine ring and stablization resulted from β,γ-methylene substitutions in the phosphate group.

AZD6140 is an active drug that does not require hepatic conversion like the thienopyridines. One active metabolite AR-C124910XX is present in the blood at about one-third the concentration of the parent drug. Both the parent drug and the metabolite are equally potent in specifically blocking the $P2Y_{12}$ receptor.[21] Even at concentrations >3 μmol/l

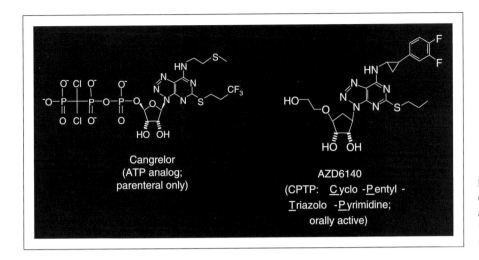

Figure 10.2
Chemical structures of the direct acting, reversible, non-thienopyridine P2Y$_{12}$ receptor antagonists. (see color plate)

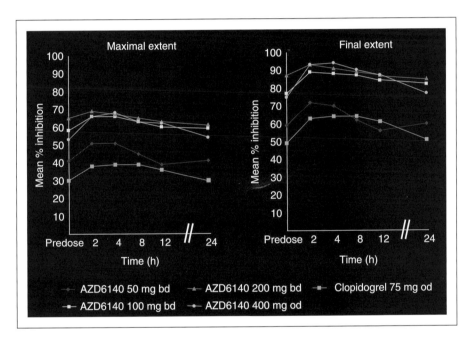

Figure 10.3
Mean inhibition of ADP-induced platelet aggregation on maximum and final response by different dosages of AZD6140 and clopidogrel standard dosage after 14 days of therapy in patients with stable atherosclerotic disease. (see color plate)

AZD6140 does not have any significant affinity towards the other P2 receptors, and in animal studies the potency (pIC$_{50}$) of AZD6140 is 7.9 in washed platelets, whereas it was 7.2 in diluted whole blood impedance aggregometry.[21] In a model of cyclic flow reductions in the femoral artery of anesthetized dogs, AZD6140 displayed a good separation between the antithrombotic effect and the prolongation of the tongue bleeding time, i.e., intermediate between that of cangrelor and that of clopidogrel.[21]

The dose-dependent effect of AZD6140 (30–400 mg single dose) was studied in healthy volunteers by measuring plasma levels of AZD6140 and the active metabolite (AR-C126910XX) together with inhibition of ADP-induced platelet aggregation ex vivo.[25] AZD6140 was rapidly absorbed and showed linear and dose-proportional pharmkokinetics best fit by a two-compartment model.

Inhibition of ADP-induced platelet aggregation was dose- and time-dependent, with maximum inhibition being observed with 300 and 400 mg doses. A high level of inhibition was maintained throughout 24 hours.[25]

In healthy volunteers, ascending single- and multiple-dose-dependent pharmacokinetic and pharmacodynamic effects of AZD6140 were compared with a 300 mg clopidogrel loading dose and a 75 mg maintenance dose.[26] Peak plasma levels of AZD6140 were obtained 1.5–3 hours post treatment, and steady state was reached after 2–3 days. Accordingly, the plasma half-life was 6–13 hours, irrespective of the dose administered. AZD6140 doses ≥100 mg twice daily and 300 mg once daily were associated with higher steady-state platelet inhibition of ADP-induced aggregation than clopidogrel. An inhibition of 97–100% (final aggregation) was achieved throughout the dosing period with 300 mg twice daily, and all of the doses were well tolerated, with adverse events comparable to those of clopidogrel.

In a randomized, double-blind, parallel-group phase IIa study, DISPERSE (Dose confirmation Study assessing anti-Platelet Effects of AZD6140 vs clopidogRel in NSTEMI), AZD6140 was compared with clopidogrel in 200 patients with confirmed stable atherosclerotic disease in any vascular bed.[27]

The study involved both males and females aged 25–85 years, who were randomized to one of four different dose regimens of AZD6140 (50, 100, or 200 mg twice daily, or 400 mg once daily) or clopidogrel (75 mg once daily) for 28 days, without any loading dose in the treatment groups. All patients also received low-dose aspirin 75–100 mg once daily. A superior platelet inhibition (>90%; final extent) was obtained with AZD6140 (≥100 mg twice

daily) treatment, whereas clopidogrel was associated with only about 60% platelet inhibition (Figure 10.3). In addition, inhibition of platelet aggregation by AZD6140 was very rapid, with a maximum 2 hours post dose (Figure 10.4), and showed less variability compared with that of clopidogrel (Figure 10.5). There was no substantial difference between the three highest doses of AZD6140 with respect to mean percentage of inhibition of platelet aggregation (IPA).

AZD6140 treatment was well tolerated across the dose range, with an increased bleeding time compared with clopidogrel, which was not AZD6140 dose-related. Only one major bleeding event occurred in a patient receiving 400 mg once daily, whereas other bleeding events were of minor or mild to moderate severity. An increase in dyspnea was associated with increasing dose; however, none of the incidents were considered serious.

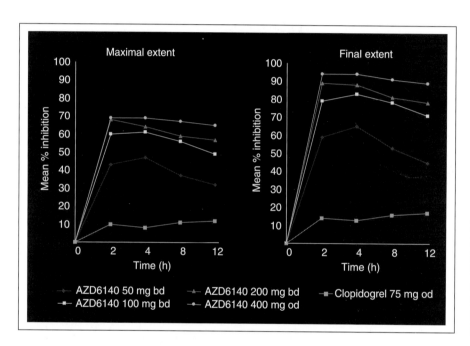

Figure 10.4
Mean inhibition of ADP-induced platelet aggregation on maximum and final response following one single oral dosage of AZD6140, 50–400 mg and clopidogrel 75 mg in patients with stable atherosclerotic disease. (see color plate)

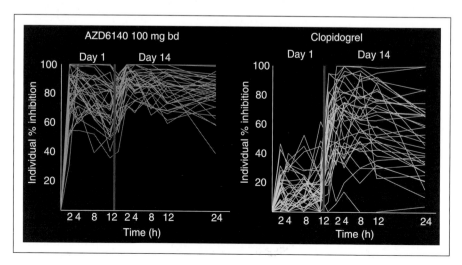

Figure 10.5
Individual inhibitory effect on response to ADP-induced platelet aggregation by AZD6140, a direct acting, reversible P2Y$_{12}$ receptor antagonist, 100 mg twice daily and clopidogrel 75 mg daily in patients with stable atherosclerotic disease after one single dosage and after 14 days of therapy. (see color plate)

Pharmacokinetic data were comparable to those obtained in normal human volunteers.

Overall, DISPERSE demonstrates that AZ6140 is well tolerated and gives a rapid, consistent and high level of IPA during treatment of patients with stable atherosclerotic disease .

DISPERSE2 was a double-blind phase IIb trial that randomized 990 patients with non-ST elevation (NSTE) acute coronary syndrome (ACS) to receive AZD6140 at 90 or 180 mg twice daily or a clopidogrel loading dose of 300 mg followed by 75 mg daily for 4–12 weeks, with the option to give an additional double-blind clopidogrel 300 mg dose before PCI.[28] Half of the AZD6140 patients received a loading dose of 270 mg. Clopidogrel-pretreated patients did not receive a loading dose of clopidogrel. All patients were treated with aspirin (325 mg loading dose followed by 75–100 mg once daily) and in addition unfractionated heparin/low-molecular-weight heparin and a glycoprotein (GP) IIb/IIIa receptor antagonist as selected by the local physician.

Clinical outcomes (cardiovascular death, myocardial infarction, and stroke) together with ex vivo platelet inhibition were studied. The AZD6140 180 mg dose was associated with a decrease in MI (2.5% compared to 5.6% with clopidogrel and 3.8% with AZD6140 90 mg). This decrease in MI was associated with superior platelet inhibition, indicating a mechanical link between levels of platelet inhibition and occurrence of MI. There were no differences in major and minor bleeding events between groups, and major bleeding events were not influenced by dose. Overall, AZD6140 treatment was well tolerated, with no significant bleeding events, based on sex, age, weight, prior clopidogrel treatment or use of GPIIb/IIIa receptor antagonists. Ventricular pauses >2.5 s as detected on continuous ECG were more common in the AZD6140 180 mg group as compared with AZD6140 90 mg and clopidogrel groups (9.9%, 5.5%, and 4.3%, respectively). There is no known mechanism to explain this observation, although it is possible that AZD6140 may affect adenosine metabolism. The observed pauses did not lead to study-drug discontinuation and were not associated with clinical symptoms such as dizziness or syncope.

In the same study, plasma concentrations of inflammation markers were also studied. At discharge and at the 4 weeks time point, myeloperoxidase and sCD40L levels showed little change, whereas other inflammation markers such as high sensitive C-reactive protein and interleukin-6 were decreased to a similar extent in all treatment groups.[29] In a substudy of 45 patients who were not taking any clopidogrel prior to enrolment, AZD6140 treatment (90, 180, or 270 mg) was associated with more rapid, superior, and consistent ex vivo inhibition of ADP-induced platelet aggregation than a 300 mg loading dose of clopidogrel.[30] In another subgroup of 44 patients previously treated with clopidogrel, adding clopidogrel 75 mg had no additional platelet-inhibitory effect (Figure 10.6), while AZD6140

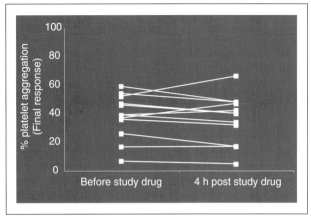

Figure 10.6
Inhibitory effect of clopidogrel 75 mg on the response to ADP-induced platelet aggregation in patients with non-ST-elevation acute coronary syndrome pretreated with clopidogrel 75 mg daily.

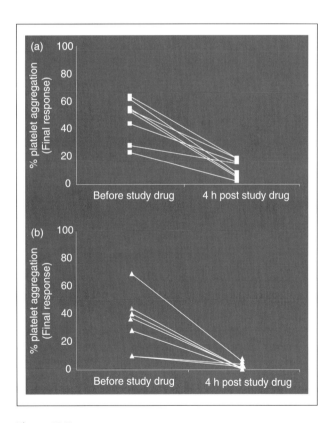

Figure 10.7
(a) Inhibitory effect of AZD6140, 90 mg on the response to ADP-induced platelet aggregation in patients with non-ST-elevation acute coronary syndrome (NSTE ACS) pretreated with clopidogrel 75 mg daily. (b) Inhibitory effect of AZD6140 180mg on the response to ADP-induced platelet aggregation in patient with NSTE ACS pretreated with clopidogrel 75 mg daily.

at 90 or 180 mg exhibited a rapid additional suppression of platelet reactivity (Figure 10.7).[30]

In conclusion, AZD6140 is a more potent and consistent inhibitor of ADP-induced platelet aggregation than clopidogrel. Since these effects are reversible, with rapid onset and offset effects, AZD6140 shows promise in the treatment of a wide variety of patients with vascular disease. Its clinical efficacy and potential adverse events are being studied in the large-scale PLATO (study of PLATelet inhibition and patients Outcomes) trial. In this study, treatment with AZD6140 will be compared with clopidogrel in 18 000 NSTE or ST-elevation ACS patients in a multinational trial.

References

1. Hechler B, Cattaneo M, Gachet C. The platelet P2 receptors in platelet function. Semin Thromb Hemost 2005; 31: 150–61.

2. Gachet C. Regulation of platelet functions by P2 receptors. Annu Rev Pharmacol Toxicol 2006; 46: 277–300.

3. Gachet C, Hechler B. The platelet P2 receptor in thrombosis. Semin Thromb Hemost 2005; 31: 162–7.

4. Storey RF, Judge HM, Wilcox RG, Heptinstall S. Inhibition of ADP-induced P-selectin expression and platelet-leucocyte conjugate formation by clopidogrel and the P2Y12 receptor antagonist AR-C69931MX but not aspirin. Thromb Haemost 2002; 88: 488–94.

5. Kunapuli SP, Dorsam RT, Kim S, Quinton TM. Platelet purinergic receptors. Curr Opin Pharmacol 2003; 3: 175–80.

6. Leon C, Ravanat C, Freund M et al. Differential involvement of the P2Y1 and P2Y12 receptors in platelet procoagulant activity. Arterioscler Thromb Vasc Biol 2003; 23: 1941–7.

7. Leon C, Alex M, Klocke A et al. Platelet ADP receptors contribute to the initiation of intravascular coagulation. Blood 2004; 103: 594–600.

8. Yusuf S, Zhao F, Mehta SR et al. Clopidogrel in Unstable angina to prevent Recurrent Events trial Investigators. Effects of clopidogrel in addition to aspirin in patients with acute coronary syndromes without ST-segment elevation. N Engl J Med 2001; 345: 494–502.

9. Steinhubl SR, Berger PB, Mann JT 3rd et al. CREDO investigators. Clopidogrel for the Reduction of Events During Observation. Early and sustained dual oral antiplatelet therapy following percutaneous coronary intervention: a randomized controlled trial. JAMA 2002; 288: 2411–20.

10. Mehta SR, Yusuf Peters RJ et al. Clopidogrel in Unstable angina to prevent Recurrent Events trial (CURE) Investigators. Effects of pre-treatment with cloidogrel and aspirin followed by long-term therapy in patients undergoing percutaneous coronary intervention: the PCI-CURE study. Lancet 2001; 358: 527–33.

11. Bertrand ME, Rupprecht HJ, Urban P, Gershlick AH. CLASSICS Investigators. Double-blind study of the safety of clopidogrel with and without a loading dose in combination with aspirin compared with ticlopidine in combination with aspirin after coronary stenting: the CLopidogrel Aspirin Stent International Cooperative Study (CLASSICS). Circulation 2000; 102: 624–9.

12. Cattaneo M. Aspirin and clopidogrel. Efficacy, safety and the issue of drug resistance. Arterioscler Thromb Vasc Biol 2004; 24: 1980–7.

13. Nguyen TA, Diodati JG, Pharand C. Resistance to clopidogrel: a review of the evidence. J Am Coll Cardiol 2005; 45: 1157–64.

14. O'Donoghue M, Wiviott SD. Clopidogrel response variability and future therapies: Clopidogrel: Does one size fit all? Circulation 2006; 114: e600–6.

15. Gurbel PA, Bliden KP, Hiatt BL, O'Connor CM. Clopidogrel for coronary stenting. Response variability, drug resistance, and the effect of pre-treatment platelet reactivity. Circulation 2003; 107: 2908–13.

16. Gurbel PA, Bliden KP, Hayes KM et al. The relation of dosing clopidogrel on responsiveness and the incidence of high post-treatment platelet aggregation in patients undergoing coronary stenting. J Am Coll Cardiol 2005; 45: 1392–6.

17. Barragan P, Bouvier JL, Roquebert PO et al. Resistance to thienopyridines: clinical detection of coronary stent thromboss by monitoring of vasodilator-stimulated phosphoprotein phosphorylation. Catheter Cardiovasc Interv 2003; 59: 295–302.

18. Matetzky S, Shenkman B, Guetta V et al. Clopidogrel resistance is associated with increased risk of recurrent atherothrombotic events in patients with acute myocardial infarction. Circulation 2004; 109: 3171–5.

19. Gurbel PA, Blinden K, Samara W et al. Clopidogrel effect on platelet reactivity in patients with stent thrombosis. J Am Coll Cardiol 2005; 46: 1827–32.

20. Jernberg T, Payne CD, Winters KJ et al. Prasugrel achieves greater inhibition of platelet aggregation and a lower rate of non-responders compared with clopidogrel in aspirin-treated patients with stable coronary artery disease. Eur Heart J 2006; 27: 1166–73.

21. Van Giezen JJJ, Humphries RG. Preclinical and clinical studies with selective reversible direct P2Y12 antagonists. Semin Thromb Hemost 2005; 31: 195–204.

22. Storey RF, Wilcox RG, Heptinstall S. Comparison of the pharmacodynamic effects of the platelet ADP receptor antagonists clopidogrel and the AR-C69931MX in patients with ischaemic heart disease. Platelets 2002; 13: 407–13.

23. Beham M, Fox S, Sanderson H et al. Efect of clopidogrel on procoagulant activity in acute coronary syndromes: evidence for incomplete P2Y12 receptor blockade. Circulation 2002; 106: II149–50.

24. GreenBaum AB, Grines CL, Bittl JA et al. Initial experience with an intravenous P2Y12 platelet receptor antagonist in patients undergoing percutaneous coronary interventon: esults from a 2-part, phase II, multicenter, randomized, placebo- and active-controlled trial. Am Heart J 2006; 151: e1–10.

25. Peters GR, Robbie G. Single dose pharmacokinetics and pharmcodynamics of AZD6140. Haematologica 2004; 89(Suppl 7): 14–15.

26. Peters GR, Butler KA, Winter HR, Mitchell PD. Multiple-dose pharmacokinetics (PK) and pharmacodynamics (PD) of the oral reversible, orally active ADP receptor antagonist AZD6140. P4556. Presented at World Congress of Cardiology, Barcelona 2006.

27. Husted S, Emanuelsson H, Heptinstall S et al. Pharmacodynamics, pharmacokinetics, and safety of the oral reversible P2Y12 antagonist AZD6140 with aspirin in patients with atherosclerosis: a double-blind comparison to clopidogrel with aspirin. Eur Heart J 2006; 27: 1038–47.

28. Cannon CP, Husted S, Harrington RA et al. Safety, tolerability, and initial efficacy of AZD6140, the first oral adenosine diphospate receptor antagonist, compared with clopidogrel in patients with non-ST segment elevation acute coronary syndrome. Primary results of the DISPERSE-2 trial. J Am Coll Cardiol 2007; 50: 1844–51.

29. Husted S, Storey RF, Harrington RA et al. The effects of AZD6140, the first oral reversible ADP receptor antagonist, compared with clopidogrel on biochemical markers in patients with acute coronary syndromes (ACS). J Am Coll Cardiol 2006; 47: 200A.

30. Storey RF, Husted S, Harrington RA et al. Inhibition of platelet aggregation by AZD6140, a reversible oral P2Y12 receptor antagonist, compared with clopidogrel in patients with acute coronary syndromes. J Am Coll Cardiol 2007; 50: 1852–6.

11

Emerging oral antiplatelet receptor inhibitors

Lori-Ann Linkins, John W Eikelboom, and Alexander G Turpie

Introduction

Aspirin remains the cornerstone of antiplatelet therapy for the prevention and treatment of coronary, cerebral, and peripheral artery disease.[1] It has several attractive properties that have contributed to its success, including (i) once-daily oral administration, (ii) the ability to permanently inactivate a platelet protein (cyclooxygenase-1) that cannot be resynthesized during the life of the platelet, (iii) lack of requirement for laboratory monitoring or dose-titration, and (iv) the ability to exert its effect through a moiety with a short half-life, which limits extra-platelet effects.[2] Despite its proven efficacy, however, aspirin is a relatively weak antiplatelet drug, as shown by persistent platelet activation and aggregation in patients taking aspirin.[3] Some patients treated with aspirin also achieve less than expected inhibition of platelet function, a phenomenon that has been termed 'aspirin resistance'.[4] Aspirin resistance has been associated with an increased risk of atherothrombotic vascular events.[4]

Recognition of the central role of platelets in atherothrombotic vascular disease and the need for more effective inhibition of platelet function has led to the development of new antiplatelet agents. These agents exert their antithrombotic effect by targeting a platelet receptor or a platelet enzyme or both. The focus of this chapter will be on oral antiplatelet agents that are in active development for prevention and treatment of coronary artery disease and that target platelet receptors.

As described in more detail in Chapter 2, platelet receptors play an important role in platelet adhesion, activation, and aggregation. By interfering with these functions, more recently developed platelet receptor antagonists have the potential to prevent acute thrombosis and to halt the progression of atherosclerosis. To date, antagonists for four main classes of platelet receptors have undergone clinical testing for prevention and treatment of coronary artery disease: $P2Y_{12}$, thromboxane/prostaglandin H_2, glycoprotein IIb/IIIa and PAR-1 (Figure 11.1). The properties of agents in advanced stages of development that target these receptors are summarized in Table 11.1.

$P2Y_{12}$ antagonists/ADP antagonists

Receptor

$P2Y_{12}$ receptors are G-protein-coupled receptors bound to the platelet surface.[5] Binding of adenosine diphosphate (ADP) released from platelet dense granules to $P2Y_{12}$ receptors reduces adenylate cyclase activity and eventually leads to activation of glycoprotein (GP) IIb/IIIa. Inhibition of the $P2Y_{12}$ receptor inhibits ADP-induced platelet aggregation.[5]

Antagonists

Thienopyridines selectively inhibit ADP-induced platelet aggregation mediated by the $P2Y_{12}$ receptor. The first-generation thienopyridine ticlopidine (Roche Pharmaceuticals) and the second-generation thienopyridine clopidogrel (Bristol-Myers Squibb/Sanofi-Aventis) have been approved for treatment of coronary artery disease[6,7] and will not be discussed in detail in this chapter. Unlike ticlopidine, clopidogrel does not cause life-threatening neutropenia and it has a more rapid onset of action. However, clopidogrel still suffers from important limitations, including a delayed onset of action, high interpatient variability of platelet inhibition, and the potential for interaction with other drugs that are metabolized via the cytochrome P450 CYP3A4 pathway (e.g., lipophilic statins).[8] A third-generation thienopyridine, prasugrel, is currently under development.

Prasugrel

Like its predecessors, prasugrel (Eli Lilly) is a prodrug that requires hepatic metabolism by cytochrome P450 to generate an active metabolite.[9] R-138727, the active metabolite of prasugrel, competes with ADP to bind with the $P2Y_{12}$ receptor. Once bound, R-138727 induces formation of a disulfide bridge between its sulfhydryl moiety and cysteine residues of the receptor.[9] These alterations are irreversible and

Table 11.1	*Properties of emerging oral antiplatelet receptor antagonists*				
Antiplatelet agent	Target receptor	Administration	Prodrug?	Reversible?	Status
Prasugrel	P2Y$_{12}$	Once daily	Yes	No	Phase III
AZD-6140	P2Y$_{12}$	Twice daily	No	Yes, within 48 h of drug withdrawal	Phase III
S-18886	Thromboxane	Once daily	No	Yes, within 48 h of drug withdrawal	Phase III
SCH-530348	PAR-1	Once daily	No	Yes	Phase III
E-5555	PAR-1	Unclear	No	Unknown	Phase II

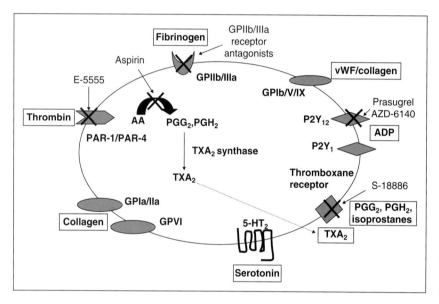

Figure 11.1
Emerging oral antiplatelet receptor inhibitors. Natural agonists for the receptors are in boxes. GP, glycoprotein; TXA$_2$, thromboxane A$_2$; PAR, protease-activated receptors; AA, arachidonic acid; PG, prostaglandin.

inactivate the receptor for the lifetime of the platelet. Prasugrel is given once daily, and although a loading dose is still required, it is more rapidly converted to its active metabolite than clopidogrel. Animal studies suggest that prasugrel achieves a greater degree of platelet inhibition and may therefore be more potent than clopidogrel.[10]

Prasugrel was evaluated in a phase II clinical trial (JUMBO-TIMI 26) of patients who underwent elective or urgent percutaneous coronary interventions (PCI).[11] In this trial, 904 patients were randomized to receive clopidogrel or one of three doses of prasugrel. The first dose of the antiplatelet agent was given either immediately before or after the procedure and continued for 30 days. The primary endpoint – clinically significant (TIMI (Thrombolysis in Myocardial Infarction) minor plus major) bleeding at 30 days (other than bleeding with coronary artery bypass grafting) – occurred in 1.7% of patients (11/650) who received prasugrel and 1.2% of patients (5/254) who received clopidogrel (hazard ratio (HR) 1.42; 95% confidence interval (CI) 0.40–5.08; $p = 0.59$). A non-significant trend toward increased bleeding with the highest dose of prasugrel was noted. The secondary endpoint – the combined rate of major adverse cardiac events (defined as death, target vessel revascularization or occlusion,

Myocardial infarction (MI), stroke, and recurrent ischemia at 30 days) – occurred in 7.2% of patients (47/650) who received prasugrel and 9.4% of patients (24/254) who received clopidogrel (HR 0.76; 95% CI 0.46–1.24, $p = 0.26$).

A phase III trial (TRITON-TIMI 38) comparing prasugrel to clopidogrel with respect to cardiovascular death, MI, or ischemic stroke in patients with acute coronary syndromes (ACS) who undergo PCI has recently been published.[12] The primary efficacy endpoint occurred in 12.1% of patients receiving clopidogrel and 9.9% of patients receiving prasugrel ($p < 0.001$). Major bleeding was observed in 2.4% of patients receiving prasugrel and in 1.8% of patients receiving clopidogrel ($p = 0.03$). (For further details see Chapter 9). Several phase II trials, including a study comparing the effect of prasugrel with clopidogrel on platelet activity in patients with ACS, approximately 1 week after the first dose of study drug, and a study comparing the effect of prasugrel with clopidogrel on platelet function and inflammation in patients undergoing elective PCI, are ongoing.[13]

AZD-6140

AZD-6140 (AstraZeneca), a cyclopentyltriazolopyrimidine, is the first oral reversible P2Y$_{12}$ antagonist.[14] This agent binds directly to the $P2Y_{12}$ receptor and does not require metabolic activation. AZD-6140 has one known active metabolite, which is found in about one-third the concentration of the parent compound and has approximately the same potency as the latter. AZD-6140 has a half-life of 12 hours and is administered twice daily. The antithrombotic effect of this agent is reversed 48 hours after drug withdrawal.

AZD-6140 was evaluated in a phase II clinical trial of patients with stable atherosclerosis (DISPERSE).[15] In this trial, 200 patients who had received daily aspirin for at least 2 weeks before randomization for evidence of coronary artery disease, peripheral vascular disease, or cerebrovascular disease were randomized to clopidogrel or one of four doses of AZD-6140 for 28 days. The trial showed that AZD-6140 at doses above 50 mg twice daily inhibited platelet aggregation as measured by optical aggregometry more effectively and with less variability than clopidogrel. In addition, the inhibition of platelet aggregation was more rapid than with clopidogrel. The incidence of bleeding events was higher in patients treated with the higher doses of AZD-6140, and one major bleed occurred in a patient who received the highest dose of this agent. Unexpectedly, there was a relatively high frequency of dose-dependent dyspnea and bradycardia noted in patients who received AZD-6140.

In DISPERSE-2,[16] another phase II clinical trial, 900 patients with non-ST elevation MI (NSTEMI) were randomized to AZD-6140 plus aspirin (at one of two doses of AZD-6140) or clopidogrel plus aspirin for 12 weeks (in addition, half of the patients who received AZD-6140 were randomized to receive a loading dose of this agent). Preliminary results presented at the American College of Cardiology in 2006 revealed that the primary endpoint – major plus minor bleeding at 4 weeks – occurred in 9.6% of patients given AZD-6140 90 mg twice daily, 7.7% of patients given AZD-6140 180 mg twice daily, and 8.0% of patients given clopidogrel.[16] The secondary endpoint – a composite of cardiovascular death, MI, and stroke – occurred in 4.8%, 3.0%, and 4.9% of patients, respectively. A trend toward reduction of MI in the AZD-6140 180 mg group was observed, but was not statistically significant. A phase III trial (PLATO) comparing AZD-6140 (180 mg initial dose followed by 90 mg maintenance dose) with clopidogrel in patients with non-ST elevation and ST-elevation ACS who are to undergo PCI was in the late stages of protocol development as of October 2006.

Thromboxane receptor (TP receptor) antagonists

Receptor

Thromboxane receptors (TP receptors) are G-protein-coupled receptors found on vascular smooth muscle cells and platelets.[17] When bound to an agonist, these receptors activate phospholipase C, resulting in mobilization of second-messenger molecules, including intracellular calcium, to induce platelet aggregation. One agonist of these receptors is thromboxane A_2 (TXA_2), a metabolite of arachidonic acid that is formed via the cyclooxygenase pathway within activated platelets. Binding of TXA_2 to platelet TP receptors causes platelet aggregation primarily by acting as an amplifying signal for other strong agonists, such as thrombin and ADP. TXA_2 also binds to TP receptors on vascular smooth muscle cell membranes, to cause vasoconstriction. Other agonists that are capable of binding to TP receptors include prostaglandin H_2 (PGH_2) and isoprostanes.

Antagonists

TP receptor antagonists were first evaluated for management of patients with atherothrombosis in the early 1990s (e.g. vapiprost and sulotroban), but they fell out of favor when phase II clinical trials failed to demonstrate a clear benefit of these agents over aspirin.[18,19] More recent observations about the potential advantages of selective TP receptor antagonists over aspirin, including (i) the ability to block all TP receptor agonists (not just TXA_2) and (ii) the induction of an antiplatelet effect without interfering with beneficial endothelial prostacyclin production, has renewed interest in development of this class of antiplatelet agents.[20]

S-18886

S-18886 (Servier), the active isomer of S-18204, is a specific TP receptor antagonist.[21] It is given once daily and its inhibition of platelet aggregation persists for up to 36 hours after an oral dose of 10–30 mg. Reversibility of inhibition of platelet aggregation is dose-dependent and occurs within 24–48 hours of drug withdrawal.

S-18886 has been evaluated in small phase II clinical trials in patients with coronary artery disease, and in patients with peripheral vascular disease.[22,23] These studies suggest that this agent induces flow-mediated vasodilation and improves endothelial function – a potentially beneficial effect for patients with cardiovascular disease that is outside of its effect on platelet aggregation. The safety profile of S-18886 has been reported as excellent, with no attributable adverse events in the small trials completed to date. Phase III trials of S18886 are awaited.

Combined thromboxane synthase inhibitor and TP receptor antagonists

Several agents that inhibit both the enzyme thromboxane synthase and TP receptors have been evaluated, but only a few are orally available and have undergone clinical testing in patients with coronary artery disease (as outlined below).

Picotamide, a derivative of methoxyisophthalic acid, was compared with aspirin in 101 patients taking low-intensity oral anticoagulation for acute MI.[24] The primary endpoint – the incidence of death, reinfarction, postinfarction angina, and heart failure at 6 months – occurred in 40% in the picotamide–anticoagulant group compared with 61% of the aspirin–anticoagulant group ($p < 0.05$). The cumulative incidence of major clinical events plus major hemorrhagic episodes was lower in the picotamide–anticoagulant group than the aspirin–anticoagulant group (28 and 48, respectively; $p < 0.001$). This agent has also been evaluated in patients with peripheral arterial disease (with or without diabetes), carotid atherosclerosis, and severe congestive heart failure. Although picotamide is commercially available in a few European countries, due to limited data on efficacy and safety it is not currently recommended for management of atherosclerotic cardiovascular disease in expert guidelines.[2]

Ramatroban (BAY u3405) has been evaluated in patients with severe limb arteriopathy,[25] and in canine and porcine models of coronary artery disease, but there are no published trials using this agent for treatment of patients with coronary artery disease to date. The primary focus of development of this drug appears to be treatment of allergic rhinitis.

Glycoprotein IIb/IIIa (GPIIb/IIIa) antagonists

Receptor

The GPIIb/IIIa receptor, the most abundant receptor on the platelet surface, is a member of the integrin receptor family.[26] These receptors are in an inactive conformation until the platelet to which they are bound is activated. When platelets are activated, a calcium-dependent conformational change occurs in GPIIb/IIIa receptors that allows them to bind to fibrinogen with high affinity. Fibrinogen bound to GPIIb/IIIa receptors is able to crosslink nearby platelets, resulting in platelet aggregation. Activation of GPIIb/IIIa receptors is the final common pathway mediating platelet aggregation, regardless of the agonist.

Antagonists

Several oral GPIIb/IIIa antagonists have been developed in the hope of extending the benefit seen with intravenous GPIIb/IIIa antagonists to the long-term management of patients with acute coronary syndromes. Unfortunately, large-scale clinical trials with these agents (xemilofiban, orbofiban, sibrafiban, lotrafiban, and roxifiban) failed to show that they are more effective than aspirin.[27] Two meta-analyses of these trials have reported a lack of benefit with

respect to the composite endpoint of death, recurrent MI, or other recurrent ischemic events.[28,29] In addition, the mortality rate was 30–35% higher in patients who received oral GPIIb/IIIa antagonists. It has been proposed that these agents paradoxically activate platelets, resulting in a prothrombotic state that increases the risk of thrombotic events and mortality. In vitro studies have suggested that binding of a GPIIb/IIIa antagonist to a receptor followed by dissociation of the antagonist from the receptor leaves the receptor open for binding to fibrinogen. Regardless of the mechanism, development of oral GPIIb/IIIa antagonists for long-term management of coronary artery disease has been abandoned. There was a suggestion that Virtual Drug Development was considering evaluating their oral GPIIb/IIIa antagonist xemilofiban for short-term treatment post-PCI, but no further information on development of this agent is available.

Protease-activated receptor (PAR) antagonists

Receptor

Protease-activated receptors (PARs) are expressed on endothelial cells, smooth muscle cells, and platelets.[30] PAR-1 and PAR-4 act as thrombin receptors on platelets. PAR-1, a high-affinity receptor, is cleaved by thrombin (even if the latter is present only in subnanomolar concentrations). Once cleaved, PAR-1 rapidly transmits a signal to the internally located G-proteins that results in platelet shape change, release of platelet dense granules, and activation of the GPIIb/IIIa fibrinogen receptor. PAR-1-dependent formation of platelet–platelet aggregates is transient unless strengthened by additional inputs from the P2Y$_{12}$ receptor or the PAR-4 receptor. PAR-4 is a low-affinity receptor for thrombin. Like PAR-1, it is cleaved by thrombin and signals through G proteins, but the signal travels significantly slower than with activation of PAR-1. Unlike PAR-1, PAR-4 does not require input from other platelet receptors to form stable platelet–platelet aggregates.

Antagonists

SCH-530348

SCH-530348 (Schering-Plough) blocks the platelet PAR-1 receptor to which thrombin binds (Figure 1), thus inhibiting thrombin-induced activation and aggregation of platelets. Since a PAR-1 receptor antagonist does not inhibit the ability of thrombin to catalyze the production of fibrin, agents in this class may have a lower rate of hemorrhagic side-effects than conventional anticoagulants. Clinical studies to date have shown no increase in bleeding time or prolongation in coagulation times (activated partial thromboplastin time or prothrombin time) with SCH-530348, indicative of a selective antiplatelet effect with this agent.

A pharmacokinetic study in healthy individuals indicated that single-dose oral SCH-530348 was well tolerated and caused a significant dose-related inhibition of thrombin receptor–activating peptide-induced platelet aggregation, with maximum effects (> 90% inhibition) achieved as early as 1 hour after administration.[32] SCH-530348 was rapidly absorbed and slowly eliminated (terminal half-life > 72 hours). In the phase II TRA–PCI trial, 1031 patients scheduled for angiography and possible elective stenting were randomized equally to receive one of three oral loading doses of SCH-530348 (10, 20, or 40 mg) or a placebo.[33] The patients who subsequently underwent PCI (n = 573) or CABG (n = 382) were randomized to receive one of three oral daily maintenance doses of SCH-530348 (0.5, 1.0, or 2.5 mg) if they received an SCH-530348 loading dose, or standard care if they received a placebo loading dose. The total duration of treatment was 60 days, and patients were followed for an additional 60 days after treatment. All patients also received aspirin, clopidogrel, and antitcoagulant therapy. No increase in major and minor bleeding was observed when SCH-530348 was added to standard dual antiplatelet therapy (including aspirin and clopidogrel) among patients undergoing PCI (primary endpoint). Although this study was not powered to establish efficacy, it showed a non-statistically significant 46% reduction in cardiovascular events at the highest SCH-530348 dose tested compared with standard antiplatelet therapy. The phase III clinical development program will include two large clinical trials (TRACER and TRA 2P) to evaluate the risk reduction provided by SCH-530348 plus standard antiplatelet therapy compared with placebo plus standard antiplatelet therapy. The trials will be conducted in approximately 30 countries at more than 800 sites for each trial. The phase TRACER trial will be a multinational, randomized, double-blind, placebo-controlled study in approximately 10,000 patients with NSTE-ACS. The TRA 2P–TIMI 50 trial will be a multinational, randomized, double-blind, placebo-controlled study in approximately 19,500 patients with prior MI or stroke, or who have existing peripheral arterial disease.

E-5555

E-5555 (Eisai) is an oral PAR-1 antagonist that has been shown to inhibit platelet aggregation and vascular smooth muscle proliferation in preclinical trials. A phase II clinical trial designed to evaluate the safety and tolerability of E-5555 in patients with coronary artery disease is expected to begin recruitment shortly.[31] SCH-205831, an orally active PAR-1 antagonist based on the natural product himbacine, is also reported to be in the early stages of clinical development.

Other platelet receptor antagonists

Other platelet receptors have the potential to serve as targets for parenteral and oral antiplatelet agents.[34] However, little or no clinical data on development of these antagonists for treatment of cardiovascular disease is available in the public domain.

P2Y$_1$

This is a G-protein-coupled platelet receptor that is activated by ADP. Activation of this receptor initiates platelet aggregation and ADP-induced platelet shape change. In contrast to the previously described ADP receptor P2Y$_{12}$, P2Y$_1$ receptors are ubiquitously expressed. The limited distribution of the P2Y$_{12}$ receptor makes it a better target for antiplatelet agents; however, selective parenteral P2Y$_1$ antagonists (e.g., MRS2500) have been shown to inhibit platelets in knockout mice and experimental thrombosis models.[34] Interestingly, early observations suggest that P2Y$_1$ antagonists may prolong bleeding time less than P2Y$_{12}$ antagonists. Whether this difference translates into a lower risk of bleeding while retaining antithrombotic efficacy remains to be seen.

GPIb

This is a platelet adhesion receptor.[35] Under high-shear conditions, binding of von Willebrand factor (vWF) to GPIb triggers platelet adhesion. Snake venom proteins that bind to GPIb and interfere with its ability to bind to vWF have been shown to have antithrombotic potential in animal studies (e.g., agkistin and crotalin). Recombinant vWF fragments that compete with native vWF to bind to GPIb (e.g., RG12986) may also have potential as antithrombotic agents.

5-HT$_2$

These are G-protein-coupled receptors found in the central nervous system, on smooth vascular muscle, and on platelets.[36] Serotonin (5-hydroxytryptamine, 5-HT), synthesized in neuronal cells in the brain and enterochromaffin cells in the gastrointestinal tract, is taken up by platelet transporters and stored in dense granules. Serotonin is released from activated platelets and binds to 5-HT$_{2A}$ receptors on platelets and vascular smooth muscle, resulting in amplification of platelet activation and vasoconstriction. The primary focus of development of selective 5-HT$_{2A}$ receptor antagonists to date has been treatment of peripheral vascular disease (e.g., R-102444, naftidrofuryl, sarpogrelate, and AT-1015).[36]

GPIa/IIa and GPVI

These serve as the main collagen receptors on platelets. Examples of antagonists for these receptors include EMS16, a protein isolated from snake venom (a GPIa/IIa antagonist), and monoclonal antibodies against GPVI receptors.[36]

Conclusions

The crucial role played by membrane-bound receptors in platelet adhesion, activation and aggregation make platelet receptors attractive targets for new oral antiplatelet agents. Two of these new agents, prasugrel and AZD-6140 (P2Y$_{12}$ antagonists), aspire to replace clopidogrel in the prevention and treatment of ACS, and are in the more advanced stages of clinical testing. Both agents appear to exhibit a more rapid onset of action, less inter-patient variability, and a higher level of inhibition of platelet aggregation than clopidogrel. Another new antiplatelet agent under development, S-18886 (thromboxane receptor/prostaglandin H$_2$ receptor antagonist), has been shown not only to inhibit platelet aggregation, but also induce flow-mediated vasodilation and improve endothelial function in early clinical trials. These properties suggest this agent may have benefits for patients with coronary artery disease in addition to its effect on platelets. Although the benefits of parenteral GPIIb/IIIa receptor antagonists are clear, further development of oral agents in this class has largely been abandoned due to the failure of clinical trials to show benefit over aspirin with respect to efficacy and safety. Irrespective of the receptor targeted, emerging oral platelet receptor antagonists will need to be shown to be superior to aspirin (or synergistic with aspirin) with respect to efficacy and risk of bleeding before they will gain widespread acceptance for prevention and treatment of coronary artery disease.

References

1. Antithrombotic Trialists' Collaboration. Collaborative meta-analysis of randomised trials of antiplatelet therapy for prevention of death, myocardial infarction, and stroke in high risk patients. BMJ 2002;324:71–86.
2. Patrono C, Bachman F, Baigent C et al. Expert consensus document on the use of antiplatelet agents. The task force on the use of antiplatelet agents in patients with atherosclerotic cardiovascular disease of the European Society of Cardiology. Eur Heart J 2004;25:166–81.
3. Pulcinelli FM, Riondino S, Celestini A et al. Persistent production of platelet thromboxane A2 in patients chronically treated with aspirin. J Thromb Haemost 2005;3:2784–9.
4. Hankey GJ, Eikelboom JW. Aspirin resistance. Lancet 2006;367:606–17.
5. Cattaneo M. P2Y12 receptor antagonists: a rapidly expanding group of antiplatelet agents. Eur Heart J 2006;27:1010–12.
6. Janzon L. The STIMS trial: the ticlopidine experience and its clinical applications. Swedish Ticlopidine Multicenter Study. Vasc Med 1996;1:141–3.
7. Yusuf S, Zhao F, Mehta SR et al. Effects of clopidogrel in addition to aspirin in patients with acute coronary syndromes without ST-segment elevation. N Engl J Med 2001;345:494–502.
8. Steinhubl SR, Akers WS. Clopidogrel–statin interaction: a mountain or a mole hill? Am Heart J 2006;152:200–3.
9. Niitsu Y, Jakubowski JA, Sugidachi A et al. Pharmacology of CS-747 (prasugrel, LY640315), a novel, potent antiplatelet agent with in vivo P2Y12 receptor antagonist activity. Semin Thromb Hemost 2005;31:184–94.
10. Sugidachi A, Asai F, Ogawa T et al. The in vivo pharmacological profile of CS-747, a novel antiplatelet agent with platelet ADP receptor antagonist properties. Br J Pharmacol 2000;129:1439–46.
11. Wiviott SD, Antman EM, Winters KJ et al. Randomized comparison of prasugrel (CS-747, LY640315), a novel thienopyridine P2Y12 antagonist, with clopidogrel in percutaneous coronary intervention: results of the Joint Utilization of Medications to Block Platelets Optimally (JUMBO)-TIMI 26 trial. Circulation 2005;111:3366–73.
12. Wiviott SD, Braunwald E, McCabe CH et al. TRITON-TIMI 38 Investigators. Prasugrel versus clopidogrel in patients with acute coronary syndromes. NEJM 2007;357:2001–15.
13. ClinicalTrials.gov. Available at http://www.clinicaltrials.gov/ct/search?term=prasugrel (Accessed October 14, 2006).
14. van Giezen JJ, Humphries RG. Preclinical and clinical studies with selective reversible direct P2Y12 antagonists. Semin Thromb Hemost 2005;31:195–204.
15. Husted S, Emanuelsson H, Heptinstall S et al. Pharmacodynamics, pharmacokinetics, and safety of the oral reversible P2Y12 antagonist AZD6140 with aspirin in patients with atherosclerosis: a double-blind comparison to clopidogrel with aspirin. Eur Heart J 2006;27:1038–47.
16. Cannon CP, Husted S, Storey RF et al. Safety, tolerability and preliminary efficacy of AZD6140, the first oral reversible ADP receptor antagonist compared with clopidogrel in patients with non-ST segment acute coronary syndrome. J Am Coll Cardiol 2006;47 (Suppl A):Abst 2906.
17. FitzGerald GA. Mechanisms of platelet activation: TXA$_2$ as an amplifying signal for other agonists. Am J Cardiol 1991;68:B11–15.
18. Serruys PW, Rutsch W, Heyndrickx GR et al. Prevention of restenosis after percutaneous transluminal coronary angioplasty with thromboxane A2-receptor blockade. A randomized, double-blind, placebo-controlled trial. Coronary Artery Restenosis Prevention on Repeated Thromboxane-Antagonism Study (CARPORT). Circulation 1991;84:1568–80.
19. Savage MP, Goldberg S, Bove AA et al. Effect of thromboxane A2 blockade on clinical outcome and restenosis after successful coronary angioplasty. Multi-Hospital Eastern Atlantic Restenosis Trial (M-HEART II). Circulation 1995;92:3194–200.
20. Pratico D, Cheng Y, FitzGerald GA. TP or not TP: primary mediators in a close runoff? Arterioscler Thromb Vasc Biol 2000;20:1695–8.
21. Cayatte AJ, Du Y, Oliver-Krasinki J et al. The thromboxane receptor antagonist S18886 but not aspirin inhibits atherogenesis in apo E-deficient mice: evidence that eicosanoids other than thromboxane contribute to atherosclerosis. Arterioscler Thromb Vasc Biol 2000;20:1724–8.
22. Belhassen L, Pelle G, Dubois-Rande JL et al. Improved endothelial function by the thromboxane A2 receptor antagonist S 18886 in patients with coronary artery disease treated with aspirin. J Am Coll Cardiol 2003;41:1198–204.
23. Gaussem P, Reny JL, Thalamas C et al. The specific thromboxane receptor antagonist S18886: pharmacokinetic and pharmacodynamic studies. J Thromb Haemost 2005;3:1437–45.
24. Vetrano A, Milani M, Corsini G. Effects of aspirin or picotamide, an antithromboxane agent, in combination with low-intensity oral anticoagulation in patients with acute myocardial infarction: a controlled randomized pilot trial. G Ital Cardiol 1999;29:524–8.

25. Bellucci S, Kedra W, Groussin H et al. Ex vivo inhibition of platelet aggregation in patients with severe limb arteriopathy treated with BAY U3405, a specific TX A2 receptor antagonist. Thromb Haemost 1994;72:659–62.

26. Cannon CP. Oral platelet glycoprotein IIb/IIIa receptor inhibitors – Part I. Clin Cardiol 2003;26:358–64.

27. Cannon CP. Oral platelet glycoprotein IIb/IIIa receptor inhibitors – Part II. Clin Cardiol 2003;26:401–6.

28. Chew DP, Bhatt DL, Sapp S et al. Increased mortality with oral platelet glycoprotein IIb/IIIa antagonists: a meta-analysis of phase III multicenter randomized trials. Circulation 2001;103:201–6.

29. Newby LK, Califf RM, White HD et al. The failure of orally administered glycoprotein IIb/IIIa inhibitors to prevent recurrent cardiac events. Am J Med 2002;112:647–58.

30. Leger AJ, Covic L, Kuliopulos A. Protease-activated receptors in cardiovascular diseases. Circulation 2006;114:1070–7.

31. ClinicalTrials.gov. Study of E5555 and its effects on markers of intravascular inflammation in subjects with coronary artery disease. Available from http://www.clinicaltrials.gov/ct/show/NCT00312052 (Accessed October 14, 2006).

32. Kosoglou T, Reyderman L. Pharmacodynamics and pharmacokinetics of a novel protease-activated receptor (PAR-1) antagonist SCH-530348. Circulation 2005; 112(suppl):II-32.

33. Moliterno DJ, Becker RC, Jennings LK et al. Results of a multinational randomized double-blind, placebo-controlled study of a novel thrombin receptor antagonist in percutaneous coronary intervention. Presented at the Late Breaking Clinical Trials at the American College of Cardiology Scientific Sessions, New Orleans, Louisiana, 2007.

34. Messmore HL, Jeske W, Wehrmacher W et al. Antiplatelet agents: current drugs and future trends. Hematol Oncol Clin North Am 2005;19:87–117.

35. Phillips DR, Conley PB, Sinha U et al. Therapeutic approaches in arterial thrombosis. J Thromb Haemost 2005;3:1577–89.

36. Horiuchi H. Recent advance in antiplatelet therapy: the mechanisms, evidence and approach to the problems. Ann Med 2006;38:162–72.

Section II.B

Antithrombotic drugs: intravenous antiplatelet drugs

12

Platelet glycoprotein IIb/IIIa receptor antagonists: fundamental and pharmacological aspects

Joseph Jozic and David J Moliterno

Biology of platelet function

In the setting of plaque rupture, an early step in platelet activation is adhesion of the platelet to the subendothelial matrix. Intimal injury during an acute coronary syndrome or angioplasty disrupts the endothelium and leads to exposure of collagen and other subendothelial molecules. Initial contact of the platelet and the exposed endothelium is via von Willebrand factor (vWF) and the platelet surface molecule glycoprotein (GP) Ib, which helps initiate the intracellular messengers of platelet activation.[1]

The main adhesion mechanism binding the platelet to the subendothelial matrix is via collagen. There are two main collagen receptors on the platelet membrane, GPIa/IIa and GPVI. GPIa/IIa serves as an anchor for platelets to connect to exposed collagen,[2] while GPVI activates adhesive receptors, including GPIa/IIa, which strengthen collagen–platelet adherence.[3] Collagen, while serving as the scaffolding for platelet adherence, also activates platelets by intracellular second messengers.[4] Other molecules that activate platelets include epinephrine (adrenaline), serotonin, and adenosine diphosphate (ADP), as well as vWF.[5]

One of the most potent activators of the platelet is thrombin. The primary thrombin receptor on the platelet is protease-activated receptor 1 (PAR-1). Thrombin, thromboxane A_2 (TXA_2), and ADP directly activate the platelet through G-protein-coupled receptors, leading to platelet aggregation and granule release.[6] The ADP receptors on the platelet are $P2Y_1$ and $P2Y_{12}$.[7]

The final step of activation is platelet aggregation to form a platelet plug. In their resting state, platelets are freely circulating, but activated platelets bound to extracellular matrix proteins and soluble factors initiate an inside-to-outside signal. This signal causes a conformational change in the GPIIb/IIIa receptor, allowing it to bind with specific ligands.[8] The main ligand that binds to GPIIb/IIIa is fibrinogen, but fibronectin, vWF, and vitronectin are also able to bind to the receptor.[9] The binding of the GPIIb/IIIa receptor initiates an outside-to-inside signal that causes platelets to secrete the contents of their cytoplasmic granules – which include adhesive molecules, growth factors, and procoagulants[10] – as well as to synthesize and release TXA_2.[5] This leads to further recruitment and activation of adjacent platelets. Platelet-activated second-messenger signals also cause a structural change in the platelet, transforming it from a discoid shape to an irregular form with multiple projections.[11] As platelets continue to aggregate, further changes to the cytoskeleton occur.[12] These changes in the platelet cytoskeleton are involved in reinforcement and contraction of the clot.

Figure 12.1 is a schematic summary of the mechanisms activating the platelet GPIIb/IIIa receptor.

GPIIb/IIIa receptor

The GPIIb/IIIa receptor is a member of the integrin family of cell surface adhesion receptors. Integrins are heterodimers consisting of non-covalently associated α and β subunits.[13] There are at least six different β subunits and various α subunits. Combinations of these subunits form receptors with specificities for individual ligands.[14] The GPIIb/IIIa receptor consists of the α_{IIb} and β_3 subunits (Figure 12.2). The α subunit is a 136 kDa molecule with a light and a heavy chain. The light chain contains a short cytoplasmic tail, a transmembrane region, and a short extracellular domain. The heavy chain is entirely extracellular.[15] The β subunit is a 84.5 kDa molecule with a short intracellular tail, a transmembrane region, and a large extracellular domain.[16] There are approximately 80 000 receptors on the platelet surface.[17] Platelet activation leads to a conformational change in the GPIIb/IIIa receptor, markedly increasing its affinity for its major ligand, fibrinogen.[18]

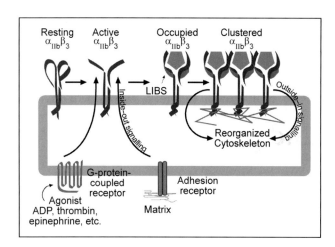

Figure 12.1
Platelet GPIIb/IIIa receptor activation. LIBS, ligant-induced binding site. With permission from Topol et al.[41]

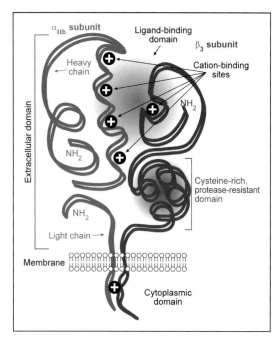

Figure 12.2
Structure of the GPIIb/IIIa receptor. With permission from Topol et al.[41]

There are two main binding sites on the GPIIb/IIIa receptor. One recognizes the amino acid sequence Arg-Gly-Asp (RGD). This sequence is found on multiple ligands (fibronectin, vWF, and vitronectin) but most notably on fibrinogen, in which it occurs twice.[19] The other peptide sequence is Lys-Gln-Ala-Gly-Asp-Val (KQAGDV), is only located at the C-terminus of the γ chain of fibrinogen.[20] The relationship between these two sites is not fully understood. One theory is that ligands containing either one of these sequences have shared contact sites on the GPIIb/IIIa receptor. This would help explain the high affinity of fibrinogen to the receptor.[21]

GPIIb/IIIa antagonists

Irrespective of the initiating agonist, the final common step for platelet aggregation is fibrinogen binding. This makes GPIIb/IIIa inhibitors many times more effective in inhibiting platelets than other agents (i.e., aspirin, clopidogrel, and ticlopidine). Parenteral GPIIb/IIIa inhibitors inhibit ADP-induced platelet aggregation in vitro by approximately 80–90%. This is in contrast to 10% for aspirin and 30–40% for the thienopyridines.[22]

The three GPIIb/IIIa inhibitors in clinical use are the chimeric antibody abciximab, the peptide-based antagonist eptifibatide, and the non-peptide-based molecule tirofiban (Table 12.1). At therapeutic doses, these GPIIb/IIIa antagonists achieve ≥80% inhibition of available platelet-bound receptors, which appears to be necessary for inhibition of platelet-dependant thrombus formation.[23]

Abciximab

Abciximab (Reopro, Centocor BV/Eli Lilly and Co.) was the first GPIIb/IIIa antagonist to the approved for clinical use. Coller et al[24] first described a mouse monoclonal antibody against GPIIb/IIIa inhibiting fibrinogen binding to platelets. The Fc portion of the antibody was removed to decrease immunogenicity and the Fab portion was attached to the constant regions of a human immunoglobulin.[9] Abciximab has a high affinity for its receptor, with a dissociation constant (K_D) of 5nmol/l.[25] Abciximab binding is specific for the β_3 subunit. This explains its ability to bind other β_3 receptors as well. It has an almost equal potency for inhibition of the vitronectin ($\alpha_V\beta_3$) receptor[26] and a lower affinity for the MAC-1 receptor found on leukocytes. The mechanism of action is the large antibody fragment, which causes a steric hindrance of access of ligands to their binding sites. After bolus infusion, 50% of the compound is bound to platelets in the first 10 minutes. Abciximab has a short plasma half-life secondary to proteolysis of the unbound antibody. However, it has a very long half-life of dissociation from the platelet GPIIb/IIIa receptor, which can be up to 4 hours.[23] Abciximab also redistributes from platelet to platelet, as well as from platelet to vascular cells bearing the β_3 chain.[26] This slow rate of dissociation and receptor redistribution allows platelet-inhibiting effects to be measured days after drug administration.[25] In fact, an estimated 29% of GPIIb/IIIa receptors are still occupied by abciximab 8 days after completion of infusion.[23]

Given that abciximab is a chimeric antibody possessing a human and a mouse portion, there is potential for induction of human anti-chimeric antibody formation. Despite this, no anaphylactic events have been reported. Bleeding is noted to be higher with abciximab infusion than with placebo infusion, with a major bleeding event rate modestly higher in the abciximab-treated groups versus

Table 12.1 *List of FDA-approved indications and dosing of glycoprotein IIb/IIIa inhibitors*

Agent	FDA-approved Indications	Dose	Trials
Abciximab	• PCI	• PCI: Bolus 0.25 mg/kg 10–60 min prior to PCI Infusion 0.125 μg/kg/min (maximum of 10 μg/min) × 12 h	EPIC[27] EPISTENT[39]
	• UA not responding to conventional medical therapy when PCI is planned within 24 h hours	• UA: Bolus 0.25 mg/kg Infusion 10 μg/min × 18–24 h concluding 1h after PCI	CAPTURE[28]
Eptifibatide	• ACS (UA/NSTEMI), including patients managed medically and those undergoing PCI	• ACS: Bolus 180 μg/kg Infusion 2.0 μg/kg/min up to 72 h *Renal dysfunction:[a]* Bolus 180 μg/kg Infusion 1.0 μg/kg/min	PURSUIT[40]
	• PCI, including intracoronary stenting	• PCI: Bolus double bolus 180 μg/kg 10 min apart Infusion 2.0 μg/kg/min × 18–24h *Renal dysfunction:[a]* Bolus double bolus 180 μg/kg 10 min apart Infusion 1.0 μg/kg/min	ESPRIT[34]
Tirofiban	• ACS, including patients managed medically and those undergoing PCI[c]	• ACS: [c]Bolus 0.4 μg/kg/min for 30 min Infusion 0.1 μg/kg/min 36–10 h *Renal dysfunction:[b]* Bolus 0.2 μg/kg/min for 30 min Infusion 0.05 μg/kg/min 36–108 h	PRISM-PLUS[37] RESTORE[38]
	• PCI	• PCI:[c] Bolus 10–25μg/kg Infusion 0.15 μg/kg/min × 12–24 h	

PCI, percutaneous coronary intervention; UA, unstable angina, ACS, acute coronary syndrome; NSTEMI, non-ST-elevation myocardial infarction.
[a]Serum creatinine >2 mg/dl.
[b]Creatinine clearance <30 ml/min.
[c]Not an FDA-approved indication or dose.

placebo.[27,28] Any drop in the platelet count below laboratory normal values occurred in 4.7–6.5% of patients in the early large abciximab trials. Although unclear, thrombocytopenia was suggested to be secondary to drug-dependant antibodies.[23] Clinically meaningful thrombocytopenia (platelet counts <100 000/mm³) reportedly occurred in <2% of patients.

Eptifibatide

Viper venom-derived disintegrins are peptide molecules containing the amino acid sequence RGD and are potent inhibitors of ligand binding to GPIIb/IIIa. Eptifibatide (Integrilin, COR Therapeutics, Inc.; Figure 12.3) is a synthetic cyclic peptide based on barbourin, a unique member of the disintegrin family, which contains a novel Lys-Gly-Asp (KGD) sequence making it highly specific for the GPIIb/IIIa receptor.[29] Secondary to its low molecular weight, eptifibatide is non-immunogenic.[30]

Eptifibatide has high specificity for the GPIIb/IIIa receptor. It has a low affinity for the receptor (K_D=120 nmol/l) and rapidly dissociates from it.[25] Eptifibatide has a mean plasma half-life of 1.13 hours. Renal clearance accounts for 40% of total body clearance.[31] Plasma clearance is 1.0–1.2 ml/min/kg.[32] Nearly complete inhibition of ADP-induced platelet aggregation is seen within 15 minutes of bolus infusion. Bleeding times increase to greater than two times baseline with standard infusion, and return to near-baseline levels within 1 hour of infusion discontinuation.[33]

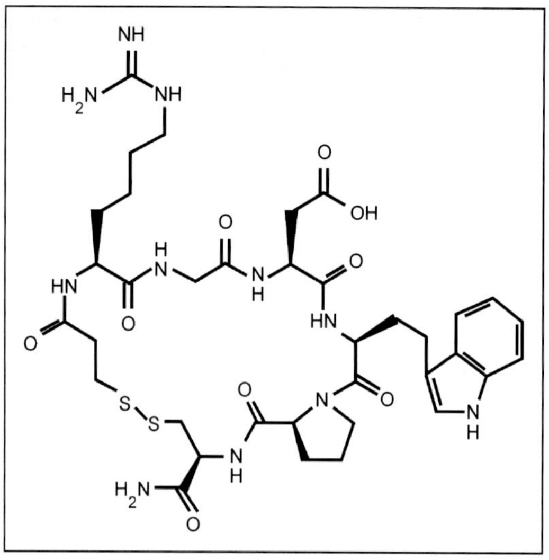

Figure 12.3
Structure of eptifibatide. With permission from Topol et al.[41]

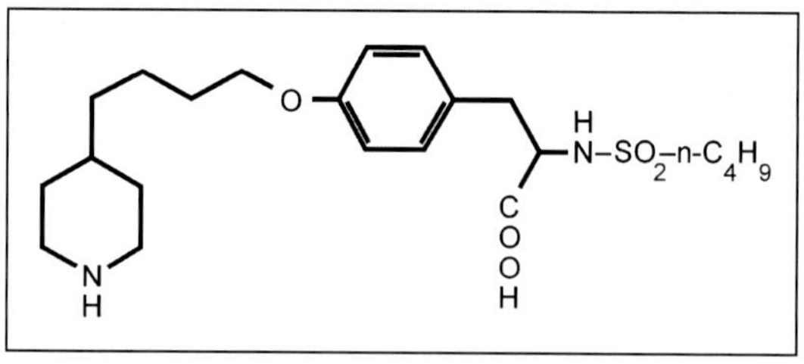

Figure 12.4
Structure of tirofiban. With permission from Topol et al.[41]

Platelet aggregation returns toward normal within 2–4 hours after the infusion has been terminated.[30] In the ESPRIT trial, higher TIMI (Thrombolysis is Myocardial Infarction) major bleeding rates with eptifibatide were not statistically significant: 1% eptifibatide versus 0.4% placebo.[34] Rates of thrombocytopenia are also not significantly elevated with the use of eptifibatide.

Eptifibatide has a unique dosing regimen. An initial bolus is followed by an infusion, which is followed 10 minutes later by another bolus. This dosing schedule was developed after less than excepted efficacy was observed in the IMPACT-II trial. The lower efficacy was determined to be due to overestimated pharmacodynamics of eptifibatide secondary to effects of calcium chelation by the anticoagulant sodium citrate.[32] The ESPRIT trial, which evaluated the new dosing regimen, was terminated early, as efficacy was achieved versus placebo.[34]

Tirofiban

Tirofiban (Aggrastat, Merck & Co. Inc.; Figure 12.4) is a non-peptide tyrosine derivative that functions as a mimic of the RGD sequence. It is highly specific for the GPIIb/IIIa receptor,[35] and does not apparently bind any other integrins. Unlike a monoclonal antibody agent, tirofiban is also far less likely to induce an immune response.

Tirofiban has a relatively short half-life of only about 2 hours.[35] Greater than 80% inhibition of ADP-induced platelet aggregation is achieved after 5 minutes of a high-dose bolus. Bleeding time exhibits a twofold prolongation with infusion;[36] however, it returns to baseline levels 3–4 hours after discontinuation of the drug.[35] The molecule rapidly dissociates from the GPIIb/IIIa receptor, with a half-time for dissociation rate constant of $0.062 \, s^{-1}$.[25] Platelet aggregation

inhibition decreases to less than 50% approximately 4 hours after cessation of infusion.[36]

The plasma clearance of the drug is 173.5–562.0 ml/min, with renal clearance ranging from 25% to 54%.[35] Therefore, patients with severe renal insufficiency should receive a reduced infusion rate. The most common adverse event reported with tirofiban use is bleeding. In administration with heparin, TIMI major bleeding occurred in 1.4% and 2.2% of patients in the PRISM-PLUS and RESTORE trials, respectively.[37,38] Thrombocytopenia is seen at a higher but not statistically significant rate than for heparin infusion alone: 1.9% for tirofiban with heparin versus 0.8% for heparin alone.[37]

References

1. Kroll MH, Harris TS, Moake JL, Handin RI, Schafer AI. von Willebrand factor binding to platelet GpIb initiates signals for platelet activation. J Clin Invest 1991;88:1568–73.
2. Holtkotter O, Nieswandt B, Smyth N et al. Integrin α_2-deficient mice develop normally, are fertile, but display partially defective platelet interaction with collagen. J Biol Chem 2002;277:10789–94.
3. Nieswandt B, Brakebusch C, Bergmeier W et al. Glycoprotein VI but not $\alpha_2\beta_1$ integrin is essential for platelet interaction with collagen. EMBO J 2001;20:2120–30.
4. Clemetson KJ, Clemetson JM. Platelet collagen receptors. Thromb Haemost 2001;86:189–97.
5. Schafer AI, Ali NM, Levine GN. Hemostasis, thrombosis, fibrinolysis, and cardiovascular disease. In: Braunwald E, Zipes DP, Libby P, eds. Heart Disease: A Textbook of Cardiovascular Medicine. 6th edn. Philadelphia: WB Saunders, 2001:2099–32.
6. Hourani SM, Cusack NJ. Pharmacological receptors on blood platelets. Pharmacol Rev 1991;43:243–98.
7. Kunapuli SP, Dorsam RT, Kim S, Quinton TM. Platelet purinergic receptors. Curr Opin Pharmacol 2003;3:175–80.
8. Shattil SJ, Ginsberg MH. Integrin signaling in vascular biology. J Clin Invest 1997;100(11 Suppl):S91–5.
9. Lefkovits J, Plow EF, Topol EJ. Platelet glycoprotein IIb/IIIa receptors in cardiovascular medicine. N Engl J Med 1995;332:1553–9.
10. Harrison P, Cramer EM. Platelet alpha-granules. Blood Rev 1993;7:52–62.
11. Ma AD, Abrams CS. Pleckstrin homology domains and phospholipid-induced cytoskeletal reorganization. Thromb Haemost 1999;82:399–406.
12. Fox JE. The platelet cytoskeleton. Thromb Haemost 1993;70:884–93.
13. Buck CA, Horwitz AF. Cell surface receptors for extracellular matrix molecules. Annu Rev Cell Biol 1987;3:179–205.

14. Albelda SM, Buck CA. Integrins and other cell adhesion molecules. FASEB J 1990;4:2868–80.

15. Poncz M, Eisman R, Heidenreich R et al. Structure of the platelet membrane glycoprotein IIb. Homology to the alpha subunits of the vitronectin and fibronectin membrane receptors. J Biol Chem 1987;262:8476–82.

16. Fitzgerald LA, Steiner B, Rall SC Jr, Lo SS, Phillips DR. Protein sequence of endothelial glycoprotein IIIa derived from a cDNA clone. Identity with platelet glycoprotein IIIa and similarity to 'integrin.' J Biol Chem 1987;262:3936–9.

17. Wagner CL, Mascelli MA, Neblock DS et al. Analysis of GPIIb/IIIa receptor number by quantification of 7E3 binding to human platelets. Blood 1996;88:907–14.

18. Hughes PE, Pfaff M. Integrin affinity modulation. Trends Cell Biol 1998;8:359–64.

19. Pytela R, Pierschbacher MD, Ginsberg MH, Plow EF, Ruoslahti E. Platelet membrane glycoprotein IIb/IIIa: member of a family of Arg-Gly-Asp-specific adhesion receptors. Science 1986;231:1559–62.

20. Kloczewiak M, Timmons S, Hawiger J. Recognition site for the platelet receptor is present on the 15-residue carboxy-terminal fragment of the gamma chain of human fibrinogen and is not involved in the fibrin polymerization reaction. Thromb Res 1983;29:249–55.

21. Plow EF, D'Souza SE, Ginsberg MH. Ligand binding to GPIIb–IIIa: a status report. Semin Thromb Hemost 1992;18:324–32.

22. Duval WL, Vorchheimer DA, Fuster V. Thrombogenesis and antithrombotic therapy. In: Fuster V, Alexander RW, O'Rourke RA et al, eds. Hurst's The Heart, 11th edn. New York: McGraw-Hill, 2004;1361–1418.

23. Schror K, Weber AA. Comparative pharmacology of GP IIb/IIIa antagonists. J Thromb Thrombolysis 2003;15:71–80.

24. Coller BS, Peerschke EI, Scudder LE, Sullivan CA. A murine monoclonal antibody that completely blocks the binding of fibrinogen to platelets produces a thrombasthenic-like state in normal platelets and binds to glycoproteins IIb and/or IIIa. J Clin Invest 1983;72:325–38.

25. Scarborough RM, Kleiman NS, Phillips DR. Platelet glycoprotein IIb/IIIa antagonists. What are the relevant issues concerning their pharmacology and clinical use? Circulation 1999;100:437–44.

26. Tam SH, Sassoli PM, Jordan RE, Nakada MT. Abciximab (ReoPro, chimeric 7E3 Fab) demonstrates equivalent affinity and functional blockade of glycoprotein IIb/IIIa and $\alpha_v\beta_3$ integrins. Circulation 1998;98:1085–91.

27. Use of a monoclonal antibody directed against the platelet glycoprotein IIb/IIIa receptor in high-risk coronary angioplasty. The EPIC Investigation. N Engl J Med 1994;330:956–61.

28. Randomised placebo-controlled trial of abciximab before and during coronary intervention in refractory unstable angina: the CAPTURE study. Lancet 1997;349:1429–35.

29. Scarborough RM, Naughton MA, Teng W et al. Design of potent and specific integrin antagonists. Peptide antagonists with high specificity for glycoprotein IIb–IIIa. J Biol Chem 1993;268: 1066–73.

30. Phillips DR, Scarborough RM. Clinical pharmacology of eptifibatide. Am J Cardiol 1997;80:11B–20B.

31. Alton KB, Kosoglou T, Baker S et al. Disposition of ^{14}C-eptifibatide after intravenous administration to healthy men. Clin Ther 1998;20:307–23.

32. Gilchrist IC, O'Shea JC, Kosoglou T et al. Pharmacodynamics and pharmacokinetics of higher-dose, double-bolus eptifibatide in percutaneous coronary intervention. Circulation 2001;104:406–11.

33. Harrington RA, Kleiman NS, Kottke-Marchant K et al. Immediate and reversible platelet inhibition after intravenous administration of a peptide glycoprotein IIb/IIIa inhibitor during percutaneous coronary intervention. Am J Cardiol 1995;76:1222–7.

34. The ESPRIT Investigators. Novel dosing regimen of eptifibatide in planned coronary stent implantation (ESPRIT): a randomised, placebo-controlled trial. Lancet 2000;356:2037–44.

35. Barrett JS, Murphy G, Peerlinck K et al. Pharmacokinetics and pharmacodynamics of MK-383, a selective non-peptide platelet glycoprotein-IIb/IIIa receptor antagonist, in healthy men. Clin Pharmacol Ther 1994;56:377–88.

36. Kereiakes DJ, Kleiman NS, Ambrose J et al. Randomized, double-blind, placebo-controlled dose-ranging study of tirofiban (MK-383) platelet IIb/IIIa blockade in high risk patients undergoing coronary angioplasty. J Am Coll Cardiol 1996;27:536–42.

37. Platelet Receptor Inhibition in Ischemic Syndrome Management in Patients Limited by Unstable Signs and Symptoms (PRISM-PLUS) Study Investigators. Inhibition of the platelet glycoprotein IIb/IIIa receptor with tirofiban in unstable angina and non-Q-wave myocardial infarction. N Engl J Med 1998;338:1488–97.

38. The RESTORE Investigators. Randomized Efficacy Study of Tirofiban for Outcomes and REstenosis. Effects of platelet glycoprotein IIb/IIIa blockade with tirofiban on adverse cardiac events in patients with unstable angina or acute myocardial infarction undergoing coronary angioplasty. Circulation 1997;96:1445–53.

39. The EPILOG Investigators. Platelet glycoprotein IIb/IIIa receptor blockade and low-dose heparin during percutaneous coronary revascularization. N Engl J Med 1997;336:1689–96.

40. The PURSUIT Trial Investigators. Platelet Glycoprotein IIb/IIIa in Unstable Angina: Receptor Suppression Using Integrilin Therapy. Inhibition of platelet glycoprotein IIb/IIIa with eptifibatide in patients with acute coronary syndromes. N Engl J Med 1998;339:436–43.

41. Topol EJ; Byzova TV, Plow EF. Platelet GP116–111a blockers. Lancet 1999;353:227–31.

13

Platelet glycoprotein IIb/IIIa receptor antagonists: a guide to patient selection and optimal use

Dirk Sibbing, Melchior Seyfarth, and Peter B Berger

Overview of platelet glycoprotein IIb/IIIa receptor antagonists in clinical use

Platelet membrane glycoprotein (GP) IIb/IIIa inhibitors are potent antiplatelet agents that block what has been termed 'the final common pathway' of platelet aggregation by inhibiting the binding of the GPIIb/IIIa integrin receptor with its primary ligand, fibrinogen. Several types of GPIIb/IIIa inhibitors exist; three are currently available for clinical use.

Abciximab (ReoPro) (Centocor, Malvern, PA and Eli Lilly, Inc., Indianapolis, IN) is a monoclonal antibody that is a Fab (fragment antigen binding) fragment of a chimeric human–mouse genetic reconstruction of 7E3. It was generated in 1985[1] and is a non-competitive inhibitor of the GPIIb/IIIa receptor with a biological half-life of 8–12 hours. Although frequently described an irreversible inhibitor, it is not; when a patient who has received abciximab receives a platelet transfusion, abciximab molecules leave many of the platelets they are bound to and redistribute throughout the entire platelet pool. The recommended dose for abciximab is 0.25 mg/kg bolus followed by an intravenous infusion with 0.125 µg/kg/min for 12 hours.

Eptifibatide (Integilin) (COR Therapeutics, South San Francisco, CA and Key Pharmaceuticals, Kenilworth, NJ), a synthetic peptide, is a competitive antagonist to fibrinogen with a biological half-life of approximately 2.5 hours. The recommended dose for eptifibatide depends of its indication for use. The initial bolus treatment ranges from 135 µg/kg when administered for the treatment of an acute coronary syndrome (ACS)[2] to a double bolus of 180 µg/kg when administered for a percutaneous coronary intervention (PCI).[3] The recommended continuous infusion dosing regimen ranges from 0.5 µg/kg/min to 2.0 µg/kg/min for 20–24 hours.

Tirofiban (Aggrastat) (Merck and Co., White House Station, NJ), a non-peptide mimetic, is also, similarly to eptifibatide, a competitive antagonist to fibrinogen, with a

biological half-life of approximately 2.5 hours. It is more similar to abciximab than to eptifibatide, however, in the strength of its bond to the GPIIb/IIIa receptor. The recommended dosing regimen for an ACS is 0.4 µg/kg/min for 30 minutes followed by 0.10 µg/kg/min for 48 hours; it is not currently approved in the USA for PCI, although it is both approved and widely used throughout Europe for this indication. Doses for both eptifibatide and tirofiban need adjustments for patients with renal insufficiency. All three agents inhibit in vitro platelet aggregation by approximately 80% when large doses of strong agonists for thrombosis are used. Orally active GPIIb/IIIa inhibitors including xemilofiban, sibrafiban, and orbofiban, have been tested in large clinical trials, but all were found to increase the risk of death, myocardial infarction (MI), or both, and are not available for use. As a result, as a class, oral GPIIb/IIIa inhibitors are no longer being studied.

GPIIb/IIIa receptor antagonists in patients with stable coronary artery disease

In the last decade, our knowledge about antiplatelet therapy following PCI has improved considerably. With intensification of antiplatelet treatment, the rate of postprocedural major adverse cardiovascular events (MACE) has decreased in patients scheduled for PCI regardless of the clinical setting in which it is performed. The use of optimal antithrombotic and antiplatelet regimens is critical in reducing adverse events among patients undergoing PCI. In particular, dual antiplatelet therapy with aspirin and a thienopyridine has markedly improved both the efficacy and safety of PCI.[4–6] Nowadays, pretreatment with clopidogrel using loading doses ranging from 300 to 600 mg administered prior to PCI is routinely performed, whenever possible, to achieve the maximal inhibition of platelets possible with the drug by the time the coronary intervention is performed.

Pretreatment with a thienopyridine hours before a coronary intervention significantly reduces the rate of adverse events among those patients who demonstrated maximal inhibition of platelet aggregation.[4,7]

Prior to the era of pretreatment with large loading doses of a thienopyridine, the safety and efficacy of GPIIb/IIIa inhibition using different inhibitors was tested in several studies that included patients with stable coronary artery disease (CAD). The first study was the EPIC (Evaluation of 7E3 for the Prevention of Ischemic Complications) trial,[8] which compared three different treatment regimens. In this trial, 2099 patients undergoing balloon angioplasty were randomly assigned in a double-blinded manner to receive placebo, an abciximab bolus, or an abciximab bolus plus infusion. A 35% reduction in the combined endpoint of death, non-fatal MI, unplanned surgical revascularization, unplanned repeat percutaneous procedure, unplanned implantation of a coronary stent, or insertion of an intra-aortic balloon pump for refractory ischemia was found at 30 days after PCI in the group of patients treated with abciximab bolus plus infusion,[8] and remarkably persisted for 3 years.[9] However, there was a doubling (a 100% increase) in major bleeding with abciximab, and the use of the drug did not become common. Subsequently, the EPILOG (Evaluation in PTCA to Improve Long-term Outcome with abciximab GP IIb/IIIa blockade) trial[10] was performed among patients who were also undergoing balloon angioplasty but who were at a somewhat lower risk than patients in EPIC were.[8,10] In this trial, two different lower doses of weight-adjusted heparin were administered with abciximab than had been administered in EPIC; a lower weight-adjusted infusion dose of abciximab was also implemented. This study was stopped prematurely due to efficacy when a large and highly significant reduction in the incidence of death and acute MI (AMI) was observed in patients who received abciximab ($p < 0.001$). Bleeding was lowest, however, in the patients who received the lower dose of heparin, and so this became the preferred way in which to administer abciximab. And again, as in EPIC, the reduction in ischemic events remained evident 6 and 12 months following PCI.[10] Similar results were reported from the EPISTENT (Evaluation of Platelet GP IIb/IIIa Inhibition in Stenting) trial,[11,12] the first randomized trial examining the use of GPIIb/IIIa inhibitors among patients undergoing stent placement. Again, the frequencies of death and AMI were significantly lower at follow-up (30 days, 6 months, and 12 months) in the group of patients who received abciximab during PCI.

The first major trial to investigate eptifibatide was the IMPACT-II (Integrilin to Minimize Platelet Aggregation and Prevent Coronary Thrombosis-II) trial.[2] A significant reduction of major adverse cardiac events was found 24 hours after PCI, although by 30 days, the difference was no longer statistically significant. It was later determined that the wrong dose of eptifibatide had been selected based on an anomaly of platelet function testing brought about by calcium chelation resulting from the EDTA anticoagulant in test tubes used to perform aggregometry.[13] The ESPRIT (Enhanced Suppression of the Platelet IIb/IIIa Receptor with Integrilin) trial[3] used a higher dose of eptifibatide than was used in IMPACT-II; the proportion of patients who received a stent was higher as well. ESPRIT was stopped prematurely due to efficacy; the composite endpoint of death, AMI, and urgent target vessel revascularization (TVR) was significantly reduced both 48 hours and 30 days after PCI in the group of patients who received eptifibatide.

On the basis of these trials, GPIIb/IIIa inhibitors became a cornerstone in the treatment of patients undergoing PCI because of their ability to improve short- and long-term outcome – largely (although not exclusively) by reducing the occurrence of procedural MI. Subsequently, however, an observational study and a retrospective analysis of the EPIC trial suggested that a GPIIb/IIIa inhibitor may no longer offer benefit if patients have been adequately pretreated with a thienopyridine.[14,15] Because it took so long for patients to reach the maximal level of platelet inhibition with ticlopidine (5–7 days) and large loading doses invariably caused nausea and vomiting, the issue remained largely moot, however, until clopidogrel became available and largely replaced ticlopidine for PCI and eventually all other indications. Large loading doses of clopidogrel are well tolerated, and can reduce the time required to achieve maximal inhibition of platelet aggregation to hours. In the first ISAR-REACT (Intracoronary Stenting and Antithrombotic Regimen: Rapid Early Action for Coronary Treatment) trial, 2159 low to intermediate-risk patients, all of whom had been pretreated with 600 mg of clopidogrel for at least 2 hours, were randomized to receive either abciximab therapy or placebo in a double-blinded manner.[16] The trial was designed to determine whether the administration of abciximab reduces the incidence of ischemic complications in patients undergoing elective PCI after pretreatment with a high loading dose of 600 mg of clopidogrel at least 2 hours before the intervention. The composite endpoint (death, MI, and urgent TVR at 30 days after PCI) was reached in 4% (45 patients) in the group treated with abciximab and in 4% (43 patients) in the group treated with placebo ($p = 0.82$).

In conclusion, the ISAR-REACT trial suggested that abciximab offers no further clinical benefit within the first 30 days after PCI in low to intermediate-risk patients scheduled for coronary intervention if they have been pretreated with 600 mg of clopidogrel for at least 2 hours (Figure 13.1). Analysis of 1-year outcome of ISAR-REACT similarly revealed no benefit of abciximab after pretreatment with 600 mg of clopidogrel.[17] Despite the lack of a measurable benefit for adjunctive abciximab treatment in patients with stable CAD, it has to be emphasized that results of the ISAR-REACT trial, in which low to intermediate-risk patients were included, cannot be projected to high-risk patients presenting with an ACS, or to patients in whom pretreatment with 600 mg of clopidogrel for at least 2 hours has not

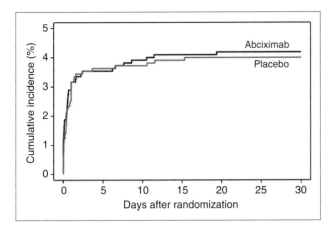

Figure 13.1
Kaplan–Meier event curves for the 30-day cumulative incidence of the primary endpoint – death, myocardial infarction, or urgent revascularization – in the group of patients who received abciximab or placebo. (Adapted from Kastrati A et al.[16])

been accomplished. Moreover, diabetic patients taking insulin were excluded from ISAR-REACT.

Diabetic patients with CAD who undergo PCI, particularly those requiring insulin, present a special group of patients characterized by a worse outcome after PCI due to an increased risk of both thrombosis and restenosis.[18] Several randomized trials demonstrated a reduction in the incidence of adverse events in the subgroup of diabetic patients following PCI when GPIIb/IIIa receptor antagonists in patients with an ACS, were administered during coronary intervention.[19] However, few, if any, diabetic patients included in these trials were adequately pretreated with a thienopyridine.

The ISAR-SWEET (Intracoronary Stenting and Antithrombotic Regimen: Is Abciximab a Superior Way to Eliminate Elevated Thrombotic Risk in Diabetics?) trial, the first dedicated randomized trial evaluating GPIIb/IIIa blockade in diabetic patients scheduled for elective PCI, was designed similarly to ISAR-REACT and sought to determine whether the administration of abciximab to diabetic patients taking insulin who had been pretreated with 600 mg of clopidogrel was beneficial. In the trial, abciximab did not reduce adverse events at 30 days or 1 year.[20] The 1-year cumulative incidence of the primary endpoint (death or MI) occurred in 8.3% of patients who received abciximab versus 8.6% of those who did not ($p=0.91$). Surprisingly, angiographic restenosis and target vessel revascularization (TVR) was significantly lower in the group of diabetic patients who received abciximab ($p=0.01$ and $p=0.03$, respectively). The impact of abciximab on the reduction of restenosis was also investigated in the ISAR-SMART 2 (Intracoronary Stenting or Angioplasty for Restenosis in SMall ARTeries 2) trial.[21] In this study, abciximab failed to reduce the incidence of angiographic restenosis following PCI of small coronary arteries.[21] Other studies have also

subsequently failed to confirm the ability of abciximab to reduce restenosis.[22–24]

In conclusion, the ISAR-REACT, ISAR-SWEET, and ISAR-SMART 2 trials all demonstrated that in patients with stable CAD, abciximab does not provide additional clinical benefit when administered to patients who had been pretreated with 600 mg of clopidogrel for at least 2 hours.

GPIIb/IIIa receptor antagonists in patients with an ACS

ACS are a frequent cause of hospital admission and are associated with an increased risk of death.[25] PCI is an established treatment of proven benefit for patients who present with an ACS,[26] and almost three-fourths of all patients scheduled for coronary intervention worldwide present with the diagnosis of an ACS.[27] Platelet activation and aggregation are enhanced in ACS patients compared with patients with stable CAD.[28,29] Consequently, inhibition of both platelet activation and aggregation – using aspirin, thienopyridines such as clopidogrel, and GPIIb/IIIa inhibitors – is pivotal in the treatment of patients with ACS, whether or not they undergo PCI. But, as was the case with patients undergoing elective PCI described above, the clinical experience and proven utility of GPIIb/IIIa inhibitors in ACS patients began in the era before pretreatment of ACS patients with a thienopyridine prior to PCI was able to be performed easily.

The first trial ever to evaluate abciximab in patients with an ACS was the EPIC trial in 1994.[8] As described above, only patients undergoing PCI were included, and there was a 35% reduction in the combined endpoint for the group of patients treated with an abciximab bolus plus infusion. The second trial to investigate GPIIb/IIIa inhibition in ACS patients was the CAPTURE (c7E3 Fab Antiplatelet Therapy in Unstable Refractory Angina) trial.[30] This trial utilized an unusual design: abciximab versus placebo were administered for approximately 24 hours (beginning 18–24 hours before PCI and continuing 1 hour after PCI) in patients with an ACS only after a diagnostic angiogram confirmed anatomy suitable for PCI. Treatment with abciximab significantly reduced the primary endpoint of death, non-fatal MI, or TVR at 30 days.[30] Importantly, in a retrospective subgroup analysis of patients with an elevated and normal troponin T, it was demonstrated that only patients with an elevated troponin derived benefit from abciximab.[31] The role of abciximab in ACS patients treated medically was investigated in the GUSTO-IV ACS (Global Use of Strategies to Open Occluded Arteries IV – Acute Coronary Syndrome) trial,[32] in which PCI was actually prohibited by protocol for the first 60 hours after enrollment. In this trial, 7800 patients with non-ST-segment elevation ACS were randomized to receive placebo, abciximab for 24 hours, or abciximab for 48 hours. All patients also received heparin or dalteparin, and aspirin. This was the first study of abciximab that failed to show any benefit from the drug; in fact, not only was there no benefit, but there was a trend towards higher rates of MI and death with abciximab, and the trend was greatest with longer duration of treatment. Bleeding and thrombocytopenia were significantly increased by abciximab in the trial.

The role of eptifibatide in ACS patients was investigated in the PURSUIT (Platelet Glycoprotein IIb/IIIa in Unstable Angina: Receptor Suppression Using Integrilin Therapy) trial.[33] A total of 10 948 patients were assigned to either receive eptifibatide or placebo for 72 hours. A third arm with low-dose eptifibatide (1.3 µg/kg/min) was stopped prematurely by design after 3218 patients had been randomized, and the safety of the high-dose eptifibatide (2.0 µg/kg/min) arm was found to be acceptable. At 30 days of follow-up, eptifibatide resulted in a statistically significant, albeit modest, 10% reduction in the composite endpoint of death or non-fatal MI.

Tirofiban was studied in the PRISM (Platelet Receptor Inhibition in Ischemic Syndrome Management) trial.[34] In this trial, 3232 patients with unstable angina were assigned to receive either tirofiban or unfractionated heparin. This study differed from all previous trials of a GPIIb/III inhibitor in that heparin was not administered in conjunction with the GPIIb/IIIa inhibitor. In this trial, the incidence of death, MI, or refractory angina at 48 hours (the prespecified endpoint) was significantly lower in the tirofiban group. However, at 30 days, the frequency of these adverse events was similar in the two groups. That trial was followed by the PRISM-PLUS (Platelet Receptor Inhibition in Ischemic Syndrome Management in Patients Limited by Unstable Signs and Symptoms) trial, in which 1915 patients with unstable angina were assigned to tirofiban, tirofiban plus heparin, or heparin alone.[35] Enrollment in the arm receiving tirofiban without heparin was stopped prematurely because of excess mortality after 7 days (4.6%, as compared with 1.1% for the patients treated with heparin alone). Treatment with both tirofiban and heparin was associated with a 27% reduction in death or non-fatal MI after 30 days.

Head-to-head comparisons of the different GPIIb/IIIa inhibitor agents are scant. Two GPIIb/IIIa inhibitors, tirofiban and abciximab, were compared in the TARGET (Do Tirofiban and ReoPro Give Similar Efficacy outcomes?) trial.[24] The composite endpoint of death, MI or TVR after 30 days occurred in 7.6% of tirofiban patients versus 6.0% in the abciximab group. In this non-inferiority trial, tirofiban failed to demonstrate non-inferiority with abciximab. It was subsequently shown that the loading dose of tirofiban used in the trial was too small to inhibit platelet aggregation sufficiently in the crucial first 20 minutes after tirofiban had been given. Subsequent studies revealed that the loading dose had to be 2.5 times larger than was used in

TARGET to provide the same degree of inhibition of aggregation as abiciximab;[36,37] the infusion dose was, however, correct and able to maintain an adequate level of receptor blockade and inhibition of aggregation. Subsequent to TARGET, there have been five small randomized trials comparing tirofiban utilizing this larger loading dose with either placebo or abciximab;[37] in all of them, tirofiban was shown to be superior to placebo or approximately as effective as abciximab. These five trials were all too small to be definitive; even a recent meta-analysis of all five trials could not be considered definitive, although the results with tirofiban were very encouraging.[37]

Once a decision has been made to administer a platelet GPIIb/IIIa inhibitor, a physician must also decide when to administer it. The large randomized trials reviewed above have mainly used one of two different timing strategies. One strategy has been to administer the GPIIb/IIIa inhibitor early after the diagnosis of an ACS, prior to angiography. This strategy is usually referred to as 'upstream' treatment. A different strategy has been to treat only those patients in the cardiac catheterization laboratory who are about to undergo PCI.[3,11,38] To assess the question of the optimal timing strategy, the ACUITY (Acute Catheterization and Urgent Intervention Triage Strategy) Timing trial was performed.[39] In this very complicated large multicenter open-label trial with several different randomizations, a total of 9207 ACS patients at moderate to high risk in whom an invasive treatment strategy was planned were randomly assigned to receive either routine upstream or selective in-lab treatment with a GPIIb/IIIa inhibitor. All three GPIIb/IIIa inhibitors currently in clinical use (abciximab, tirofiban, and eptifibatide) could be used by physician preference in ACUITY. The main result of the trial is that, after 30 days, the routine upstream use of GPIIb/IIIa inhibitors in ACS patients with an invasive strategy produced a non-statistically significant 12% decrease in the combined endpoint of death, MI, or TVR. The difference (7.9% for in-lab vs 7.1% for upstream) did not meet the criterion for non-inferiority; therefore, the possibility exists that upstream use may be superior. Major bleeding rates were significantly lower in the group of patients receiving selective in-lab treatment. When analyzing the net clinical outcome (a composite including both ischemic endpoints and major bleeding), the event rates were similar in the two groups (11.7% vs 11.7%; $p = 0.93$). Another trial examining the same issue, EARLY ACS, is currently enrolling. In this trial, patients are randomized to receive either upstream eptifibatide or selective in-lab use of eptifibatide. Until the results of EARLY ACS are known, given the results of the ACUITY Timing trial, clinicians should carefully balance their decision regarding the most appropriate time of administration of a GPIIb/IIIa inhibitor for those patients with an ACS who are thought to require a GPIIb/IIIa inhibitor. The potentially lower rate of thrombotic complications associated with 'upstream' administration of a GPIIb/IIIa inhibitor must be balanced against the decreased risk of bleeding associated with the selective in-lab use of GPIIb/IIIa inhibitors.

Importantly, these trials – all of which favored GPIIb/IIIa inhibition in ACS patients, and particularly those patients who were troponin-positive and undergoing PCI – were not specifically designed to address the impact and value of GPIIb/IIIa inhibitors in ACS, especially in the era of routine treatment with a loading dose of clopidogrel prior to PCI. This important issue was assessed in the ISAR-REACT 2 (Intracoronary Stenting and Antithrombotic Regimen: Rapid Early Action for Coronary Treatment 2) trial.[38] The objective of ISAR-REACT 2 was to assess whether abciximab, administered in the catheterization laboratory, is associated with a clinical benefit in patients with an ACS undergoing PCI more than 2 hours after pretreatment with 600 mg of clopidogrel. In this double-blind randomized trial, 2022 patients were included and assigned to receive either abciximab or placebo in addition to treatment with intravenous heparin, aspirin, and the 600 mg loading dose of clopidogrel. The study revealed that the administration of abciximab significantly reduced the incidence of the primary endpoint of death, MI, or TVR at 30 days (relative risk 0.75; 95% confidence interval (CI) 0.58–0.97; $p = 0.03$). The benefit of abciximab treatment, however, was restricted only to those patients that presented with an elevated troponin (Figure 13.2). Troponin-negative patients demonstrated substantially lower and almost identical event rates with abciximab vs. placebo.

These data indirectly raise the question of whether the greater platelet activity in ACS patients requires more potent inhibition than that provided by clopidogrel alone. Based on the results of ISAR-REACT 2, and retrospective analysis of the prior randomized trials comparing GPIIb/IIIa inhibitors with placebo, troponin status should be an important

consideration (perhaps the singular most important consideration) to guide the decision about whether to administer a GPIIb/III inhibitor to an individual patient.

GPIIb/IIIa receptor antagonists in patients with ST-segment elevation myocardial infarction

Treatment of ST-segment elevation myocardial infarction (STEMI) has substantially improved over recent decades; this is mainly due to deployment of pharmacological and mechanical reperfusion therapies as well as to improvement in concomitant antiplatelet and anticoagulation regimens.[40–43] The goal of all reperfusion therapies in AMI is the rapid restoration of coronary blood flow in the culprit artery in order to reduce infarct size. Several studies have investigated the impact of GPIIb/IIIa inhibitors in STEMI patients scheduled for PCI.

The first large-scale trial to investigate the impact of abciximab treatment in STEMI patients treated with PCI was the RAPPORT (ReoPro And Primary PTCA Organization and Randomized) trial.[44] This trial included a total of 483 patients assigned to receive either abciximab or placebo during balloon angioplasty. Treatment with abciximab significantly reduced the incidence of death, reinfarction, or urgent TVR at all time points assessed (9.9% vs 3.3% ($p = 0.003$) at 7 days; 11.2% vs 5.8% ($p = 0.03$) at 30 days; and 17.8% vs 11.6% ($p = 0.05$) at 6 months). Major bleeding occurred more frequently in the abciximab group compared with placebo (16.6% vs 9.5%; $p = 0.02$). It has to be emphasized that coronary stents were not routinely used at the time the RAPPORT trial was performed. Subsequently, in the ADMIRAL (Abciximab before Direct Angioplasty and Stenting in Myocardial Infarction Regarding Acute and Long-term Follow-up) study, 300 patients with STEMI were randomly assigned to abciximab or placebo before coronary stenting.[45] All patients enrolled in the study received heparin, aspirin, and ticlopidine. A significant reduction in the primary endpoint of death, MI, and TVR was observed at 30 days in the abciximab group (6.0% vs 14.6% in the placebo group; $p = 0.01$). Six months after enrollment in the study, the primary endpoint occurred in 7.4% in the abciximab group versus 15.9% in the placebo group ($p = 0.02$). The investigators attributed the better outcome of abciximab to higher levels of Thrombolysis in Myocardial Infarction (TIMI) 3 flow in the target vessel immediately before (16.8% vs 5.4%; $p = 0.01$) and immediately after (95.1% vs 86.7%; $p = 0.04$) the procedure. The authors concluded that administration of abciximab in STEMI patients improved coronary patency, stenting success rates, and clinical outcome at follow-up. Similar results were observed in the ISAR-2

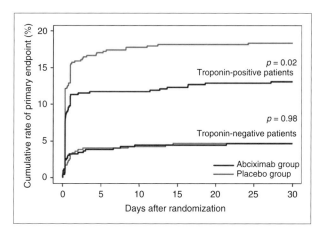

Figure 13.2
Kaplan–Meier event curves for the 30-day cumulative incidence of the primary endpoint – death, myocardial infarction, or urgent revascularization – in the group of patients who received abciximab or placebo in the subsets with or without elevated troponin levels (>0.03 μg/l). (Adapted from Kastrati A.[38])

(Intracoronary Stenting and Antithrombotic Regimen 2) trial,[46] in which 401 STEMI patients were randomized to receive either abciximab and reduced-dose heparin or full-dose heparin alone for PCI. Thirty days after PCI, the composite clinical endpoint of death, reinfarction, and TVR was reached in 5.0% of the abciximab group versus 10.5% of the control group ($p = 0.038$). After 1 year of follow-up, the absolute reduction in the composite clinical endpoint with abciximab was still 5.7%, although the difference was no longer statistically significant. The largest trial investigating the impact of GPIIb/IIIa inhibition in STEMI patients was the CADILLAC (Controlled Abciximab and Device Investigation to Lower Late Angioplasty Complications) trial.[40] In this trial, 2625 STEMI patients were randomized using a 2 × 2 factorial design to stenting versus balloon angioplasty (with bail-out stenting when needed), and to abciximab versus placebo. The principal finding was a halving in the incidence of the composite endpoint (death, MI, stroke, or TVR) at 6 months with routine stent placement, and a significant reduction in adverse events with abciximab (subacute thrombosis and recurrent ischemia leading to TVR). A major controversy in the CADILLAC trial is whether it is appropriate to look at individual parts of the 2×2 design and in particular the outcome of patients treated with stents who did or did not get abciximab. The controversy arose because in patients who received a stent, there was little reduction in MACE from the administration of abciximab (11.5% after stenting alone vs 10.2% after stenting plus abciximab; p=NS). These findings may have been related to the administration of abciximab immediately (minutes only) before the procedure, and the recruitment of a relatively low-risk population into the study.

The value of two different GP IIb/IIIa inhibitors, tirofiban and abciximab, in STEMI patients was investigated in the Single High Dose Bolus Tirofiban and Sirolimus Eluting Stent vs. Abciximab and Bare Metal Stent in Myocardial Infarction (STRATEGY) trial.[47] In this prospective, randomized and single-blind trial, 175 STEMI patients were randomized to single high-dose bolus tirofiban regimen (25 µg/kg over 3 minutes followed by 0.15 µg/kg/min for 18 to 24 hours) with sirolimus-eluting stenting vs. standard dose abciximab with bare-metal stenting. The primary endpoint of STRATEGY (composite of death, non-fatal myocardial infarction, stroke or binary restenosis at 8 months) was reached more often in the abciximab plus bare-metal stenting group (50% of patients) compared to the tirofiban plus sirolimus-eluting stenting group (19% of patients) (hazard ratio = 0.33; P<0.001). However, no differences were observed between the two groups at 30 days. Remarkably, the loading dose of tirofiban had to be higher in STRATEGY[47] compared to the TARGET trial,[24] in order to achieve a level of platelet inhibition similar to that achieved with abciximab.[36] The rationale for the study design was based on the higher costs for drug-eluting stents, which could be balanced against the lower costs for tirofiban compared to abciximab.

While ACUITY analyzed ACS patients, the optimal timing strategy of GP IIb/IIIa inhibitor treatment ("upstream" vs. "cath lab" administration) has been addressed specifically for STEMI patients by different studies. The Time to Integrilin Therapy in Acute Myocardial Infarction (TITAN)-TIMI 34 trial randomized 343 STEMI patients to early administration of eptifibatide in the emergency department (ED) vs. catheterization laboratory administration of eptifibatide following diagnostic angiography.[48] Early administration of eptifibatide in the ED resulted in superior pre-PCI TIMI frame counts (reflecting epicardial flow) and superior TIMI myocardial perfusion compared with late administration of eptifibatide in the catheterization laboratory. The benefit of early administration did not lead to higher bleeding rates. Montalescot et al investigated the optimal timing of GP IIb/IIIa inhibitors in a meta-analysis including 6 trials with a total of 931 STEMI patients treated with abciximab (3 trials) or tirofiban (3 trials).[49] Reflecting coronary patency, TIMI flow ≥ grade 2 was significantly more frequent in the early administration group compared with the late administration group (P < 0.001). For the early administration group, a 28% relative reduction in mortality (from 4.7% to 3.4%) was observed; however, this difference did not reach a level of statistical significance. In line with the results of this meta-analysis, in the Randomized Early Vs Late Abciximab in Acute Myocardial Infarction Treated With Primary Coronary Intervention (RELAx-AMI) trial, early abciximab administration improved pre-PCI angiographic findings (TIMI flow), post-PCI tissue perfusion, and 1 month left-ventricular function recovery.[50] Finally, the Facilitated Intervention with Enhanced Reperfusion Speed to Stop Events (FINESSE) trial[51] investigated the impact of the timing of drug treatment on a compact clinical endpoint. In this trial a total of 2452 STEMI patients were enrolled and randomized in a 1:1:1 fashion to primary PCI with cath lab abciximab administration, upstream abciximab-facilitated primary PCI, or half-dose reteplase/abciximab-facilitated PCI. For the primary endpoint of the study (composite of all-cause mortality, readmission for heart failure, ventricular fibrillation, or cardiogenic shock) at 3 months no differences between the treatment arms were observed. Concerning the safety endpoints, rates of TIMI nonintracranial major bleeding and minor bleeding were significantly higher for the reteplase/abciximab-facilitated PCI group as compared with primary PCI. Major and minor bleeding combined was statistically more frequent in the combination strategy as compared with primary PCI and as compared with the abciximab-only group. Taken together, a routine upstream use of GP IIb/IIIa inhibitors may have only a marginal benefit compared to a selective in cath lab administration.

For the general use of GP IIb/IIIa inhibitors, De Luca et al performed a large meta-analysis of randomized trials, indicating substantial benefits from abciximab in STEMI patients treated with PCI.[52] In this meta-analysis, a total of 11 trials in which 27 115 patients had been enrolled were analyzed. The meta-analysis demonstrated that the administration of abciximab to STEMI patients was associated with a significant reduction in 30-day (2.4% vs 3.4%, P = 0.047) and long-term (4.4% vs 6.2%, P = 0.01) mortality in patients treated with primary angioplasty. The frequency of reinfarction at 30 days was also significantly reduced by the administration of abciximab (2.1% vs. 3.3%, P<0.001). However, at present GP IIb/IIIa inhibitors have to compete with newly developed drugs being used as antithrombotic intravenous treatment during PCI. In this context, the Harmonizing Outcomes with RevascularIZatiON and Stents in Acute Myocardial Infarction (HORIZONS AMI) trial evaluated the safety and effectiveness of bivalirudin (Angiomax), an active-site directed thrombin inhibitor, compared to GP IIb/IIIa inhibitors (abciximab or eptifibatide) in STEMI patients.[53] The trial was a prospective, single-blind, randomized, multi-center study including 3 602 STEMI patients with a symptom onset ≤12 hours. The use of bivalirudin significantly reduced net adverse clinical events at 30 days (composite of major bleeding and major adverse cardiovascular events) (9.2% vs 12.1%; P = 0.006) as well as major bleeding alone (4.9% vs 8.3%; P <0.0001) compared with heparin plus a GP IIb/IIIa inhibitor. Moreover, bivalirudin significantly reduced the incidence of cardiac mortality by 38% (1.8% vs 2.9%; P = 0.035). Long-term results are outstanding and will provide further information for a possible role of bivalirudin as an alternative to GP IIb/IIIa inhibitors in STEMI patients undergoing PCI.

In conclusion, GPIIb/IIIa inhibitors improve the results of primary PCI; this has been best demonstrated with abciximab. The pretreatment regimen for clopidogrel differs in the studies investigating GP IIb/IIIa inhibitors in STEMI patients (partly no pretreatment partly pretreatment with different loading doses). Whether there is added value from administering abciximab to patients suffering a STEMI and undergoing PCI after pretreatment with a high loading dose of 600 mg clopidogrel is currently being investigated in BRAVE 3 (the third Bavarian Reperfusion Alternatives Evaluation) trial. Recruitment is expected to have been completed in 2008.

References

1. Coller BS. A new murine monoclonal antibody reports an activation-dependent change in the conformation and/or microenvironment of the platelet glycoprotein IIb/IIIa complex. J Clin Invest 1985;76:101–8.
2. The IMPACT-II Investigators. Randomised placebo-controlled trial of effect of eptifibatide on complications of percutaneous coronary intervention: IMPACT-II. Integrilin to Minimise Platelet Aggregation and Coronary Thrombosis-II. Lancet 1997;349:1422–8.
3. The ESPRIT Investigators. Novel dosing regimen of eptifibatide in planned coronary stent implantation (ESPRIT): a randomised, placebo-controlled trial. Lancet 2000;356:2037–44.
4. Steinhubl SR, Berger PB, Mann JT 3rd et al. Early and sustained dual oral antiplatelet therapy following percutaneous coronary intervention: a randomized controlled trial. JAMA 2002;288:2411–20.
5. Steinhubl SR, Charnigo R. Clopidogrel treatment prior to percutaneous coronary intervention: when enough isn't enough. JAMA 2006;295:1581–2.
6. Schömig A, Neumann FJ, Kastrati A et al. A randomized comparison of antiplatelet and anticoagulant therapy after the placement of coronary-artery stents. N Engl J Med 1996;334:1084–9.
7. Mehta SR, Yusuf S, Peters RJ et al. Effects of pretreatment with clopidogrel and aspirin followed by long-term therapy in patients undergoing percutaneous coronary intervention: the PCI-CURE study. Lancet 2001;358:527–33.
8. The EPIC Investigation. Use of a monoclonal antibody directed against the platelet glycoprotein IIb/IIIa receptor in high-risk coronary angioplasty. N Engl J Med 1994;330:956–61.
9. Topol EJ, Ferguson JJ, Weisman HF et al. Long-term protection from myocardial ischemic events in a randomized trial of brief integrin β₃ blockade with percutaneous coronary intervention. EPIC Investigator Group. Evaluation of Platelet IIb/IIIa Inhibition for Prevention of Ischemic Complication. JAMA 1997;278:479–84.
10. The EPILOG Investigators. Platelet glycoprotein IIb/IIIa receptor blockade and low-dose heparin during percutaneous coronary revascularization. N Engl J Med 1997;336:1689–96.
11. The EPISTENT Investigators. Evaluation of Platelet IIb/IIIa Inhibitor for Stenting. Randomised placebo-controlled and balloon-angioplasty-controlled trial to assess safety of coronary stenting with use of platelet glycoprotein-IIb/IIIa blockade. Lancet 1998; 352:87–92.
12. Topol EJ, Mark DB, Lincoff AM et al. Outcomes at 1 year and economic implications of platelet glycoprotein IIb/IIIa blockade in patients undergoing coronary stenting: results from a multicentre randomised trial. EPISTENT Investigators. Evaluation of Platelet IIb/IIIa Inhibitor for Stenting. Lancet 1999;354:2019–24.
13. Phillips DR, Teng W, Arfsten A et al. Effect of Ca²⁺ on GPIIb–IIIa interactions with integrilin: enhanced GPIIb–IIIa binding and inhibition of platelet aggregation by reductions in the concentration of ionized calcium in plasma anticoagulated with citrate. Circulation 1997;96:1488–94.
14. Steinhubl SR, Ellis SG, Wolski K et al. Ticlopidine pretreatment before coronary stenting is associated with sustained decrease in adverse cardiac events: data from the Evaluation of Platelet IIb/IIIa Inhibitor for Stenting (EPISTENT) Trial. Circulation 2001;103:1403–9.
15. Steinhubl SR, Lauer MS, Mukherjee DP et al. The duration of pretreatment with ticlopidine prior to stenting is associated with the risk of procedure-related non-Q-wave myocardial infarctions. J Am Coll Cardiol 1998;32:1366–70.
16. Kastrati A, Mehilli J, Schühlen H et al. A clinical trial of abciximab in elective percutaneous coronary intervention after pretreatment with clopidogrel. N Engl J Med 2004;350:232–8.
17. Schömig A, Schmitt C, Dibra A et al. One year outcomes with abciximab vs. placebo during percutaneous coronary intervention after pre-treatment with clopidogrel. Eur Heart J 2005;26:1379–84.
18. Elezi S, Kastrati A, Pache J et al. Diabetes mellitus and the clinical and angiographic outcome after coronary stent placement. J Am Coll Cardiol 1998;32:1866–73.
19. Lincoff AM. Important triad in cardiovascular medicine: diabetes, coronary intervention, and platelet glycoprotein IIb/IIIa receptor blockade. Circulation 2003;107:1556–9.
20. Mehilli J, Kastrati A, Schühlen H et al. Randomized clinical trial of abciximab in diabetic patients undergoing elective percutaneous coronary interventions after treatment with a high loading dose of clopidogrel. Circulation 2004;110:3627–35.
21. Hausleiter J, Kastrati A, Mehilli J et al. A randomized trial comparing phosphorylcholine-coated stenting with balloon angioplasty as well as abciximab with placebo for restenosis reduction in small coronary arteries. J Intern Med 2004;256:388–97.

22. The ERASER Investigators. Acute platelet inhibition with abciximab does not reduce in-stent restenosis (ERASER study). Circulation 1999;100:799–806.

23. Schühlen H, Kastrati A, Mehilli J et al. Abciximab and angiographic restenosis after coronary stent placement. Analysis of the angiographic substudy of ISAR-REACT – a double-blind, placebo-controlled, randomized trial evaluating abciximab in patients undergoing elective percutaneous coronary interventions after pretreatment with a high loading dose of clopidogrel. Am Heart J 2006;151:1248–54.

24. Topol EJ, Moliterno DJ, Herrmann HC et al. Comparison of two platelet glycoprotein IIb/IIIa inhibitors, tirofiban and abciximab, for the prevention of ischemic events with percutaneous coronary revascularization. N Engl J Med 2001;344:1888–94.

25. Braunwald E, Antman EM, Beasley JW et al. ACC/AHA 2002 guideline update for the management of patients with unstable angina and non-ST-segment elevation myocardial infarction – summary article: a report of the American College of Cardiology/American Heart Association task force on practice guidelines (Committee on the Management of Patients With Unstable Angina). J Am Coll Cardiol 2002;40:1366–74.

26. Mehta SR, Cannon CP, Fox KA et al. Routine vs selective invasive strategies in patients with acute coronary syndromes: a collaborative meta-analysis of randomized trials. JAMA 2005;293:2908–17.

27. Laskey WK, Williams DO, Vlachos HA et al. Changes in the practice of percutaneous coronary intervention: a comparison of enrollment waves in the National Heart, Lung, and Blood Institute (NHLBI) Dynamic Registry. Am J Cardiol 2001;87:964–9; A963–4.

28. Ault KA, Cannon CP, Mitchell J et al. Platelet activation in patients after an acute coronary syndrome: results from the TIMI-12 trial. Thrombolysis in Myocardial Infarction. J Am Coll Cardiol 1999;33:634–9.

29. Schulman SP. Antiplatelet therapy in non-ST-segment elevation acute coronary syndromes. JAMA 2004;292:1875–82.

30. The CAPTURE Investigator. Randomised placebo-controlled trial of abciximab before and during coronary intervention in refractory unstable angina: the CAPTURE Study. Lancet 1997;349:1429–35.

31. Hamm CW, Heeschen C, Goldmann B et al. Benefit of abciximab in patients with refractory unstable angina in relation to serum troponin T levels. c7E3 Fab Antiplatelet Therapy in Unstable Refractory Angina (CAPTURE) Study Investigators. N Engl J Med 1999; 340:1623–9.

32. Simoons ML. Effect of glycoprotein IIb/IIIa receptor blocker abciximab on outcome in patients with acute coronary syndromes without early coronary revascularisation: the GUSTO IV-ACS randomised trial. Lancet 2001;357:1915–24.

33. The PURSUIT Trial Investigators. Platelet Glycoprotein IIb/IIIa in Unstable Angina: Receptor Suppression Using Integrilin Therapy. Inhibition of platelet glycoprotein IIb/IIIa with eptifibatide in patients with acute coronary syndromes. N Engl J Med 1998;339:436–43.

34. Platelet Receptor Inhibition in Ischemic Syndrome Management (PRISM) Study Investigators. A comparison of aspirin plus tirofiban with aspirin plus heparin for unstable angina. N Engl J Med 1998;338:1498–505.

35. Platelet Receptor Inhibition in Ischemic Syndrome Management in Patients Limited by Unstable Signs and Symptoms (PRISM-PLUS) Study Investigators. Inhibition of the platelet glycoprotein IIb/IIIa receptor with tirofiban in unstable angina and non-Q-wave myocardial infarction. N Engl J Med 1998;338:1488–97.

36. Valgimigli M, Percoco G, Barbieri D et al. The additive value of tirofiban administered with the high-dose bolus in the prevention of ischemic complications during high-risk coronary angioplasty: the ADVANCE trial. J Am Coll Cardiol 2004;44:14–19.

37. Dawson CB, Valgimigli M, Charnigo R et al. Meta-analysis of high-doses single-bolus tirofiban versus abciximab in patients undergoing percutaneous coronary interventions. In: American Heart Association Scientific Sessions 2006: Abst 3071.

38. Kastrati A, Mehilli J, Neumann FJ et al. Abciximab in patients with acute coronary syndromes undergoing percutaneous coronary intervention after clopidogrel pretreatment: the ISAR-REACT 2 randomized trial. JAMA 2006;295:1531–8.

39. Stone GW, Bertrand ME, Moses JW et al. Routine upstream initiation vs deferred selective use of glycoprotein IIb/IIIa inhibitors in acute coronary syndromes: the ACUITY timing trial. JAMA 2007;297: 591–602.

40. Stone GW, Grines CL, Cox DA et al. Comparison of angioplasty with stenting, with or without abciximab, in acute myocardial infarction. N Engl J Med 2002;346:957–66.

41. Zijlstra F, Hoorntje JC, de Boer MJ et al. Long-term benefit of primary angioplasty as compared with thrombolytic therapy for acute myocardial infarction. N Engl J Med 1999;341:1413–19.

42. Schömig A, Kastrati A, Dirschinger J et al. Coronary stenting plus platelet glycoprotein IIb/IIIa blockade compared with tissue plasminogen activator in acute myocardial infarction. Stent versus Thrombolysis for Occluded Coronary Arteries in Patients with Acute Myocardial Infarction Study Investigators. N Engl J Med 2000;343:385–91.

43. Kastrati A, Mehilli J, Dirschinger J et al. Myocardial salvage after coronary stenting plus abciximab versus fibrinolysis plus abciximab in patients with acute myocardial infarction: a randomised trial. Lancet 2002;359:920–5.

44. Brener SJ, Barr LA, Burchenal JE et al. Randomized, placebo-controlled trial of platelet glycoprotein IIb/IIIa blockade with primary angioplasty for acute myocardial infarction. ReoPro and Primary PTCA Organization and Randomized Trial (RAPPORT) Investigators. Circulation 1998;98:734–41.

45. Montalescot G, Barragan P, Wittenberg O et al. Platelet glycoprotein IIb/IIIa inhibition with coronary stenting for acute myocardial infarction. N Engl J Med 2001;344:1895–903.

46. Neumann FJ, Kastrati A, Schmitt C et al. Effect of glycoprotein IIb/IIIa receptor blockade with abciximab on clinical and angiographic restenosis rate after the placement of coronary stents following acute myocardial infarction. J Am Coll Cardiol 2000;35:915–21.

47. Valgimigli M, Percoco G, Malagutti P et al. Tirofiban and sirolimus-eluting stent vs abciximab and bare-metal stent for acute myocardial infarction: a randomized trial. JAMA 2005;293: 2109–17.

48. Gibson CM, Kirtane AJ, Murphy SA et al. Early initiation of eptifibatide in the emergency department before primary percutaneous coronary intervention for ST-segment elevation myocardial infarction: results of the Time to Integrilin Therapy in Acute Myocardial Infarction (TITAN)-TIMI 34 trial. Am Heart J 2006; 152:668–75.

49. Montalescot G, Borentain M, Payot L et al. Early vs late administration of glycoprotein IIb/IIIa inhibitors in primary percutaneous coronary intervention of acute ST-segment elevation myocardial infarction: a meta-analysis. JAMA 2004;292:362–6.

50. Maioli M, Bellandi F, Leoncini M et al. Randomized early versus late abciximab in acute myocardial infarction treated with primary coronary intervention (RELAx-AMI Trial). J Am Coll Cardiol 2007;49: 1517–24.

51. Ellis SG. Final results of the FINESSE (Facilitated INtervention with Enhanced Reperfusion Speed to Stop Events) trial: evaluation of abciximab + half-dose reteplase, abciximab alone, or placebo for facilitation of primary PCI for ST elevation MI. In: ESC Congress 2007.

52. De Luca G, Suryapranata H, Stone GW et al. Abciximab as adjunctive therapy to reperfusion in acute ST-segment elevation myocardial infarction: a meta-analysis of randomized trials. JAMA 2005;293: 1759–65.

53. Stone GW. HORIZONS AMI: A Prospective, andomized comparison of bivalirudin vs heparin plus glycoprotein IIb/IIa inhibitors during primary angioplasty in acute myocardial infarction: 30-day results. In: TCT 2007.

14

Cangrelor

Thomas P Carrigan and Deepak L Bhatt

Introduction

The discovery that platelets are significant mediators of arterial thrombosis has led to the development of drugs to treat and prevent thrombosis, such as aspirin and clopidogrel. Both are used in the management of thrombotic events, particularly in the setting of acute coronary syndromes (ACS) and in the prevention of acute stent thrombosis following percutaneous interventions. Clopidogrel's mechanism of action is through the $P2Y_{12}$ receptor, preventing adenosine diphosphate (ADP) mediated platelet aggregation. However, the effect is delayed by several hours and the inhibition is irreversible. Cangrelor, on the other hand, is a new intravenous agent that rapidly and reversibly inhibits the $P2Y_{12}$ receptor, potentially ushering in a new, more flexible era in the management of acute thrombotic events. The use of cangrelor has been studied in several animal models and initial human trials. Here we present these reports and ongoing phase III trials currently in enrollment.

Background

Clopidogrel, a member of the thienopyridine class of antiplatelet drugs, has proven efficacy in the management of coronary artery disease and percutaneous interventions. However, as a pharmaceutical class, the thienopyridines have several limitations. Historically, the first thienopyridine on the market, ticlopidine, had efficacious antiplatelet activity but was also associated with a high incidence of potentially fatal hematologic dyscrasias, including thrombotic thrombocytopenic purpura. The unfavorable side-effect profile led to a decrease in its use in the United States and to widespread adoption of clopidogrel as the antiplatelet agent of choice.[1,2] As a prodrug, clopidogrel is converted into an active and irreversible platelet inhibitor by hepatic metabolization.[3] In the active form, clopidogrel binds irreversibly to the $P2Y_{12}$ platelet receptor, causing complete inhibition of platelet function until the bone marrow replaces the pharmacologically altered platelets 7–10 days later. This irreversibility presents a challenge in the management of ACS, especially in patients with unknown coronary anatomy, as surgical procedures could be delayed, or in emergent situations where significant blood loss could occur.

Despite efficacious antiplatelet activity, significant inter-individual responses to clopidogrel have been documented, prompting the coinage of the phrase 'clopidogrel resistance'. The wide variability has been associated with insufficient platelet inhibition and increased thrombotic events.[4] In the absence of a loading dose, maximum platelet inhibition takes 4–5 days to achieve, creating a lag in platelet inhibition that may explain the observation that 80% of stent thrombosis cases occur within 5 days of initiating thienopyridine treatment.[4,5] From the observed variability in achieving maximal platelet inhibition, multiple explanations have been reported, including interactions with simultaneous atorvastatin therapy,[6] differences in hepatic cytochrome function,[7] inability to convert the prodrug into an active compound,[8] and pre-existing platelet receptor variability.[9]

ADP-induced activation of the $P2Y_{12}$ receptor

Over 40 years ago, ADP was recognized as an activator of platelet aggregation and activation.[10] Since that time, the precise role that ADP plays in inducing platelet activation has been further elucidated. Under normal physiologic conditions, platelets circulate in the inactivated state (Figure 14.1a), becoming active (Figure 14.1b) in response to multiple initiators of thrombosis. One initiator is endothelial damage, which brings proaggregatory compounds, normally protected by the endothelium in the subendothelial matrix, into proximity with inactivated platelets.[11] Subsequent platelet activation – again by several different agonists – initiates shape change, aggregation, and secretion from granules of thrombogenic mediators, including ADP.[4] ADP, acting through the P2 class of platelet surface receptors, in the presence of other platelet agonists (i.e., collagen and thrombin), amplifies the activation of recruited platelets through a positive-feedback loop.[12] As platelet activation and aggregation accelerate, internalized cell surface molecules, including glycoprotein (GP) IIb/IIIa and P-selectin, are mobilized to the platelet membrane, binding to their respective receptors and stabilizing platelet aggregation.[11] The interplay of platelets and mediators continues as the thrombus grows and platelet-rich particles break off, embolizing downstream.

Three separate and distinct classes of P2 platelet transmembrane receptors exist: $P2X_1$, $P2Y_1$, and $P2Y_{12}$. Synergistic stimulation of these receptors by their respective agonists produces morphologic shape change followed by sustained aggregation. $P2X_1$ is gated ion channel receptor activated by adenosine triphosphate (ATP). Once activated, this receptor allows a rapid burst of calcium into the platelet initiating shape change.[13] Activation of $P2X_1$ is transient and rapidly reverses, thus, sustained morphologic shape change occurs only with subsequent activation of $P2Y_1$ by its agonist.[14] When activated by ADP, $P2Y_1$, a Gq-protein-coupled receptor, sustains platelet shape change by facilitating an increase of intracellular calcium. The $P2Y_1$ receptor also participates in ADP-induced platelet aggregation via a second ADP receptor $P2Y_{12}$. The $P2Y_{12}$ receptor is a Gi-coupled protein that acts through inhibition of intracellular cyclic adenosine monophosphate contributing to a complex biochemical mechanism that ends in sustained platelet aggregation.[4,12] Activation of $P2Y_{12}$ leads to downstream effects, including thrombin generation, P-selectin expression, and maintenance of GPIIb/IIIa expression, and contributing to other positive-feedback mechanisms that stimulate and sustain thrombus growth.[15,16] The $P2Y_{12}$ receptor is therefore crucial in sustaining platelet aggregation, secretion of thrombogenic mediators, and ultimately thrombus stability by affecting the quantity of GPIIb/IIIa receptors expressed on the platelet membrane.

Pharmacology

Cangrelor, known as AR-C69931MX during development, is a novel intravenously administered antithrombotic drug that reversibly inhibits the $P2Y_{12}$ platelet receptor, blocking ADP-induced platelet aggregation.[17] Its discovery came from early studies that found ATP to be a competitive inhibitor of ADP-induced platelet activation. Only much later was the ADP receptor cloned and subsequently identified as $P2Y_{12}$.[18] Since ATP is rapidly inactivated in vivo, it is not a suitable candidate for antithrombotic treatment.[19] However, chemical modification of ATP led to the discovery and development of cangrelor (Figure 14.2).

Expression of the $P2Y_{12}$ receptor is almost exclusively limited to platelets; this property made the $P2Y_{12}$ receptor an ideal target compared with the $P2Y_1$ receptor widely expressed in other tissues.[20] While the distribution of the $P2Y_{12}$ receptor is limited, it has also been found to be expressed in a subregion of the brain, resulting in increased intracellular calcium,[21] and in vascular smooth muscle, causing vasoconstriction.[22] Initial screens of the activity of cangrelor on other P2 receptors demonstrated no cross-reactivity. However, there has been a report in mice that cangrelor acts as a partial agonist of the $P2Y_{13}$ receptor, causing endocytosis of high-density lipoprotein by hepatocytes.[23]

Cangrelor is delivered intravenously, achieving near-complete platelet inactivation within minutes after a bolus dose.[24] Unlike the prodrug clopidogrel, cangrelor does not require hepatic conversion. Rather, it is immediately active upon infusion, achieving rapid steady-state concentrations.[25] Cangrelor has a very short half-life of 3.3 minutes, due to rapid and sequential dephosphorylation of the nucleoside triphosphate chain by ectonucleotidases located on endothelial and platelet surfaces.[19,26] Dephosphorylation results in metabolites that are 10 000 times less active than the parent compound.[24] Platelet function returns to preinfusion levels within 30–60 minutes after discontinuation.[24] The rapid inactivation makes cangrelor potentially very attractive for use in acute clinical situations, especially when bleeding complications may arise. The intravascular

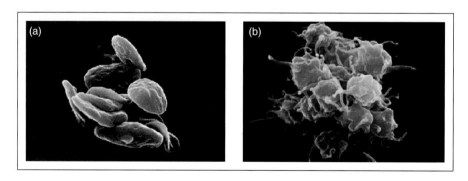

Figure 14.1
Exposure to subendothelial matrix substances convert inactive platelets (a) into a morphologically active and proaggregatory form (b). (Courtesy: Michael Rolf Mueller MD, Salat Andreas MD, Losert Udo MD; Medical University of Vienna.)

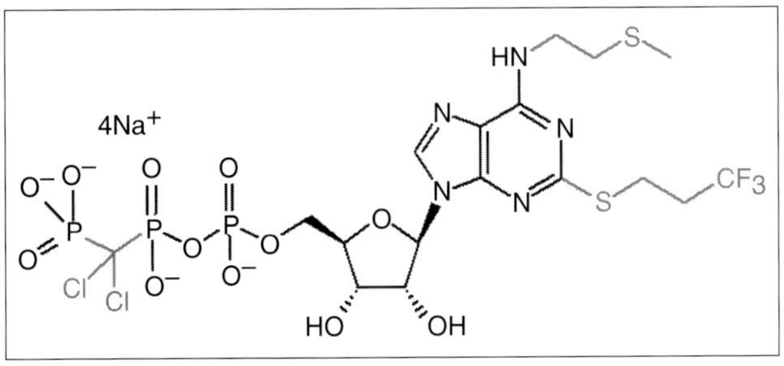

Figure 14.2
The inhibitory effects of cangrelor come from its molecular structure, which is analogous to that of the competitive antagonist ATP. During development, cangrelor was referred to as AR-C69931MX, where MX stands for the tetrasodium salt. (see color plate)

metabolism by ectonucleotidases will likely be clinically beneficial, as dose adjustments and accumulation should not be problematic when renal or hepatic dysfunction is present.[27] However, patients with underlying hepatic or renal impairment were excluded from phase II safety studies with cangrelor.[27,28] Ongoing phase III studies will help determine cangrelor's metabolic profile in these patient populations.

Animal studies

Preclinical animal studies with cangrelor demonstrated consistent and predictable antithrombotic effects. Inhibition of ex vivo ADP-induced platelet activation through the $P2Y_{12}$ receptor has been efficacious without causing excessive bleeding times at therapeutic concentrations.[17,29–32] Early animal studies demonstrated successful separation between antiplatelet function and effects on bleeding times. At supratherapeutic doses, significant fourfold increases in bleeding times were observed, but the maximum dose of cangrelor needed to achieve complete platelet inhibition was much lower.[17,32] In the first reported animal study, using canines, cangrelor prevented thrombus formation. This finding was subsequently reproduced in another dog model, thus confirming the drug's efficacy. In subsequent experiments that used rabbits and a thromboembolic model, cangrelor reduced the size and number of emboli during thromboembolism. Further investigation revealed cangrelor to be a successful adjunct to concurrent thrombolytic therapy, reducing the dose of thrombolytic needed to achieve vessel patency.

In 1999, the first reported animal study using anesthetized dogs was reported.[17] Cangrelor was compared with the glycoprotein inhibitors lamifiban, GR144053, and TP9201 in 22 dogs using a cyclic flow reduction (CFR) model originally described by Folts.[17,32,33] In this model, thrombosis is achieved via mechanical compression and partial stenosis of an artery. The glycoprotein inhibitors and cangrelor were administered as progressively increasing stepped infusions. Measurements were made of CFR (as a proxy for arterial thrombosis), ADP-induced platelet aggregation, and bleeding times, each of which was increased by all three of the glycoprotein inhibitors and by cangrelor. However, in the glycoprotein inhibitor group, statistically significant ($p < 0.05$) increases in bleeding times (fold increases from baseline: lamifibanm $= 4.0 \pm 0.9$ minutes; GR144053 $= 4.3 \pm 0.5$ minutes; TP9201 $= 3.7 \pm 0.8$ minutes) were observed at doses required to achieve complete CFR inhibition. On the other hand, significant increases in bleeding times of 4.3 ± 0.5-fold over baseline ($p < 0.01$) were also observed in the cangrelor group. However, this was only at the extreme upper end of dosing, 71–98 times higher than the dose needed to achieve maximal platelet inhibition.[17,32] At lower dosing schemes needed to achieve total platelet inhibition, only trends towards higher bleeding times were observed: 1.4 ± 0.3-fold over baseline.

Another important finding of this study was the drug's rapid reversal. Baseline platelet function returned within 10 minutes after discontinuing the study drug infusion. Antithrombotic medications that completely and specifically inhibit the $P2Y_{12}$ receptor without increasing the risk of hemorrhage are needed in the clinical setting. Future animal and human studies would build on the observed separation of bleeding times and antiplatelet effects.

A second investigation of cangrelor using electrically injured carotid dog arteries as a nidus for arterial thrombosis confirmed the separation of antiplatelet effects and bleeding time.[31] In this investigation, endothelial injury was elicited by an electric current applied to the intimal surface, which exposed the subendothelial thrombogenic matrix to circulating blood products causing progressive thrombus formation. The current was then applied to the vessel wall continuously for 3 hours while the carotid artery flow rate was observed simultaneously and for 3 hours post procedure. Eleven dogs were randomized to receive either intravenous cangrelor ($n = 6$) or a saline placebo ($n = 5$). The cangrelor group received a 6-hour infusion (4 μg/kg/min), beginning 15 minutes prior to application of the current. Bleeding times were also recorded in both groups by periodic tongue and buccal mucosal incisions using a reproducible SurgiCut device. Each dog underwent a postmortem carotid artery examination and concomitant thrombus dissection and weighing.

In the treatment group, only one dog (16.7%) had complete arterial occlusion, versus all five dogs (100%) in the placebo group. Cangrelor infusion doubled the length of time to thrombus formation in the one animal that developed complete occlusion (106 minutes vs 195 minutes) The antithrombotic effects of cangrelor significantly decreased the weight of thrombus by 83% (47 mg vs 8 mg; $p < 0.05$). Buccal and tongue bleeding times were significantly elevated in the cangrelor group, with a time-dependent increase noted from study hour 1 through

6, 2–3.4-fold and 3.5–4.4-fold ($p < 0.05$) increases respectively. Ex vivo ADP-induced aggregation was prevented with near-complete inhibition at doses of 4 µg/kg/min. Cangrelor was well tolerated in the dogs; no hematologic or physiologic abnormalities were observed during the study. Bleeding parameters returned to preinfusion levels within 1 hour of infusion cessation, further supporting the reversible nature of cangrelor.

Another study investigated the role of the P2Y$_{12}$ receptor in embolic events using a rabbit model ($n = 65$). At the time of this study, ADP had been identified as a key moderator of thrombosis, yet its role in embolic events had not been explored.[29] Rabbit mesenteric arteries were dissected through an abdominal incision, and the microvasculature was visualized via microscopy. Using the tip of a micropipette, the arterioles were punctured, causing white (platelet-rich) thrombus formation and subsequent downstream embolization of platelet-rich emboli. The optimal dose that achieved maximal platelet inhibition was 3 µg/kg/min, which reduced aggregation by 71% ± 6% and ex vivo thrombin generation by 25% ± 7% ($p = 0.06$). Higher doses of cangrelor did not reduce levels of thrombin production. Following puncture of the arteriole, thrombus formation occurred within 1–2 s. The height of the primary thrombus was calculated as a percentage of vessel diameter. Cangrelor significantly decreased the height of the thrombus by 20% ($p < 0.005$). Vessel bleeding times, however, were not affected (4.9 minutes in controls ($n = 29$) vs 2.9 minutes with the study drug ($n = 36$); $p = 0.57$). The occurrence of rebleeding was similar between the controls and the study drug group (24% vs 28%). Steady-state doses of clopidogrel were also studied, with results similar to those of cangrelor, confirming blockade of the P2Y$_{12}$ receptor.

Downstream emboli were observed on average to last 469 s in the control group, with 11 rabbits having embolic events lasting > 600 s. Comparatively, the embolization time lasted for 228 s in the cangrelor group and only one rabbit had emboli occurring after 600 s. Significant qualitative differences in embolic phenomena were observed between the treatment and control groups ($p = 0.001$). The control group had, on average, 14 emboli, with a median size of 10–15 µm, whereas the cangrelor group had an average of 8 emboli ($p = 0.01$), with a median size of 5–10 µm ($p < 0.01$). Similar results were seen in the clopidogrel group.

Comparing the sizes of emboli by study arm revealed significantly smaller emboli in the cangrelor group ($p \leq 0.05$). Adherence rates were similar between groups (4.8 platelets/min vs 3.9 platelets/min; $p = 0.39$), despite the smaller emboli in the cangrelor group. The similar adherence rates suggest that while the overall rate of emboli formation was unchanged, cangrelor reduced the size of the thrombus, and the resultant embolic platelet aggregates were too small to be detected. Furthermore, cangrelor could potentially preserve downstream tissue perfusion through a reduced number and smaller emboli. Measured bleeding times in the cangrelor-treated group were prolonged when compared with controls (7.0 minutes vs 20.5 minutes) consistent with previous studies.

In another study, cangrelor (4 µg/kg/min) or saline placebo was combined with thrombolytics tissue-type plasminogen activator (tPA), aspirin, and heparin in a dog coronary thrombosis model.[30] Mechanical occlusion and partial stenosis of the coronary artery caused thrombosis in coronary arteries. The arteries were monitored for complete occlusion using CFR. When complete stenosis was achieved, thrombolytic treatment was infused. Combination treatment with cangrelor significantly prevented reocclusion ($p < 0.05$) in all study animals. Interestingly microvascular perfusion measured with contrast echocardiography significantly improved at 20 minutes ($p = 0.01$) and 120 minutes ($p = 0.001$). Postmortem exam showed that the total infarct size was significantly reduced by 51% ($p < 0.05$) in the cangrelor-treated group. In second phase of this study, the dose of tPA was reduced by 50% with identical findings. Bleeding times were again noted to be significantly prolonged in the cangrelor group (1.8–2.8-fold; $p < 0.001$).

An important implication of this study is that tissue perfusion was restored at the microvascular level. Taken in combination with previous findings, cangrelor has the potential to prevent thrombus formation and embolic phenomena, and, when combined with thrombolytics, to restore vessel patency, reverse microvascular ischemia, and improve blood flow in downstream capillary beds.

The human experience

The first study of cangrelor in healthy humans was reported by Nassim et al in 1999.[25] Male and female volunteers received four 1-hour escalating dose range infusions of cangrelor (over the dose range 10–4000 µg/kg/min), with the maximum dose extending for 19 hours. Cangrelor infusion, measured ex vivo, caused dose-dependent inhibition of ADP-induced platelet aggregation. Pharmacologic parameters were favorable, with cangrelor achieving rapid steady-state concentrations with a clearance of 50 liters/h and a short half-life of 2.6 minutes. Infusions were well tolerated, with only minor increases of petechiae or bruising in the cangrelor group. Once the infusion was discontinued, rapid and complete reversal of platelet inhibition occurred after 20 minutes, with no observed rebound effect in platelet activity. Importantly, there was an observed separation between antiplatelet activity and bleeding times, which were increased by 3.2-fold over baseline in males and 2.9-fold over baseline in females. There were no pharmacokinetic differences in cangrelor metabolism between sexes. This study confirmed the previously observed separation of bleeding times and antiplatelet activity reported in the animal models, suggesting that cangrelor would be similarly well tolerated in humans.

A subsequent study compared cangrelor in eight healthy male subjects with in vitro administered cangrelor.[34] Subjects received clopidogrel administered at 75 mg daily with serially measured ADP-induced platelet aggregation (APA) at days 0, 1, 2, 3, and 11. The observed ex vivo antiplatelet effects of clopidogrel slowly increased over this time period, with considerable interindividual variability. None of the study subjects had complete inhibition of APA over the 11-day period until cangrelor was added in vitro. The addition of cangrelor achieved rapid and complete platelet inhibition, conversely by day 11: APA was only 46% ± 10% of baseline. In this study, clopidogrel as monotherapy demonstrates slow and incomplete inhibition of the $P2Y_{12}$ receptor that, despite proven efficacy, leaves functionally active receptors available for platelet aggregation.

Cangrelor as an adjunct to thrombolysis improves TIMI 3 flow during STEMI

In animals, cangrelor demonstrated sustained arterial patency when used adjunctively with intravenous thrombolytics in the setting of experimentally induced thrombosis.[30] Overall, thrombus burden, size of emboli, and downstream tissue perfusion were favourable over platelets in the cangrelor-treated group. However, whether these positive effects would translate to humans receiving similar therapy in acute thrombosis was unknown.

In an early report, the STEP-AMI (Safety, Tolerability, and Effect on Patency in Acute Myocardial Infarction) trial investigated cangrelor as adjunctive therapy with thrombolytics in patients presenting with ST-segment-elevation myocardial infarction (STEMI).[35] During the study, (tPA) was used as the thrombolytic in 101 patients presenting with STEMI. In each of the five different treatment arms, patients received a 280 µg/min cangrelor infusion alone, a full dose of thrombolytic alone, or a reduced dose (50 mg) of thrombolytic plus three different continuous-infusion doses of cangrelor (35, 140, or 280 µg/kg/min) over a 60-minute period.

Angiographic evidence of intracoronary reperfusion showed no significant differences in the primary endpoint, Thrombolysis in Myocardial Infarction (TIMI) 3 flow, when thrombolytics with or without cangrelor were given. In patients receiving full-strength thrombolytic alone, 50% of patients achieved TIMI 3 flow. Similarly, on combining reduced-strength thrombolytic, with any dose of cangrelor, TIMI 3 flow occurred in 57% of patients. However, cangrelor, without thrombolytic, offered no reperfusion benefit, and was, in fact, worse than thrombolytic alone with only 19% of patients attaining TIMI 3 Flow. On electrocardiography (EKG), patients with >70% ST-segment elevation showed trends toward improved ST-segment recovery in the groups receiving cangrelor. Across treatment groups, cangrelor was well tolerated, with no differences in 30-day major adverse cardiovascular events (MACE) or non-coronary artery bypass graft (CABG)-related TIMI major bleeds[36] (cangrelor + reduced dose tPA = 20% and tPA alone = 17%; p = NS). With cangrelor infusion, a reduction in thrombolytic dose achieved similar rates of TIMI 3 flow. This suggests that there would be no treatment tradeoff with reduced doses of thrombolytic and concurrent cangrelor infusion. This could have the dual benefit of improving myocardial perfusion without the risk of serious bleeding complications such as intracranial hemorrhage.

Phase II cangrelor studies have demonstrated safety and efficacy

The first safety assessment of cangrelor came from an open-label study in 39 patients presenting with ACS in the UK and the Netherlands.[27] All patients received ascending stepped dose infusions of cangrelor plus aspirin, as-needed nitrate therapy, and anticoagulation with unfractionated heparin (UFH) or low-molecular-weight heparin (LMWH). Cangrelor demonstrated a consistent dose-dependent effect on platelet inhibition, with steady-state plasma concentrations being achieved within 30 minutes of continuous infusion. When platelet aggregation was measured ex vivo, the average level of inhibition was similar between doses ranging from 0.2 to 2.0 µg/kg/min. Only when plateau infusions were increased to greater than 2.0 µg/kg/min did all patients achieve >80% inhibition. From the dose range between 2.0 and 4.0 µg/kg/min, variability in platelet inhibition between patients was decreased, with 74% of patients having 100% inhibition of platelet aggregation. Independent of the dose received, a rapid decline in inhibition occurred upon cessation. Within 1 hour after discontinuing the infusion, platelet function had recovered to >60% of baseline levels in 70% of the patients. Despite increases in bleeding times, there were no severe bleeds by TIMI minor or major criteria.[36] However, trivial bleeding was frequently reported. Measured bleeding times increased as the length of infusion was extended from 24 to 72 hours and the plateau dose doubled to 4.0 µg/kg/min. Further analysis between cangrelor plasma concentration and bleeding times revealed no correlation. The authors cited variations in the pharmacokinetic profiles of LMWH and UFH for the increases in bleeding times, which were not seen with cangrelor.

Adverse events were common in this study. At least one adverse event was reported in 85% of study patients. The most frequent event occurred at the injection site. One patient experienced phlebitis at the cannulation site and nine others reported slight bleeding. The second most common adverse event was elevations in alanine aminotransferase occurring in eight patients; abnormalities in aspartate aminotransferase were less common, in four patients. Purpura, dyspnea, and hematuria were equally the next most reported events. In 38% of patients, elevations in creatinine or urea occurred at some point during the study. Hematologic parameters showed no effect from the study drug infusion. There were no reports of thrombocytopenia or drops in hemoglobin. While adverse events were frequent, this was an open-label study without a placebo group for comparison.

A second phase II Swedish study assessed the safety and tolerability of cangrelor in 91 patients with unstable angina and non-ST-segment-elevation myocardial infarction (NSTEMI) randomized to cangrelor or placebo.[28] In addition to the study compound, patients received aspirin or LMWH. Patients were included if they had unstable angina plus new ischemic EKG changes, known ischemic heart disease, or elevation of cardiac biomarkers consistent with MI. Patients were excluded on presentation if they were hemodynamically unstable, presented with STEMI, required thrombolytics, percutaneous intervention, or had an increased risk of bleeding, kidney impairment, or known liver disease. Cangrelor was administered as a continuous infusion of $4 \mu g/kg/min$ for 72 hours and was initiated as an ascending dose over 19 hours. Despite randomization, the two groups were not identical. Patients in the cangrelor group were more likely to be older or female, and had lower body weights. Measured pharmacokinetic parameters were similar to those in previous studies. Cangrelor was rapidly cleared (44.3 ± 6.4 liters/h) from a small volume of distribution (5.10 ± 1.77 liters). At a concentration of $4.0 \mu g/kg/min$, cangrelor achieved a calculated steady-state plasma concentration of 401 ng/ml.

Cangrelor was well tolerated, with a side-effect profile mirroring that of the placebo group. Rates of adverse bleeding events were similar between the groups. During the index hospital admission, there were no major bleeds occurring in either group during infusion of either the study drug or placebo. Following discharge, one patient experienced a major gastrointestinal bleed 15 days after receiving cangrelor, which, given cangrelor's short half-life, is likely unrelated. The rates of minor bleeding events were slightly higher in the cangrelor group (38% vs 26%), but did not achieve statistical significance.

Other reported adverse events included one death during the study. A patient receiving cangrelor acutely decompensated 24 hours following infusion, when a papillary muscle ruptured. There was also a significantly ($p < 0.05$) higher rate of mild respiratory disorders during the cangrelor infusion. These symptoms were not present during follow-up 1 month later. Patients randomized to the study drug reported statistically significant lower rates of angina compared with placebo. Conversely, one patient developed unstable angina 27 hours after the infusion. The authors suggest that this could be explained by a reactivation phenomenon in which, following reversal of $P2Y_{12}$ blockade by cangrelor, the platelets through an unknown pathway became active again, precipitating an ischemic event. Although not powered to assess efficacy, there were no differences in the number of endpoints, including percutaneous transluminal coronary angiography (PTCA), CABG, myocardial infarction (MI), death, or angina at 1 month.

The randomization process helped clarify the observed elevations in laboratory values. Elevations in liver function tests, creatinine, and blood urea seen previously were likely from variation and not the study drug. Hematologic parameters, including hemoglobin and hematocrit, showed no significant differences between groups. The report did not mention the presence or absence of thrombocytopenia.

Cangrelor is safe and effective during PCI

During coronary interventions, the vascular endothelium underlying the stent is universally damaged. Exposing the underlying prothrombotic subendothelial matrix necessitates antiplatelet therapy to prevent acute vessel closure and stent thrombosis. To date, clopidogrel has been used for preventing these dire complications. However, its pharmacologic profile combined with patient variability can be problematic. Even with high loading doses of clopidogrel, maximum and timely inhibition is not guaranteed. Cangrelor, on the other hand, rapidly blocks ADP-induced platelet aggregation, which might make it an ideal agent during PCI.

The safety and tolerability of cangrelor was reported in a two-part study, demonstrating favorable results.[37] In both parts, patients undergoing PCI received 325 mg of aspirin and weight-adjusted UFH. In part 1, 200 patients were randomized to three different continuous cangrelor infusions of 1.0, 2.0, or $4.0 \mu g/kg/min$ or placebo. The infusions began just prior to the coronary intervention and were continued for 18–24 hours after PCI.

In the first group, four patients (8%) receiving the highest concentration of cangrelor experienced a major bleed, compared with none in the placebo group ($p = 0.052$). Attributing the trend towards increased rate of major bleeds to cangrelor alone was confounded by the presence of other patient-specific bleeding risks, including concommittant surgical revascularization, simultaneous glycoprotein inhibitor therapy, or patient non-compliance following left heart catheterization (premature ambulation). At lower infusion doses, there was no observed dose–response relationship between rates of minor bleeds and infusion concentration. There was also no statistical difference in thrombocytopenia (defined by a drop in platelets to $100 000/mm^3$ or less) between cangrelor and placebo, occurring in 1% and 0%, respectively. Secondary endpoints, measured by a composite of clinical outcomes (MI, death, and reintervention) at 2-, 7-, and 30-day intervals between groups were similar between cangrelor and placebo. The authors noted that patients randomized to placebo had a higher rate of reinterventions between 1 week and the end of the study. Despite the short half-life of cangrelor, the authors hypothesize a possible delayed benefit from acutely inhibiting proinflammatory growth factors. In another study, the proinflammatory interactions of platelet–leukocyte conjugate formation were decreased by cangrelor, which may be one possible mechanism contributing to the observed benefit.[38]

With the positive safety results, part 2 of the study included 199 patients undergoing PCI, who were randomized to cangrelor or abciximab. Patients received infusions of either cangrelor ($4\,\mu g/kg/min$) or abciximab ($0.25\,mg/kg$) throughout the procedure. Patients' anticoagulation with heparin was adjusted down in an attempt to avoid the major bleeds experienced during part 1.

Cangrelor was well tolerated throughout the study, with no statistically significant TIMI major or minor bleeds reported. Bleeding times, as a ratio of the baseline, were almost double in the cangrelor group (2.07) and triple in the abciximab group (3.05) when compared with placebo alone (1.14). In a head to head comparison between abciximab and cangrelor, at steady state concentrations, abciximab had a bleeding time 1.6 times higher than any dose of cangrelor. Thrombocytopenia occurred in 1% of patients receiving cangrelor, but this was significantly less often when compared with the 7% of abciximab-treated patients ($p = 0.025$).

Platelet function measured ex vivo demonstrated rapid platelet inhibition and reversal in both parts of the study. Within 15 minutes after discontinuing cangrelor, mean platelet aggregation began to return to baseline, whereas patients receiving abciximab had persistent inhibition of mean platelet aggregation beyond 24 hours. There were no significant differences in 30-day outcomes as measured by a composite of death, MI, or reintervention in part 2.[37] While the secondary endpoints were comparable independent of antiplatelet agent, the study was not designed or powered to assess outcomes.[37]

In another study, the pharmacodynamic effects of cangrelor during PCI were compared with those of clopidogrel in patients with known ischemic heart disease.[39,40] A small group of 13 patients with NSTEMI received open-label cangrelor at $2.0\,\mu g/kg/min$ ($n = 8$) or $4.0\,\mu g/kg/min$ ($n = 5$). A second group of patients undergoing coronary stenting were loaded with 300 mg clopidogrel at implantation and maintained on 75 mg daily. Platelet function was then measured ex vivo using whole-blood single-platelet counting. Doubling the dose of cangrelor showed no differences in inhibition of ADP-induced platelet aggregation ($p = 0.22$). However, when comparing any dose of cangrelor with clopidogrel, a higher level of inhibition occurred in cangrelor-treated individuals. Plasma samples from the clopidogrel group were then inoculated with cangrelor in vitro. Not only did this addition demonstrate superior antiplatelet effects compared to clopidogrel alone, but also the antiplatelet effect was additive ($p < 0.05$) when cangrelor was given after clopidogrel.

Clopidogrel and cangrelor block thrombosis by similarly inhibiting the P2Y$_{12}$ receptor, preventing platelet-induced amplification from ADP induced segregation. However, both agents have uniquely different biochemical affinities for the active receptor site. Clopidogrel irreversibly binds the P2Y$_{12}$ receptor and cangrelor reversibly blocks it. Furthermore, at therapeutic doses of clopidogrel, active P2Y$_{12}$ receptors remain.[41] During a pharmacodynamic comparison, cangrelor demonstrated superior platelet inhibition over clopidogrel even when an effective loading dose was employed.[39] Defining the potential pharmacological interaction between clopidogrel and cangrelor is paramount in optimizing antiplatelet function when transitioning from acute to chronic settings.

With simultaneous administration, cangrelor interferes with the mechanism of action of clopidogrel

A recent study in 20 healthy volunteers explored the treatment strategy when transitioning from cangrelor to clopidogrel.[42] In this two-arm study, each group of 10 subjects received cangrelor as a $30\,\mu g/kg$ intravenous bolus followed by a continuous $4\,\mu g/kg/min$ infusion for 1–2 hours and a 600 mg loading dose of clopidogrel. The loading dose was given either at the beginning of the infusion or immediately upon discontinuation. Platelet activity was then measured ex vivo by whole-blood impedance aggregometry, light transmittance aggregometry, and flow cytometry. Each experimental methodology has been previously validated to accurately measure platelet function.[43]

In all study subjects, cangrelor was well tolerated, with no adverse events. When given alone, cangrelor and clopidogrel each demonstrated consistent levels of platelet inhibition measured across all ex vivo diagnostic modalities. By itself, cangrelor achieved >83% inhibition within 2–5 minutes of dosing and returned to 60–95% baseline platelet activity within 20–40 minutes, depending on the diagnostic modality. When clopidogrel was given at the end of cangrelor infusion, complete inhibition of platelet function occurred between 3 and 6 hours later. Despite recent P2Y$_{12}$ blockade by cangrelor, the measured length of time to complete platelet inhibition by clopidogrel was identical when compared with subjects receiving oral doses of clopidogrel only. This suggests that when transitioning from intravenous to oral P2Y$_{12}$ receptor inhibitors, there may be a temporary 'unprotected window' of unblocked P2Y$_{12}$ receptor activity that lasts from as little as 2 hours to as many as 6 hours.

When cangrelor and clopidogrel are administered at the same time, maximal blockade of platelet function is achieved within minutes of starting the cangrelor infusion and continues until the infusion is stopped. However, the long lasting effect of clopidogrel is delayed and is not as robust when compared to sequential administration of the two drugs.

If cangrelor is present in the circulation when clopidogrel is given, the level of long term platelet inhibition is only about 25% of that achieved when clopidogrel is given as monotherapy. The authors note that clopdigrel metabolism undergoes a first-pass effect in the portal system. When cangrelor is present in the portal circulation, irreversible binding of the active clopidogrel metabolite to the $P2Y_{12}$ receptor does not occur. Conversely, when clopidogrel is given immediately after cangrelor infusion, long term and maximum platelet inhibition is achieved. These findings demonstrate not only that cangrelor limits the long term irreversible effects on platelet function, but also, that cangrelor does not have long lasting metabolites that interfere with clopidogrel's mechanism of action.

This study has important implications regarding the timing of clopidogrel administration following cangrelor infusion. These findings strongly support sequencing the use of $P2Y_{12}$ receptor inhibitors as opposed to simultaneous administration. In the acute setting, administering cangrelor would result in immediate antiplatelet inactivity. Following the acute management, patients could then transition to chronic treatment with clopidogrel. However, in patients already at a steady-state level of clopidogrel, use of cangrelor would not be expected to be problematic. Problems would only arise in clopidogrel naive populations during simultaneous administration. If cangrelor passes Phase 3 clinical testing, prior clopidogrel use will be critical component of the patient's history prior to PCI.

Phase III

Two phase III trials are currently enrolling patients for further evaluation of cangrelor. The CHAMPION (Cangrelor versus standard tHerapy to Achieve optimal Management of Platelet InhibitiON), Platform study is a prospective, randomized controlled trial to evaluate the efficacy of cangrelor in clopidogrel-naive patients undergoing PCI.[44] Over 200 clinical sites worldwide will be involved, enrolling more than 4000 patients. This double-blind study will randomize patients to a 30 µg/kg bolus and 4 µg/kg/min infusion of cangrelor. Following the cangrelor bolus, the infusion will last for a minimum of 2 hours or the length of the procedure. Patients will then receive a 600 mg loading dose of clopidogrel, followed by 75 mg daily. The primary endpoints are efficacy and a clinical composite of death, MI, or ischemia-driven revascularization within 48 hours of cangrelor infusion.

A second phase III trial, CHAMPION PCI, is currently enrolling patients to evaluate the efficacy of cangrelor in patients requiring PCI.[45] More than 400 centers worldwide are enrolling patients in this prospective, double-dummy, double-blind, active control study. Patients will be randomized to one of two study arms. The first arm will consist of a cangrelor bolus (30 µg/kg) and infusion (4 µg/kg/min)

given immediately prior to the index procedure. The study drug will run during the length of the intervention for at least 2 hours, or the duration of the procedure if it is longer. Study center physicians will have the option to continue the infusion after the procedure for a maximum length of 4 hours, after which a 600 mg clopidogrel loading dose will be given. The second study arm will receive a placebo bolus/infusion and a loading dose of clopidogrel during PCI, with infusion lasting up to 4 hours. The study endpoints are measurements of safety and efficacy at 48 hours.

Conclusions

Cangrelor is a novel intravenous ADP receptor antagonist with a very short half-life. Early animal studies demonstrated that cangrelor, which is specific for the $P2Y_{12}$ receptor, had a low risk of bleeding, with the benefit of complete inhibition of platelet function that helped define the threshold of separation between antiplatelet function and bleeding times. Initial human testing seems promising. In phase I and II studies, cangrelor has been shown to achieve superior levels of antiplatelet function when compared with clopidogrel. Cangrelor has also demonstrated improved performance when compared with glycoprotein inhibitors, without the increased risk of bleeding and long duration of action. Ongoing phase III trials will determine the ultimate role of cangrelor in clinical practice. The drug seems to be an ideal treatment for patients presenting with ACS or undergoing PCI who need quick and effective antithrombotic therapy that is easily reversible if bleeding complications develop. Should cangrelor prove to be efficacious, the management of ACS and PCI could be significantly improved. Furthermore, the drug holds potential appeal in STEMI, stroke, and a variety of other situations where quick, effective, and safe antithrombotic therapy is warranted.

References

1. Boeynaems JM, van Giezen H, Savi P, Herbert JM. P2Y receptor antagonists in thrombosis. Curr Opin Invest Drugs 2005;6:275–82.
2. Paradiso-Hardy FL, Angelo CM, Lanctot KL, Cohen EA. Hematologic dyscrasia associated with ticlopidine therapy: evidence for causality. CMAJ 2000;163:1441–8.
3. Savi P, Combalbert J, Gaich C et al. The antiaggregating activity of clopidogrel is due to a metabolic activation by the hepatic cytochrome P450-1A. Thromb Haemost 1994;72:313–17.
4. Cattaneo M. P2Y12 receptor antagonists: a rapidly expanding group of antiplatelet agents. Eur Heart J 2006;27:1010–12.
5. Cutlip DE, Baim DS, Ho KK et al. Stent thrombosis in the modern era: a pooled analysis of multicenter coronary stent clinical trials. Circulation 2001;103:1967–71.
6. Neubauer H, Mugge A. Thienopyridines and statins: assessing a potential drug–drug interaction. Curr Pharm Des 2006;12:1271–80.
7. Lau WC, Gurbel PA, Watkins PB et al. Contribution of hepatic cytochrome P450 3A4 metabolic activity to the phenomenon of clopidogrel resistance. Circulation 2004;109:166–71.

8. Heestermans AA, van Werkum JW, Schomig E et al. Clopidogrel resistance caused by a failure to metabolize clopidogrel into its metabolites. J Thromb Haemost 2006;45:1143–5.

9. Michelson AD, Linden MD, Furman MI et al. Evidence that pre-existent variability in platelet response to ADP accounts for 'clopidogrel resistance'. J Thromb Haemost 2006.

10. Gaarder A, Jonsen J, Laland S et al. Adenosine diphosphate in red cells as a factor in the adhesiveness of human blood platelets. Nature 1961;192:531–2.

11. Bhatt D, Topol EJ. Scientific and therapeutic advances in antiplatelet therapy. Nat Rev Drug Discov 2003;2:15–28.

12. Kunapuli SP, Ding Z, Dorsam RT et al. ADP receptors – targets for developing antithrombotic agents. Curr Pharm Des 2003;9:2303–16.

13. Mahaut-Smith MP, Ennion SJ, Rolf MG, Evans RJ. ADP is not an agonist at $P2X_1$ receptors: evidence for separate receptors stimulated by ATP and ADP on human platelets. Br J Pharmacol 2000;131:108–14.

14. Maayani S, Patel ND, Craddock-Royal BD et al. Concurrent responses elicited by isolated activation of platelet Gq-coupled receptors, in vitro: a novel approach for their separation and analysis. Platelets 2003;14:89–102.

15. Kuijpers MJ, Nieuwenhuys CM, Feijge MA et al. Regulation of tissue factor-induced coagulation and platelet aggregation in flowing whole blood. Thromb Haemost 2005;93:97–105.

16. Goto S, Tamura N, Ishida H, Ruggeri ZM. Dependence of platelet thrombus stability on sustained glycoprotein IIb/IIIa activation through adenosine 5′-diphosphate receptor stimulation and cyclic calcium signaling. J Am Coll Cardiol 2006;47:155–62.

17. Ingall AH, Dixon J, Bailey A et al. Antagonists of the platelet P2T receptor: a novel approach to antithrombotic therapy. J Med Chem 1999;42:213–20.

18. Hollopeter G, Jantzen H, Vincent D et al. Identification of the platelet ADP receptor targeted by antithrombotic drugs. Nature 2001;409:202–7.

19. van Giezen JJ, Humphries RG. Preclinical and clinical studies with selective reversible direct P2Y12 antagonists. Semin Thromb Hemost 2005;31:195–204.

20. von Kugelgen I. Pharmacological profiles of cloned mammalian P2Y-receptor subtypes. Pharmacol Ther 2006;110:415–32.

21. Lechner SG, Dorostkar MM, Mayer M et al. Autoinhibition of transmitter release from PC12 cells and sympathetic neurons through a P2Y receptor-mediated inhibition of voltage-gated Ca^{2+} channels. Eur J Neurosci 2004;20:2917–28.

22. Wihlborg AK, Wang L, Braun OO et al. ADP receptor P2Y12 is expressed in vascular smooth muscle cells and stimulates contraction in human blood vessels. Arterioscler Thromb Vasc Biol 2004;24:1810–15.

23. Jacquet S, Malaval C, Martinez LO et al. The nucleotide receptor P2Y13 is a key regulator of hepatic high-density lipoprotein (HDL) endocytosis. Cell Mol Life Sci 2005;62:2508–15.

24. The Medicines Company. Data on File

25. Nassim MA, Sanderson JB, Clarke C et al. Investigation of the novel P2T receptor antagonist AR-C69931MX on ex vivo adenosine diphosphate-induced platelet aggregation and bleeding time in healthy volunteers. J Am Coll Cardiol 1999;33(2 Suppl A):A254.

26. Cauwenberghs S, Feijge MA, Hageman G et al. Plasma ectonucleotidases prevent desensitization of purigenic receptors in stored platelets: importance for platelet activity during thrombus formation. Transfusion 2006;46:1018–28.

27. Storey RF, Oldroyd KG, Wilcox RG. Open multicentre study of the P2T receptor antagonist AR-C69931MX assessing safety, tolerability and activity in patients with acute coronary syndromes. Thromb Haemost 2001;85:401–7.

28. Jacobsson F, Swahn E, Wallentin L, Ellborg M. Safety profile and tolerability of intravenous AR-C69931MX, a new antiplatelet drug, in unstable angina pectoris and non-Q-wave myocardial infarction. Clin Ther 2002;24:752–65.

29. van Gestel MA, Heemskerk JW, Slaaf DW et al. In vivo blockade of platelet ADP receptor P2Y12 reduces embolus and thrombus formation but not thrombus stability. Arterioscler Thromb Vasc Biol 2003;23:518–23.

30. Wang K, Zhou X, Zhou Z et al. Blockade of the platelet P2Y12 receptor by AR-C69931MX sustains coronary artery recanalization and improves the myocardial tissue perfusion in a canine thrombosis model. Arterioscler Thromb Vasc Biol 2003;23:357–62.

31. Huang J, Driscoll EM, Gonzales ML et al. Prevention of arterial thrombosis by intravenously administered platelet P2T receptor antagonist AR-C69931MX in a canine model. J Pharmacol Exp Ther 2000;295:492–9.

32. Humphries RG, Nicol AK, Tomlinson W et al. Effect of the novel P2T receptor antagonist, AR-C69931MX, on thrombosis and hemostasis in the dog: comparison with GPIIb/IIIa antagonists. Haematologica 2000;85(Suppl):91–2.

33. Folts JD, Crowell EB Jr, Rowe GG. Platelet aggregation in partially obstructed vessels and its elimination with aspirin. Circulation 1976;54:365–70.

34. Jarvis GE, Nassim MA, Humphries RG et al. The P2T antagonist AR-C69931MX is a more effective inhibitor of ADP-induced platelet aggregation than clopidogrel. Blood 1999;94(Suppl 1):22a.

35. Greenbaum AB, Ohman EM, Gibson MS et al. Intravenous adenosine diphosphate P2T platelet receptor antagonism as an adjunct to fibrinolysis for acute myocardial infarction. J Am Coll Cardiol 2002; 39(Suppl 2):281A.

36. Rao AK, Pratt C, Berke A et al. Thrombolysis in Myocardial Infarction (TIMI) trial – phase I: hemorrhagic manifestations and changes in plasma fibrinogen and the fibrinolytic system in patients treated with recombinant tissue plasminogen activator and streptokinase. J Am Coll Cardiol 1988;11:1–11.

37. Greenbaum AB, Grines CL, Bittl JA et al. Initial experience with an intravenous P2Y12 platelet receptor antagonist in patients undergoing percutaneous coronary intervention: results from a 2-part, phase II, multicenter, randomized, placebo- and active-controlled trial. Am Heart J 2006;151:689e1–10.

38. Storey RF, Judge HM, Wilcox RG, Heptinstall S. Inhibition of ADP-induced P-selectin expression and platelet-leukocyte conjugate formation by clopidogrel and the P2Y12 receptor antagonist AR-C69931MX but not aspirin. Thromb Haemost 2002;88: 488–94.

39. Storey RF, Wilcox RG, Heptinstall S. Comparison of the pharmacodynamic effects of the platelet ADP receptor antagonists clopidogrel and AR-C69931MX in patients with ischaemic heart disease. Platelets 2002;13:407–13.

40. Storey RF, Henderson RA, Wilcox RG, Heptinstall S. Superior antiplatelet effects of AR-C69931MX compared to clopidogrel in patients with ischemic heart disease. Haematologica 2000; 85(Suppl):92.

41. Jarvis GE, Nassim MA, Humphries RG et al. Clopidogrel produces incomplete inhibition of [^{33}P]-2MeSADP binding to human platelets and less inhibition of ADP-induced platelet aggregation than the P_2T antagonist AR-C69931MX. Haematologica 2000;85(Suppl):92–3.

42. Steinhubl S, Oh J, Oestreich J et al. Transitioning patients from cangrelor to clopidogrel: Pharmacodynamic evidence of a competitive effect. Thromb Res. 2007 Jul 11.

43. Nylander S, Johansson K, Van Giezen JJ, Lindahl TL. Evaluation of platelet function, a method comparison. Platelets 2006;17:49–55.

44. Clinical Study Protocol CHAMPION Platform (TMC-CAN-05-03). The Medicines Company, 2006.

45. Clinical Study Protocol CHAMPION PCI (TMC-CAN-05-02). The Medicines Company, 2005.

Section II.c

Antithrombotic drugs: thrombin inhibitors and thrombin generation inhibitors

15

Indirect thrombin inhibitors: fundamentals and guide to optimal therapy using unfractionated heparin and low-molecular-weight heparins

Raphaelle Dumainev and Gilles Montalescot

Introduction

Mural thrombus formation may be the consequence either of the spontaneous disruption of an atherosclerotic plaque or of an endothelial denudation following percutaneous coronary intervention (PCI) with or without stent implantation. An acute coronary syndrome (ACS) is usually the clinical manifestation of spontaneous plaque disruption, and endothelial denudation during PCI may lead to acute or subacute stent thrombosis or to distal embolization.

The plaque disruption results in (1) platelet activation and aggregation, due to pathological contact between circulating blood procoagulant molecules and structures of the vessel wall such as fibronectin, collagen, and von Willebrand factor, and (2) activation of tissue factor and coagulation factors. Thrombin (or activated factor II: factor IIa) is a key enzyme of the coagulation cascade, as it controls the ultimate step: the conversion of fluid-phase fibrinogen into fibrin, which polymerizes into crosslinked fibrin polymers, the basis of the clot. Furthermore, thrombin sustains the clotting process by two mechanisms: (i) amplification of its own production by activating the intrinsic pathway – particularly factors XI, IX, VIII, and X – (ii) and platelet activation. Thrombin binds to fibrin and fibrin degradation products, as well as to the subendothelial matrix, and remains active once bound.

Indirect thrombin inhibitors such as unfractionated heparin (UFH) and low-molecular-weight heparins (LMWH) are essential in limiting the coagulation process following a spontaneous or provoked plaque disruption. The present chapter will discuss the mechanisms of action, properties and optimal management of UFH and LMWH in the setting of ACS as well as PCI.

Mechanisms of action

Figure 15.1 compares the mechanisms of action of UFH and LMWH.

Thrombin or factor IIa, has an active site and two exosites, one of which – exosite 1 – binds to its fibrin substrate, orientating it towards the active site.

UFH binds to exosite 2 on thrombin and also to antithrombin, forming a ternary complex. This ternary complex is necessary for the inhibition of thrombin by antithrombin (Figure 15.1a: left). In contrast to thrombin inhibition, inactivation of factor Xa does not require the formation of a ternary complex. UFH inhibits thrombin and factor Xa in the same proportion (the ratio of anti-Xa to anti-IIa activity is equal to 1) (Figure 15.1a: right). The interaction of the heparins (UFH as well as LMWH) with antithrombin is mediated by a unique pentasaccharide sequence, present in approximately one-third of UFH chains.[1]

In addition, UFH also binds simultaneously to fibrin and thrombin. The heparin/thrombin/fibrin complex lessens the ability of the heparin–antithrombin complex to inhibit thrombin and increases the affinity of thrombin for its fibrin substrate. This results in protection of fibrin-bound thrombin from inactivation by the heparin–antithrombin complex[2] (Figure 15.1b). Thus, thrombin-rich clot represents a powerful reservoir of prothrombotic thrombin.

LMWH are prepared by depolymerization of the benzyl ester of porcine mucosal UFH chains. The critical pentasaccharide unit needed for their interaction with antithrombin is present in about 20% of LMWH chains. Because most LMWH chains are not sufficiently long to form the ternary complex necessary for the inactivation of factor IIa, their action is primarily directed against factor Xa (Figure 15.1c). Depending on the particular LMWH,

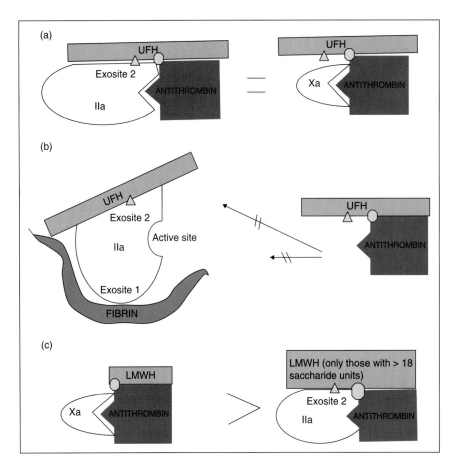

Figure 15.1
Mechanisms of action of unfractionated heparin (UFH) and low-molecular-weight heparin (LMWH). See text for details. (Adapted in part from Weitz JI, Buller HR.[2])

the ratio of anti-IIa to anti-Xa activity varies from 1.9 (tinzaparin) to 3.8 (enoxaparin).[1]

Comparison of the pharmacological properties of UFH and LMWH

The pharmacological properties of UFH and LMWH are compared in Table 15.1.

The antithrombin action of UFH is limited by variable efficacy and stability, mainly due to poor bioavailability, non-specific protein binding, neutralization by platelet factor 4 (PF4), and a lack of efficacy on fibrin-bound thrombin.[3] Moreover, UFH exhibits prothrombotic properties related to poor control of release of von Willebrand factor(vWF), as well as platelet activation, platelet aggregation through binding and upregulation of the platelet glycoprotein (GP) IIb/IIIa receptor, and rebound of thrombin generation after discontinuation.[4–8]

Fractionated LMWH have a more predictable pharmacological profile than UFH, removing the need for therapeutic

Table 15.1 *Comparison of pharmacological properties of unfractionated heparin (UFH) and low-molecular-weight heparins (LMWH)*

	UFH	LMWH
Presence of cofactor required	+++	+++
Renal clearance	±	++
Predictability in pharmacological profile	–	++
Inhibition of thrombin generation	+	++
Control of von Willebrand factor release	+	+++
Tissue factor pathway inhibitor release	+	++
Inhibition of bound thrombin	–	–
Rebound of thrombin generation after discontinuation	+++	+
Platelet activation	+++	+
Non-specific protein binding	+++	+
Neutralization by platelet factor 4	+++	+
Immunothrombocytopenia	+++	+

Table 15.2   *Contemporary guidelines for use of unfractionated heparin (UFH) in patients undergoing percutaneous coronary intervention*[33]

	No concomitant GPIIb/IIIa inhibitor use	Concomitant GPIIb/IIIa inhibitor use
Intravenous bolus	70–100 IU/kg	50–70 IU/kg
Activated clotting time	250–300 s (HemoTec device)	200 s
(ACT) to be achieved	300–350 s (Hemochron device)	
Additional bolus if target	2000–5000 IU	
ACT not achieved		
Sheath removal	When ACT < 150–180 s	

drug monitoring, except among patients with decreased renal function and elderly or extreme-weight patients (low-weight or obese patients). This predictability is mainly due to reduced non-specific protein binding and reduced neutralization by PF4. Other properties, such as reduced induction of vWF release and reduced platelet activation, are of crucial importance in the setting of ACS. The release of vWF has been shown to be a strong predictor of outcome in ACS without ST-segment elevation [5,6] as well as in acute myocardial infarction (MI) with ST-segment elevation.[9,10] LMWH have been shown repeatedly to reduce significantly this marker of outcome.[5,6,10] Furthermore, LMWH produce enhanced release of tissue factor pathway inhibitor (TFPI), a glycoprotein that forms a quaternary complex with the factor VIIa–tissue factor complex and factor Xa, thus inhibiting the factor VIIa–tissue factor complex.[3] This extended action on the coagulation cascade upstream from thrombin is a theoretical advantage over UFH, especially in the setting of ACS, where limiting the amplification of clotting formation by inhibiting thrombin generation is a key element of the treatment strategy. Heparin-induced thrombocytopenia is also less common with LMWH than UFH.[11]

UFH: Monitoring and dose adjustment

UFH and PCI

UFH has long been the only anticoagulant used during PCI. It is generally administered as weight-adjusted boluses, under activated clotting time (ACT) guidance. The main limitation on its use during PCI is the necessity for close monitoring of anticoagulant activity. This is assessed by ACT, which varies substantially in the presence of other comorbidities as well as with the devices used to measure it; higher ACT values (30–50 s) are observed using the Hemochron device than the HemoTec device.[12] Procedural anticoagulation monitoring is thus highly

dependent on the device used to guide heparin administration (Table 15.2). In addition to this variability in ACT results, the optimal range of target ACT remains uncertain. Results from retrospective studies suggest that a higher ACT may be associated with a reduction in ischemic complications, but the balance between hemorrhagic risk and thrombotic risk remains vague, and highly dependent on the PCI setting (emergent setting/thrombus-rich lesions; elective setting/low-thrombotic lesion). In a randomized study comparing a fixed dose of UFH (15 000 IU bolus) and a weight-adjusted UFH regimen (100 IU/kg), similar efficacy and safety outcomes were observed.[13] Lower fixed doses (a 5000 or 2500 IU bolus) have also been used and do not seem to be associated with an increased thrombotic risk.[14,15]

Prolonged UFH infusion after uncomplicated PCI is not recommended.

UFH and medical treatment for ACS

UFH has long been the only thrombin inhibitor used in patients with unstable angina, despite the lack of definitive proven benefit over placebo in ACS patients treated with aspirin. In a randomized trial of 479 ACS patients, although heparin therapy (1000 units per hour by intravenous infusion) was associated with a reduction of the composite of refractory angina/MI/death in the absence of aspirin, its addition to aspirin therapy did not result in a significantly greater protective effect than aspirin alone.[16] In a meta-analysis of six randomized trials comparing aspirin plus heparin versus aspirin alone, the relative risk of death or MI was 0.67 (95% confidence interval (CI) 0.44–1.02) in patients treated with aspirin plus heparin compared with those treated with aspirin alone.[17] Thus, despite the lack of conclusive evidence of benefit from adding UFH to aspirin, and because no adequately powered larger-scale trials have been conducted, clinical guidelines still recommend a strategy including administration of heparin with aspirin in ACS patients (class IB).[18]

LMWH: Monitoring and dose adjustment

LMWH in the setting of elective PCI

When patients are not pretreated with any form of anticoagulation before reaching the catheterization laboratory, rapid effective and predictable anticoagulation can be obtained with intravenous LMWH during PCI. Of the LMWH available, enoxaparin has been the most extensively studied in the setting of ACS or PCI.

In a preliminary study, Choussat et al[19] included 242 consecutive patients to receive a single intravenous bolus of enoxaparin (0.5 mg/kg) during elective PCI. A peak anti-Xa >0.5 IU/ml was obtained in 97.5% of the population (Figure 15.2); this dose allowed immediate sheath removal when used alone, and did not require dose adjustment when used with a GPIIb/IIIa inhibitor.

The large STEEPLE trial was a prospective, open-label, randomized trial in 3528 patients undergoing elective PCI. Patients were randomized to enoxaparin (0.5 or 0.75 mg/kg) or an ACT-adjusted UFH regimen, stratified by the operator's

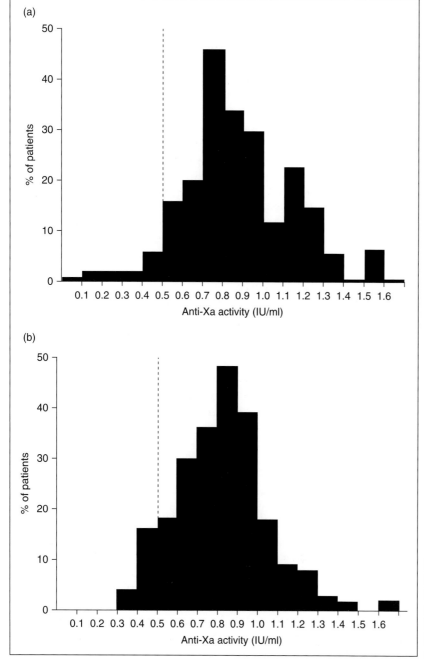

Figure 15.2
Distribution of anti-Xa activity levels at the beginning (a) and end (b) of percutaneous coronary intervention after a single intravenous dose of enoxaparin 0.5 mg/kg. (Reproduced with permission from Choussat R et al.[19])

choice of GPIIb/IIIa inhibitor use. The primary endpoint was the incidence of non-coronary artery bypass graft (CABG)-related major and minor bleeding. Enoxaparin 0.5 mg/kg was associated with a significant 31% reduction in the primary endpoint compared with UFH (6.0% vs 8.7%; $p = 0.014$), and the 0.75 mg/kg dose was associated with a 24% reduction (6.6% vs 8.7%; $p=0.052$), meeting the criteria for non-inferiority. There was a significant 57% reduction of major bleeding in both enoxaparin groups compared with UFH.

The incidence of the quadruple endpoint of death/MI/ urgent target revascularization/major bleeding at 30 days was similar between the three groups (7.2%, 7.9%, and 8.4% in the enoxaparin 0.5 mg/kg, enoxaparin 0.75 mg/kg, and UFH groups, respectively).

The sheath was immediately removed from the femoral site in the 0.5 mg/kg group without any excess bleeding.

In contrast to UFH, enoxaparin use during PCI did not require anticoagulation monitoring, and there was no dose modification with concomitant GPIIb/IIIa receptor blocker administration.[20]

LMWH in acute coronary syndromes

Comparison of LMWH with UFH without GPIIb/IIIa inhibitors and without catheterization

Several randomized clinical trials have compared the efficacy and safety of LMWH and UFH among initially medically managed patients presenting with ACS.[21–24] In these trials, enoxaparin was the only LMWH to demonstrate a significant and sustained benefit over UFH; in a meta-analysis of the TIMI 11B and ESSENCE trials, enoxaparin was associated with a significant reduction in death and MI at 8, 14, and 43 days (odds ratio (OR) 0.77, 95% CI 0.62–0.95; OR 0.79, 95% CI 0.65–0.96; and OR 0.82, 95% CI 0.69–0.97, respectively).[25]

Comparison of LMWH with UFH in combination with GPIIb/IIIa inhibitors and catheterization

More recently, the safety and efficacy of these two anti-thrombin regimens have been compared among patients receiving current antithrombotic regimens including tirofiban (A to Z[26] and ACUTE II[27]) or eptifibatide (INTERACT[28]), as well as high-risk patients undergoing an early invasive strategy (SYNERGY).[29] The SYNERGY (Superior Yield of the New Strategy of Enoxaparin Revascularization and Glycoprotein IIb/IIIa Inhibitors) trial[29] was the largest randomized, open-label, international trial comparing enoxaparin and UFH among 10 027

high-risk patients with non ST-segment elevation (NSTE) ACS to be treated with an intended early invasive strategy. The incidence of the composite primary efficacy endpoint (death/MI at 30 days) was similar in enoxaparin- and UFH-treated patients (14.0% vs 14.5%, respectively; OR 0.96; 95% CI 0.86–1.06). There was no difference in the rate of ischemic events during PCI between the two groups. The primary safety outcome (major bleeding or stroke) was similar in both groups, although there was a modest increase in the rate of major bleeding in the enoxaparin group according to the TIMI bleeding classification (9.1% vs 7.6%; $p = 0.008$), but not according to the GUSTO classification (2.7% vs 2.2%; $p = 0.08$). The need for transfusions was similar in the two groups (17.0% vs 16.0%; $p = 0.16$). However, when stratifying by pre-randomization therapy, the benefit of enoxaparin was highest among patients receiving either enoxaparin or no antithrombin therapy before randomization. The authors stated that 'as a first-line agent in the absence of changing antithrombin therapy during treatment, enoxaparin appears to be superior to UFH without an increased bleeding risk'.[29]

A pooled analysis was performed among the 21 946 patients included in the six randomized trials comparing UFH and enoxaparin in NSTE ACS.[30] Enoxaparin treatment was associated with lower incidence of death/MI at 30 days than UFH (10.1% vs 11.0%; OR 0.91; 95% CI 0.83–0.99; number needed to treat 107). The benefit of enoxaparin was even higher among patients receiving no pre-randomization antithrombin therapy (8.0% vs 9.4%; OR 0.81; 95% CI 0.70–0.94; number needed to treat 72). There was no significant difference in blood transfusion or major bleeding.

In all of these trials, enoxaparin was administered at a dose of 1 mg/kg subcutaneously every 12 hours, in order to achieve therapeutic anti-Xa levels. This is important, as it has been demonstrated that low anti-Xa activity (<0.5 IU/ml) is an independent predictor of poor outcome among ACS patients; conversely, anti-Xa activity within the target range of 0.5–1.2 IU/ml is not related to bleeding events.[31] Among patients with impaired creatinine clearance, the therapeutic range is safely achieved by reducing enoxaparin dose.[32]

PCI in patients with upstream subcutaneous LMWH

Current recommendations for antithrombin management in patients being treated with subcutaneous LMWH undergoing PCI suggest a transition to UFH, with a bolus being given immediately prior to intervention.[33] In the setting of ACS, this strategy has demonstrated at least similar safety between UFH and enoxaparin, and similar or fewer ischemic events among patients treated with enoxaparin as compared with UFH-treated patients.[26–28]

34. Collet JP, Montalescot G, Lison L et al. Percutaneous coronary intervention after subcutaneous enoxaparin pretreatment in patients with unstable angina pectoris. Circulation 2001;103:658–63.

35. Collet JP, Montalescot G, Golmard JL et al. Subcutaneous enoxaparin with early invasive strategy in patients with acute coronary syndromes. Am Heart J 2004;147:655–61.

36. Ferguson JJ, Antman EM, Bates ER et al. Combining enoxaparin and glycoprotein IIb/IIIa antagonists for the treatment of acute coronary syndromes: final results of the National Investigators Collaborating on Enoxaparin-3 (NICE-3) study. Am Heart J 2003;146:628–34.

37. Kereiakes DJ, Montalescot G, Antman EM et al. Low-molecular-weight heparin therapy for non-ST-elevation acute coronary syndromes and during percutaneous coronary intervention: an expert consensus. Am Heart J 2002;144:615–24.

16

Direct thrombin inhibitors

Rajeev Garg, Neal Kleiman, and Eli Lev

Role of thrombin in arterial thrombosis

Thrombin (factor IIa) is a serine protease that is activated at the final step of the blood coagulation cascade and converts fibrinogen to fibrin. Thrombin has multiple roles – it is the most potent known platelet agonist, it is primarily responsible for thrombus propagation through the soluble clotting cascade, and it is also responsible for both positive and negative feedback within the coagulation cascade.

Thrombin is generated by cleavage of prothrombin after activation of the direct or indirect coagulation cascade (Figure 16.1). It acts as a catalyst for converting fibrinogen to fibrin. Thrombin also activates factor (F) VIII and FV, which enhance production of thrombin through a process described as 'autocatalytic', and stimulates FXIIIa, which then stabilizes fibrin strand crosslinking.[1]

The structure of thrombin has been defined by X-ray crystallography. Thrombin is a large serine protease with high substrate specificity.[2] Various antithrombin agents block its action by binding to three distinct sites: the active or catalytic active site, which is responsible for substrate cleavage, and the two anion binding exosites 1 and 2 (Figure 16.2).[3–5]

Exosite 1 is a major docking site, which ensures that substrates are properly oriented with regard to the active site.[6] Thrombin interacts through this site with many of its physiologically relevant substrates, including protease-activated receptor (PAR-1), the primary receptor for thrombin on human platelets.

Exosite 2 is spatially distinct from exosite 1, and is believed to regulate the docking to thrombin of heparin and the serine protease inhibitor antithrombin (AT, formerly known as antithrombin III) complex.[7–9]

Thrombin activates human platelets via the cleavage of PAR-1 and PAR-4, which respond to low and high concentrations of thrombin, respectively.[10] The PARs are G-protein-coupled receptors involved in a novel mechanism in which an extracellular proteolytic cleavage event is translated into a transmembrane signal. The ligand, on the distal end of the receptor, remains cryptic until an N-terminal fragment of the receptor is cleaved by thrombin.[11] Once activated by thrombin-mediated proteolysis, the tethered ligands of these G-protein-coupled receptors bind to a separate portion of the receptor and consequently activate it.[12] PAR-1 is a high-affinity receptor for thrombin by virtue of a hirudin (Hir)-like sequence that resides in its N-terminal extracellular domain. PAR-4 lacks this Hir residue and hence requires higher concentrations of thrombin. It has also been established that PAR-1 and PAR-4 signal through different complements of G-proteins.[13] There may be a discrete signalling difference between PAR-1-mediated and PAR-4-mediated platelet activation in human platelets. Holinstat et al[14] have shown that signalling through the $P2Y_{12}$ – but not the $P2Y_1$ – receptor plays at least a partial role in PAR-4-mediated signalling, whereas no observable dependence on $P2Y_{12}$ was measured following stimulation with maximal concentrations of PAR-1-AP (20 µmol/l). Therefore, inhibition of signalling by ADP through $P2Y_{12}$ may affect platelet aggregation by attenuating the PAR-4 signalling pathway while having little effect on PAR-1-mediated thrombin signalling. If this is the case, a specific inhibitor of PAR-4 signalling may result in a more desirable side-effect profile compared with clopidogrel. Further understanding of these signalling differences may also provide insight into targets that lend themselves to the development of better antiplatelet therapies and possibly a whole new paradigm in the management of acute coronary syndromes (ACS).[15,16]

Unfractionated heparin / LMWH and its limitations

Heparin (both unfractionated and low-molecular-weight: UFH and LMWH) binds endogenous AT to exert its antithrombotic effect. AT is an endogenous anticoagulant, and heparin binding leads to an increase in its level of activity. Therefore, it is termed an indirect anticoagulant. Heparin has certain limitations:

• When heparin is bound to AT, it cannot inhibit thrombin bound to fibrin, fibrin degradation products, or the subendothelial matrix. This is because it attaches

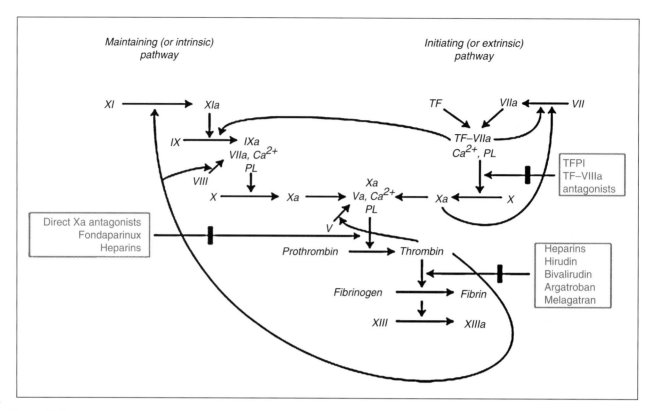

Figure 16.1
Schematic depiction of the coagulation system with its various inhibitors. Adapted from: Conde et al.[16a]

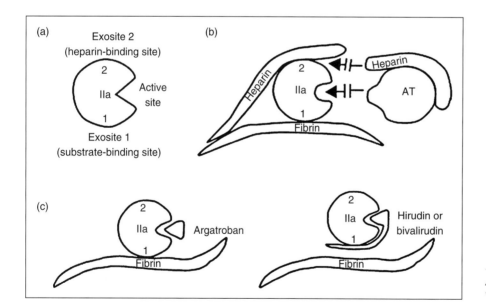

Figure 16.2
Depiction of the binding of heparin and DTIs to thrombin.
AT, Antithrombin. Adapted from: Weitz et al.[16]

to exosite 2 in order to enhance the binding of AT to thrombin (Figure 16.2) While circulating thrombin is inactivated by indirect anticoagulants, the clot-bound thrombin is able to continue catalyzing fibrinogen, activating platelets, and amplifying its own generation by activating FV, FVIII, and FXI.

- Heparin has a highly variable dose response and anticoagulant effect among individual patients.[17]

- Heparin has a consistent proaggregant effect on platelets (mainly unfractionated heparin).[18,19]
- It undergoes inactivation by platelet factor 4 (PF4).[20]
- These is a rebound prothrombotic effect after cessation of therapy.[21,22]
- Both UFH and LMWH can cause heparin-induced thrombocytopenia (HIT), with its attendant hazard of thrombosis, although the risk may be less with LMWH.[23]

Therefore, direct thrombin inhibitors (DTIs) were developed to overcome the inability of the heparin/AT complex to inactivate clot-bound thrombin and to allow more precise regulation of anticoagulation. The DTIs, such as hirudin and bivalirudin, directly inhibit soluble and clot-bound thrombin without depending on AT for anticoagulant activity. They have high specificity and potency for thrombin inhibition, and do not promote platelet aggregation. At therapeutic concentrations that prolong the activated partial thromboplastin time (aPPT) to twice normal, heparin inhibits only 20–40% of clot-bound thrombin activity, whereas DTIs achieve at least 70% inhibition.[24]

Given their potential benefits over heparin, parenteral DTIs have undergone extensive appraisal in patients with ACS or HIT, and those undergoing percutaneous coronary intervention (PCI). In current practice, parenteral DTIs are most commonly used for anticoagulation for patients undergoing PCI.

Direct thrombin inhibitors

Currently, three parenteral DTIs are available for clinical use: hirudin, argatroban, and bivalirudin.

Mechanism of action

DTIs as a class can inhibit both circulating and clot-bound thrombin because they are physically small molecules and do not interact with exosite 2. They bind directly to the active site of thrombin and inhibit all its proteolytic activity without the need for AT as an intermediary molecule.

Hirudin and bivalirudin bind in a bivalent fashion to both the catalytic site and exosite 1, while argatroban binds only to the catalytic site (Figure 16.2). Hirudin binds to thrombin with very high affinity, while binding of bivalirudin to thrombin is reversible and is associated with the eventual cleavage near the N-terminus of bivalirudin by thrombin itself.[25,26] When bivalirudin is cleaved, the bond between exosite 1 and the N-terminus of the bivalirudin segment is weakened, leading to their dissociation and to restoration of normal thrombin activity. This process may play an important role in the recovery of normal hemostatic function after bivalirudin use.

Hirudin

Hirudin was originally isolated from the salivary tissue of the medicinal leech, *Hirudo medicinalis*. It is a 65-amino-acid peptide that binds thrombin with high specificity. Recombinant hirudins (r-hirudins) lack a sulfated tyrosine residue at position 63 and hence are known as desulfato-hirudins or desirudins. Desirudins have a 10-fold lower affinity for thrombin than hirudin does, but are still potent

inhibitors. They are the largest of the DTI molecules (7 kDa).[27] Currently, r-hirudin is available as Lepirudin and is approved in the USA for anticoagulation in patients with HIT. Lepirudin is cleared primarily by the kidneys; consequently, patients with renal dysfunction require careful monitoring.[28] Overdosage of hirudin in patients with renal insufficiency can be treated with hemodialysis using polymethyl methylacrylate membranes, which have high avidity for hirudin.[29]

Argatroban

Argatroban, a synthetic competitive inhibitor of thrombin, is a heterocyclic peptide that binds to a site near the catalytic site. Because of its small size, argatroban does not face steric hindrance and can neutralize clot-bound thrombin in vitro.[30] It has a short half-life (approximately 45 minutes) and is metabolized principally by the liver. Therefore, it does not accumulate in patients with renal failure, but requires dose adjustment in patients with hepatic dysfunction.[31]

Bivalirudin

Bivalirudin is a 20-amino-acid polypeptide that binds bivalently to thrombin. Its structure was originally derived from hirudin: bivalirudin shares the same N- and C-termini, but they are linked by a Gly_4 'spacer' to maintain steric configuration. It has been studied extensively for use in coronary and peripheral intervention. In patients undergoing PCI, bivalirudin is administered intravenously as a bolus of 0.75 mg/kg followed by an infusion of 1.75 mg/kg for the duration of the procedure. Its distribution is predominantly intravascular and it does not bind to plasma proteins or blood cells. The clearance of bivalirudin is primarily via proteolysis, with renal excretion accounting for <20% of its degradation. The half-life of bivalirudin is 25 minutes in individuals with normal kidney function[32] and is prolonged by renal insufficiency. The bolus dose does not need reduction in patients with renal failure, but a dose-reduction algorithm for the maintenance infusion is available for such patients. In patients on dialysis, the half-life is about 3.5 hours, and the infusion must be reduced by 90%. Approximately 25% of a bivalirudin dose is cleared by hemodialysis.[33]

Clinical application of DTIs in PCI

Hirudin and argatroban are approved in the USA for treatment of patients with HIT, whereas bivalirudin has been approved as a heparin substitute or 'foundation anticoagulant' in patients undergoing PCI.

Hirudin in PCI

Early phase II PCI trials comparing hirudin with heparin suggested a reduction in ischemic events among patients treated with hirudin.[34,35] Subsequently, the Helvetica trial[36] examined 1141 patients with unstable angina undergoing coronary angioplasty (treated with aspirin) and randomized participants to UFH or one or two different doses of hirudin. Hirudin reduced early ischemic events, which occurred in 11.0%, 7.9%, and 5.6% of patients in the respective groups (UFH group, intravenous hirudin, and intravenous followed by subcutaneous hirudin for 3 days) ($p = 0.023$). However, there was no difference in survival free of myocardial infarction (MI) or revascularization at 7 months with hirudin ($p = 0.61$). No studies have evaluated the role of hirudin in contemporary PCI.

Argatroban in PCI

Argatroban was evaluated by Lewis et al[37] in 91 HIT patients who underwent 112 PCIs; there were no procedural deaths, but there was a 7.7% rate of occurrence of MI or urgent revascularization.[37] Overall, outcomes were comparable with those historically reported for heparin. Therefore, it was concluded that argatroban is a reasonable anticoagulant option in this setting, where current options are limited.

Two recent studies from Japan have examined the role of argatroban in angioplasty. One reported that the local delivery of argatroban is safe and effective in preventing restenosis after balloon angioplasty in patients with chronic coronary artery disease.[38] Another study reported that argatroban provides similar prevention of acute thrombotic events compared with heparin in patients undergoing PCI for acute MI, with the additional benefit of reduced bleeding complications in the argatroban group.[39]

Bivalirudin in PCI

Bivalirudin is currently the only DTI that has been evaluated extensively in clinical trials with respect to its use in coronary and peripheral intervention (Table 16.1).

In the first large-scale study of bivalirudin in PCI,[40] 4098 patients undergoing balloon angioplasty (without stents or glycoprotein (GP) IIb/IIIa receptor inhibitors) for unstable angina or post-MI angina were randomized to either UFH or bivalirudin (1 mg/kg bolus followed by a 4-hour infusion at a rate of 2.5 mg/kg/h and a 14–20-hour infusion at a rate of 0.2 mg/kg/h). Patients randomized to UFH received a high-dose UFH bolus (175 IU/kg bolus followed by a 15 IU/kg/h infusion for 18–24 hours). The primary endpoint of death, MI, or need for emergency bypass surgery was similar in the two groups. An intention-to-treat re-analysis of the data from this study including the full cohort of enrolled patients using a contemporary composite endpoint of death, MI, or repeat revascularization[41] demonstrated event rates at 7 days of 6.2% in the bivalirudin group and 7.9% in the UFH group ($p = 0.032$), as well as reduced bleeding in bivalirudin-treated patients. These differences persisted at 90 and 180 days.

REPLACE-1 (Randomized Evaluation of PCI Linking Angiomax to reduced Clinical Events 1) was an open-label study comparing heparin and bivalirudin in 1056 patients undergoing PCI.[42] GPIIb/IIIa inhibitors were used at the discretion of the investigator. There was no difference between the two arms in the incidence of the composite of death, MI, and repeat revascularization before hospital discharge or within 48 hours (5.6% vs 6.9%; $p = 0.40$). Major bleeding occurred in 2.1% of those assigned to bivalirudin and 2.7% of those assigned to heparin. Although not significant, the reduction in ischemic events was seen both among patients who received GPIIb/IIIa inhibitors and among those who did not receive them. Bleeding events were less common among patients receiving bivalirudin than those receiving heparin, but only in the subset not treated with GPIIb/IIIa inhibitors – suggesting that the benefits of bivalirudin with respect to bleeding were negated by routine GPIIb/IIIa inhibitor use.

REPLACE-2 was a randomized, double-blind, active-controlled trial with patients receiving either heparin and a planned GPIIb/IIIa inhibitor or bivalirudin with *provisional* GPIIb/IIIa inhibitor in the setting of non-emergency PCI.[43] The investigators randomized 6010 patients with stable or unstable angina undergoing PCI to receive intravenous bivalirudin (0.75 mg/kg bolus followed by an infusion of 1.75 mg/kg/h for the duration of the PCI) with provisional GPIIb/IIIa inhibitor or UFH (65 IU/kg bolus) plus a GPIIb/IIIa inhibitor (either abciximab or eptifibatide).

Provisional GPIIb/IIIa inhibitor use was permitted for abrupt or side-branch closure, obstructive dissection, suspected thrombus, slow flow, distal embolization, persistent stenosis, or at the discretion of the operator for clinical or angiographic instability. An additional bivalirudin (0.3 mg/kg) or heparin (20 U/kg) bolus was given if the activated clotting time (ACT) was ≤225 s; a matching saline placebo bolus was administered if the ACT was >225 s. Of the patients randomized to receive bivalirudin, 7.2% required provisional GPIIb/IIIa inhibitor treatment – a proportion that has remained very consistent across multiple studies. In this trial, the primary endpoint was a composite of major bleeding (typically a 'safety' endpoint) as well as the 'classic' ischemic end points of death, MI, or urgent repeat revascularization. At 30 days, bivalirudin with provisional GPIIb/IIIa blockade was statistically not inferior to UFH plus planned GPIIb/IIIa blockade in terms of suppression of the acute ischemic endpoints (9.2% vs 10%, respectively), and was superior to a 'virtual' heparin control group. Bivalirudin was associated with less major bleeding (2.4% vs 4.1%; $p < 0.001$) and fewer transfusions (1.7% vs 2.5%; $p = 0.02$). These results were maintained over 12 months.[44] The investigators concluded that substituting bivalirudin for routine GPIIb/IIIa inhibition for low- or medium-risk patients undergoing elective PCI provides protection from ischemic events with a low risk of bleeding. A subsequent cost analysis of US patients randomized in REPLACE-2 comparing the two treatment strategies[45] revealed that, compared with routine GPIIb/IIIa, in-hospital and 30-day costs were reduced by $405 (95% confidence interval (CI) $37–773) and $374 (95% CI $61–688) per patient with bivalirudin ($p < 0.001$ for both). Further regression modelling demonstrated that, in addition to the costs of the anticoagulants themselves, hospital savings were due primarily to reductions in major bleeding (cost savings $107/patient), minor bleeding ($52/patient), and thrombocytopenia ($47/patient).

High-risk patients with acute coronary syndromes undergoing PCI were excluded from REPLACE-2, as were those with angiographic thrombus and those in whom GPIIb/IIIa inhibitors were required. The efficacy of bivalirudin monotherapy in high-risk ACS was therefore, assessed in the subsequent ACUITY (Acute Catheterization and Urgent Intervention Triage Strategy) trial.[46]

This trial compared heparin plus GPIIb/IIIa inhibitors begun before PCI, bivalirudin plus GPIIb/IIIa inhibitors before PCI, and bivalirudin alone in 13 819 patients with moderate- or high-risk ACS undergoing an early invasive strategy. Bivalirudin plus GPIIb/IIIa inhibitors, compared with heparin plus GPIIb/IIIa inhibitors, was associated with non-inferior rates of the composite ischemic endpoint (7.7% vs 7.3%) and major bleeding (5.3% vs 5.7%) at 30 days. Bivalirudin alone was non-inferior to heparin plus GPIIb/IIIa inhibitors (composite ischemic endpoint rates 7.8% vs 7.3%) and significantly reduced rates of major bleeding (3.0% vs 5.7%; $p < 0.001$).[43] However, in a prespecified subgroup analysis, patients assigned to bivalirudin alone in whom clopidogrel therapy was not begun at least 6 hours before PCI had an increase in ischemic events compared with those treated with heparin plus GPIIb/IIIa inhibitors. In a postrandomization analysis of ACUITY (ACUITY-PCI),[47] anticoagulation with bivalirudin was assessed during PCI in 7789 individuals who underwent PCI. There were no differences in the rates of the composite ischemic endpoint, major bleeding, or net clinical outcomes at 30 days between those who received bivalirudin plus GPIIb/IIIa inhibitors and those who received heparin plus GPIIb/IIIa inhibitors. However, fewer patients who received bivalirudin alone experienced major bleeding compared with those who received heparin plus GPIIb/IIIa inhibitors, resulting in a trend toward better 30-day net clinical outcomes.

Despite such caveats, and controversies surrounding the study (a wide non-inferiority margin and the use of a composite endpoint), the ACUITY trial indicates that a treatment strategy of bivalirudin alone is acceptable in patients with ACS undergoing contemporary PCI, particularly when pretreatment with thienopyridine is administered. However, for high-risk patients, such as those with positive troponin values, the use of GPIIb/IIIa inhibitors should be still be strongly considered.

Bivalirudin in ST-elevation myocardial infarction

Overall, bivalirudin has emerged as a useful alternative to heparin with or without GPIIb/IIIa inhibitors among both low- and high-risk patients undergoing PCI. It has been shown to yield event rates compared with UFH plus GPIIb/IIIa inhibitors, but with less bleeding. Its role in ST-elevation myocardial infarction (STEMI) is not clear. Theoretically, it might be more effective than heparin, since its small size and lack of fibrinogen binding might result in greater activity against the large thrombus that undergoes disruption during primary PCI or thrombolysis. However, in one large trial in which it was combined with streptokinase (HERO-2), bivalirudin did not result in either increased survival or reduced bleeding risk.[48] The lack of benefit among patients treated with a non-fibrin-specific thrombolytic drug also does not necessarily imply that the drug is likely to be efficacious during primary PCI. The role of bivalirudin in primary PCI has been recently evaluated in the HORIZONS-AMI trial, which assessed the use of bivalirudin as an adjunctive therapy in modern primary PCI for STEMI, comparing bivalirudin plus bail-out GPIIb/IIIa inhibitor with heparin plus planned GPIIb/IIIa inhibitor treatment. The trial was a prospective, single-blind, randomized, multicenter study in 3 602 patients presenting with STEMI. Patients undergoing angioplasty were randomly assigned to receive either bivalirudin with provisional use of GP IIb/IIIa inhibitor or UFH plus GP IIb/IIIa inhibitor. Patients enrolled in the HORIZONS-AMI trial were also assigned randomly to receive either TAXUS drug-eluting stents or bare-metal stents; this component of the trial is still ongoing. The two primary endpoints were major bleeding and net adverse clinical events, a composite of major adverse cardiovascular events (death, reinfarction, stroke, or ischemic target vessel revascularization) and major bleeding at 30 days. For the primary endpoint, the incidence of net adverse clinical events at 30 days, bivalirudin significantly reduced the composite of major adverse cardiac events or major bleeding by 24% (9.2% vs 12.1%, $p = 0.006$). Bivalirudin also significantly reduced the incidence of major bleeding by 40% (4.9% vs 8.3%, $p < 0.0001$). There were comparable rates of major adverse cardiac events in the two groups (5.4% vs 5.5%, $p = 1.0$). At 30 day follow-up, bivalirudin significantly reduced the incidence of cardiac-related mortality by 38% (1.8% vs 2.9%, $p = 0.035$). There was no significant difference in stent thrombosis at 30 days between the groups (2.5% with bivalirudin vs 1.9% with UFH plus GP IIb/IIIa inhibitor, $p = 0.33$), but rates of acute stent thrombosis within 24 hours were higher in the bivalirudin

Table 16.1 *Bivalirudin in PCI*

Trial	Sample size	Study population	Comparison drugs	Primary endpoints	Safety (bleeding) endpoints
Bivalirudin Angioplasty Trial[40,41]	4098	Post-MI angina or UA undergoing balloon angioplasty	UFH vs bivalirudin	Any of the following: death, MI, abrupt closure of the dilated vessel, or rapid clinical deterioration of cardiac origin. (11.4% vs 12.2%) for bivalirudin vs. heparin	Retroperitoneal hemorrhage, blood transfusion or major bleeding (3.0% vs 11.1%; $p<0.001$) for bivalirudin vs heparin
CACHET[55]	268	Elective coronary stenting	Heparin + abciximab vs bivalirudin ± abciximab (in three different strategies)	Composite of death, MI, repeat revascularization. On pooled analysis, primary endpoint was 3.4% vs 10.6% ($p=0.018$) in the three bivalirudin arms vs heparin+abciximab	Major bleeding occurred less frequently in bivalirudin group
REPLACE-1[42]	1056	Low-risk PCI	Heparin vs bivalirudin ± GPIIb/IIIa inhibitor	Composite of death, MI, repeat revascularization (5.6% and 6.9% of patients in the bivalirudin and heparin groups, respectively; ($p=0.40$)	Major bleeding occurred in 2.1% vs 2.7% of patients randomized to bivalirudin or heparin, respectively ($p=0.52$)
REPLACE-2[43–45]	6010	Elective PCI	Heparin + GPIIb/IIIa inhibitor vs bivalirudin ± GPIIb/IIIa inhibitor	Composite of 30-day incidence of death, MI, urgent repeat revascularization, or in-hospital major bleeding. 9.2% of patients in the bivalirudin group vs 10.0% of patients in the heparin + GPIIb/IIIa group ($p=0.32$)	Bleeding rates: 2.4% vs 4.1% ($p<0.001$ in bivalirudin vs heparin + GPIIb/IIIa inhibitor
ACUITY[46]	13819	High-risk ACS undergoing early invasive strategy	Heparin + GPIIb/IIIa inhibitor begun before PCI (a), bivalirudin + GPIIb/IIIa inhibitor before PCI (b), and bivalirudin (c)	The primary endpoints were a composite ischemia endpoint (death, MI, or unplanned revascularization for ischemia), major bleeding, and the net clinical outcome, defined as the combination of composite ischemia or major bleeding. Composite ischemia endpoint for (a) and (b) was 7.3% and 7.7%, respectively and the net clinical outcome endpoint was 11.7% and 11.8%, respectively	Major bleeding (5.3% and 5.7%), in bivalirudin + GPIIb/IIIa inhibitor vs heparin + GPIIb/IIIa inhibitor

141

Study	N	Setting	Intervention	Results	Bleeding
ACUITY-PCI[47]	7789	High-risk ACS undergoing PCI	Heparin + GPIIb/IIIa inhibitor begun before PCI, bivalirudin + GPIIb/IIIa inhibitor before PCI, and bivalirudin	Primary endpoints were a composite ischemia endpoint, major bleeding, and the net clinical outcome, defined as the combination of composite ischemia or major bleeding at 30 days. Heparin + GPIIb/IIIa inhibitor vs bivalirudin + GPIIb/IIIa inhibitor: composite ischemia 9% vs 8% ($p=0.16$); net clinical outcomes 15% vs 13%, ($p=0.1$). Bivalirudin alone vs heparin + GPIIb/IIIa inhibitor: 9% vs 8% ($p=0.45$); 30-day net clinical outcomes 12% vs 13% ($p=0.057$)	Major bleeding: heparin + GPIIb/IIIa inhibitor vs bivalirudin + GPIIb/IIIa inhibitor (8% vs 7%; $p=0.32$) Bivalirudin alone vs heparin plus GPIIb/IIIa inhibitor: 92 (4%) patients vs 174 (7%) patients, ($p<0.0001$)
HORIZONS-AMI[56]	3400	Primary PCI in STEMI	Bivalirudin + bail-out GPIIb/IIIa inhibitor vs heparin + planned GPIIb/IIIa inhibitor	Primary endpoints were major bleeding and net adverse clinical events, a composite of major adverse cardiovascular events (death, reinfarction, stroke, or ischemic target vessel revascularization) and major bleeding at 30 days. The bivalirudin significantly reduced the incidence of net adverse clinical events at 30 days, the composite of major adverse cardiac events or major bleeding by 24% (9.2% vs. 12.1%, $p=0.006$). There were comparable rates of major adverse cardiac events in the two groups (5.4% vs. 5.5%, $p=1.0$). At a 30 day follow-up, bivalirudin significantly reduced the incidence of cardiac-related mortality by 38% (1.8% vs. 2.9%, $p=0.035$). There was no significant difference in stent thrombosis at 30 days between the groups (2.5% with bivalirudin vs. 1.9% with UFH plus GPIIb/IIIa inhibitor, $p=0.33$), but rates of acute stent thrombosis within 24 hours were higher in the bivalirudin group (1.3% vs. 0.3%, $p=0.0009$)	Major bleeding (4.9% vs. 8.3%; $p<0.0001$) in bivalirudin alone vs. heparin plus GPIIb/IIIa inhibitor

ACS, acute coronary syndrome; CVA, cerebrovascular accident; GPIIb/IIIa, glycoprotein IIb/IIIa; MI, myocardial infarction; PCI, percutaneous coronary intervention; STEMI, ST-elevation myocardial infarction; TVR, target vessel revascularization; UA, unstable angina; UFH, unfractionated heparin.

group (1.3% vs 0.3%, $p = 0.0009$). In summary, among patients undergoing planned primary PCI for STEMI, use of a strategy of bivalirudin was associated with a reduction in the composite endpoint of death, MI, target vessel revascularization, stroke, and major bleeding at 30 days compared with UFH plus GP IIb/IIIa inhibitors, driven by a reduction in major bleeding with no difference in major adverse cardiac events.

Use of bivalirudin in other patient populations

Bivalirudin may be particularly valuable for patients with HIT or those with renal insufficiency. In a study of 52 patients with HIT, successful PCI was performed in 98%, with no occurrence of thrombocytopenia with only one episode of major bleeding and death.[49]

Renal dysfunction is prevalent among patients undergoing PCI and is associated with an increased risk of bleeding as well as ischemic complications.[50] In a meta-analysis of trials comparing heparin with bivalirudin in patients undergoing angioplasty, the benefit of bivalirudin was maintained across patients with low creatinine clearance; the largest absolute benefit was in patients in the lowest quartile of creatinine clearance.[51] Preliminary analysis of REPLACE-2 suggests a similar benefit across the continuum of creatinine clearance.

Similar data regarding the benefit of bivalirudin over heparin in peripheral interventions has emerged from small series of patients undergoing peripheral angioplasty.[52,53] Although limited in number, these series suggest that bivalirudin may be of value in selected patients undergoing peripheral interventions.

Cases of acute closure or threatened closure during γ-brachytherapy have been reported, and probably relate to the prolonged dwell time, with resultant stasis contributing to bivalirudin proteolysis and thrombin recovery.[54]

References

1. Badimon L, Meyer BJ, Badimon JJ. Thrombin in arterial thrombosis. Haemostasis 1994;24:69–80
2. Stubbs MT, Oschkinat H, Mayr I et al. The interaction of thrombin with fibrinogen. A structural basis for its specificity. Eur J Biochem 1992;206:187–95.
3. Rydel TJ, Ravichandran KG, Tulinsky A et al. The structure of a complex of recombinant hirudin and human alpha-thrombin. Science 1990;249:277.
4. Grutter MG, Priestle JP, Rahuel J et al. Crystal structure of the thrombin–hirudin complex: a novel mode of serine protease inhibition. EMBO J 1990;9:2361.
5. Sheehan JP, Sadler JE. Molecular mapping of the heparin-binding exosite of thrombin. Proc Natl Acad Sci U S A 1994;91:5518.

6. Hirsh J, Weitz JI. New antithrombotic agents. Lancet 1999;353:1431.
7. Bode W, Stubbs MT. Spatial structure of thrombin as a guide to its multiple sites of interaction. Semin Thromb Hemost 1993;19:321–33.
8. Stubbs MT, Bode W. A player of many parts: the spotlight falls on thrombin's structure. Thromb Res 1993;69:1–58.
9. Stubbs MT, Bode W. A model for the specificity of fibrinogen cleavage by thrombin. Semin Thromb Hemost 1993;19:344–51.
10. Chung AW, Jurasz P, Hollenberg MD, Radomski MW. Mechanisms of action of proteinase-activated receptor agonists on human platelets. Br J Pharmacol 2002;135:1123–32.
11. Coughlin SR. Thrombin signalling and protease-activated receptors. Nature 2000;407:258–64.
12. Callahan KP, Malinin AI, Gurbel PA et al. Platelet function and fibrinolytic agents: two sides of a coin? Cardiology 2001;95:55–60.
13. Graff J, Klinkhardt U, Harder S. Thromb Res 2004;113:295–302.
14. Holinstat M, Voss B, Bilodeau ML et al. PAR4, but not PAR1, signals human platelet aggregation via Ca^{2+} mobilization and synergistic P2Y12 receptor activation. J Biol Chem 2006;281:26665–74.
15. Maroo A, Lincoff AM. Bivalirudin in PCI: an overview of the REPLACE-2 trial. Semin Thromb Hemost 2004;30:329–36.
16. Ali A, Hashem M, Rosman HS et al. Glycoprotein IIb/IIIa receptor antagonists and risk of bleeding: a single-center experience in 1020 patients. J Clin Pharmacol 2004;44:1328–32.
16a. Conde ID, Kleiman NS. Arterial thrombosis for the interventional cardiologist: from adhesion molecules and coagulation factors to clinical therapeutics. Catheter Cardiovasc Interv 2003;60:236-46.
16b. Weitz JI, Buller HR. Direct thrombin inhibitors in acute coronary syndromes: present and future. Circulation 2002;105:1004–11.
17. Hirsh J. Heparin. N Engl J Med 1991;324:1565–74.
18. Xiao Z, Theroux P. Platelet activation with unfractionated heparin at therapeutic concentrations and comparisons with a low-molecular-weight heparin and with a direct thrombin inhibitor. Circulation 1998;97:251–6.
19. Aggarwal A, Sobel BE, Schneider DJ. Decreased platelet reactivity in blood anticoagulated with bivalirudin or enoxaparin compared with unfractionated heparin: implications for coronary intervention. J Thromb Thrombolysis 2002;13:161–5.
20. Eitzman DT, Chi L, Saggin L et al. Heparin neutralization by platelet-rich thrombi. Role of platelet factor 4. Circulation 1994;89:1523–9.
21. Theroux P, Waters D, Lam J et al. Reactivation of unstable angina after the discontinuation of heparin. N Engl J Med 1992;327:141–5.
22. Lauer MA, Houghtaling PL, Peterson JG et al. Attenuation of rebound ischemia after discontinuation of heparin therapy by glycoprotein IIb/IIIa inhibition with eptifibatide in patients with acute coronary syndromes: observations from the Platelet IIb/IIIa in Unstable angina: Receptor Suppression Using Integrilin Therapy (PURSUIT) trial. Circulation 2001;104:2772–7.
23. Chong BH. Heparin-induced thrombocytopenia. J Thromb Haemost 2003;1:1471–8.
24. Weitz J, Hudoba M, Massel D et al. Clot-bound thrombin is protected from inhibition by heparin–antithrombin III but is susceptible to inactivation by antithrombin III-independent inhibitors. J Clin Invest 1990;86:385–91.
25. Parry MA, Maraganore JM, Stone SR. Kinetic mechanism for the interaction of Hirulog with thrombin. Biochemistry 1994;33:14807–14.
26. Witting JI, Bourdon P, Brezniak DV et al. Thrombin-specific inhibition by and slow cleavage of Hirulog-1. Biochem J 1992;283:737–43.
27. Weitz JI, Bates ER. Direct thrombin inhibitors in cardiac disease. Cardiovasc Toxicol 2003;3:13–25.
28. Nowak G, Bucha E, Goock T et al. Pharmacology of r-hirudin in renal impairment. Thromb Res 1992;66:707–15.
29. Weitz JI, Crowther M. Direct thrombin inhibitors. Thromb Res 2002;106:V275–84.
30. Walenga JM. An overview of the direct thrombin inhibitor argatroban. Pathophysiol Haemost Thromb 2002;32(Suppl 3):9–14.

31. Swan SK, Hursting MJ. The pharmacokinetics and pharmacodynamics of argatroban: effects of age, gender, and hepatic or renal dysfunction. Pharmacotherapy 2000;20:318–29.

32. Fox I, Dawson A, Loynds P et al. Anticoagulant activity of Hirulog, a direct thrombin inhibitor, in humans. Thromb Haemost 1993;69:157–63.

33. Robson R, White H, Aylward P, Frampton C. Bivalirudin pharmacokinetics and pharmacodynamics: effect of renal function, dose, and gender. Clin Pharmacol Ther 2002;71:433–9.

34. van den Bos AA, Deckers JW, Heyndrickx GR et al. Safety and efficacy of recombinant hirudin (CGP 39 393) versus heparin in patients with stable angina undergoing coronary angioplasty. Circulation 1993;88:2058–66.

35. Rupprecht HJ, Terres W, Ozbek C et al. Recombinant hirudin (HBW 023) prevents troponin T release after coronary angioplasty in patients with unstable angina. J Am Coll Cardiol 1995;26:1637–42.

36. Serruys PW, Herrman JP, Simon R et al. A comparison of hirudin with heparin in the prevention of restenosis after coronary angioplasty. Helvetica Investigators. N Engl J Med 1995;333:757–63.

37. Lewis BE, Matthai WH Jr, Cohen M et al. Argatroban anticoagulation during percutaneous coronary intervention in patients with heparin-induced thrombocytopenia. Catheter Cardiovasc Interv 2002;57:177–84.

38. Itoh T, Nonogi H, Miyazaki S et al; 3D-CAT Investigators. Local delivery of argatroban for the prevention of restenosis after coronary balloon angioplasty: a prospective randomized pilot study. Circ J 2004;68:615–22.

39. Hirahara T, Kubo N, Ohmura N et al. Prospective randomized study of argatroban versus heparin anticoagulation therapy after percutaneous coronary intervention for acute myocardial infarction. J Cardiol 2004;44:47–52.

40. Bittl JA, Strony J, Brinker JA et al. Treatment with bivalirudin (Hirulog) as compared with heparin during coronary angioplasty for unstable or postinfarction angina. Hirulog Angioplasty Study Investigators. N Engl J Med 1995;333:764–9.

41. Bittl JA, Chaitman BR, Feit R et al. Bivalirudin versus heparin during coronary angioplasty for unstable or postinfarction angina: final report reanalysis of the Bivalirudin Angioplasty Study. Am Heart J 2001;142:952–9.

42. Lincoff AM, Bittl JA, Kleiman NS et al. Comparison of bivalirudin versus heparin during percutaneous coronary intervention (the Randomized Evaluation of PCI Linking Angiomax to Reduced Clinical Events [REPLACE]-1 trial). Am J Cardiol 2004;93:1092–6.

43. Lincoff AM, Bittl JA, Harrington RA et al. Bivalirudin and provisional glycoprotein IIb/IIIa blockade compared with heparin and planned glycoprotein IIb/IIIa blockade during percutaneous coronary intervention: REPLACE-2 randomized trial. JAMA 2003;289:853–63.

44. Lincoff AM, Kleiman NS, Kereiakes DJ et al; REPLACE-2 Investigators. Long-term efficacy of bivalirudin and provisional glycoprotein IIb/IIIa blockade vs. heparin and planned glycoprotein IIb/IIIa blockade during percutaneous coronary intervention: REPLACE-2. JAMA 2004;292:696–703.

45. Cohen DJ, Lincoff AM, Lavelle TA et al. Economic evaluation of bivalirudin with provisional glycoprotein IIB/IIIA inhibition versus heparin with routine glycoprotein IIB/IIIA inhibition for percutaneous coronary intervention: results from the REPLACE-2 trial. J Am Coll Cardiol 2004;44:1792–800.

46. Stone GW, McLaurin BT, Cox DA et al; ACUITY Investigators. Bivalirudin for patients with acute coronary syndromes. N Engl J Med 2006;355:2203–16.

47. Stone GW, White HD, Ohman EM et al; Acute Catheterization and Urgent Intervention Triage Strategy (ACUITY) Trial Investigators. Bivalirudin in patients with acute coronary syndromes undergoing percutaneous coronary intervention: a subgroup analysis from the Acute Catheterization and Urgent Intervention Triage strategy (ACUITY) trial. Lancet 2007;369:907–19.

48. Hirulog and Early Reperfusion or Occlusion (HERO)-2 Trial Investigators. Thrombin-specific anticoagulation with bivalirudin versus heparin in patients receiving fibrinolytic therapy for acute myocardial infarction: the HERO-2 randomised trial. Lancet 2001;358:1855–63.

49. Mahaffey KW, Lewis BE, Wildermann NM et al. The anticoagulant therapy with bivalirudin to assist in the performance of percutaneous coronary intervention in patients with heparin-induced thrombocytopenia (ATBAT) study: main results. J Invasive Cardiol 2003;15:611–16.

50. Gurm HS, Lincoff AM, Kleiman NS et al. Double jeopardy of renal insufficiency and anemia in patients undergoing percutaneous coronary interventions. Am J Cardiol 2004;94:30–4.

51. Chew DP, Bhatt DL, Kimball W et al. Bivalirudin provides increasing benefit with decreasing renal function: a meta-analysis of randomized trials. Am J Cardiol 2003;92:919–23.

52. Shammas NW, Lemke NH, Dippel EJ et al. Bivalirudin in peripheral vascular interventions: a single center experience. J Invasive Cardiol 2003;15:401–4.

53. Allie DE, Lirtzman MD, Wyatt CH et al. Bivalirudin as a foundation anticoagulant in peripheral vascular disease: a safe and feasible alternative for renal and iliac interventions. J Invasive Cardiol 2003;15:334–42.

54. Sharma S, Bhambi B, Nyitray W et al. Bivalirudin (Angiomax) use during intracoronary brachytherapy may predispose to acute closure. J Cardiovasc Pharmacol Ther 2003;8:9–15.

55. Lincoff AM, Kleiman NS, Kotteke-Marchant K et al. Bivalirudin with planned or provisional abciximab versus low–dose heparin and abciximab during percutaneous coronary revascularization: results of the Comparison of Abciximab Complications with Hirulog for Ischemic Events Trial (CACHET). Am Heart J 2002;143:847–53.

56. http://clinicaltrials.gov/ct/show/NCT00433996order=55.

17

Fondaparinux in acute coronary syndromes

Shamir R Mehta

Pharmacology and mechanism of action

Factor Xa is located in a key position in the coagulation pathway, and is the final common element linking the intrinsic and extrinsic pathways leading to the generation of thrombin.[1] It is critical not only for the formation of thrombin itself, but also the propagation of coagulation. Thus, anticoagulants that block the activity of factor Xa inhibit the propagation of coagulation and hence the very formation of thrombin. Antithrombin, through its ability to bind to factor Xa, is able to neutralize the effect of factor Xa and hence the formation of thrombin. Fondaparinux is a synthetic analog of the antithrombin-binding pentasaccharide sequence found in heparin.[2–6] By binding to antithrombin, fondaparinux enhances the ability of antithrombin to neutralize factor Xa and hence the formation of thrombin (Figure 17.1).[2,4,5,7–9]

Fondaparinux binds to antithrombin with very high specificity.[10,11] Unlike unfractionated heparin (UFH) or low-molecular-weight heparin (LMWH), there is no detectable binding to other plasma proteins, making the interindividual anticoagulant effect of fondaparinux extremely predictable.[3] Because of this high predictability, monitoring of the anticoagulant effect is not necessary (as it is with UFH).[12] After subcutaneous injection, the bioavailability of fondaparinux approaches 100%, with a plasma half life of about 17 hours, meaning that fondaparinux can be dosed once daily.[4,11,13] Fondaparinux is not metabolized by the liver or by any other mechanism in humans, and is excreted in the urine in unchanged form. In addition, fondaparinux does not bind to platelets or to platelet factor 4 (PF4).[14] Because it does not induce the formation of heparin/PF4 complexes, heparin-induced thrombocytopenia (HIT) is unlikely to occur with fondaparinux. Studies in humans have demonstrated that effects of fondaparinux on thrombin generation time are almost completely reversible with administration of activated factor VII, which is an option for use in the rare cases of severe bleeding complications in patients receiving fondaparinux.[15,16]

Fondaparinux has a number of advantages over both UFH and LMWH.[1,3,17] It is manufactured entirely by synthetic chemical means, rather than from animal extracts. It does not interact with platelets or bind to PF4, and it does not promote HIT. The antithrombin-binding sequence of fondaparinux is the shortest fragment able to catalyze antithrombin-mediated factor Xa inhibition. The anti-factor Xa specificity of the pentasaccharide allows a more predictable anticoagulant dose and effect without necessitating safety monitoring of coagulation parameters.

Fondaparinux has been extensively studied for the prevention of venous thromboembolism (VTE) in patients undergoing major orthopedic surgery[12,18–21] or general surgery, as well as in critically ill medical patients.[22] In patients undergoing orthopedic surgery, large phase III double-blind randomized trials have shown that fondaparinux 2.5 mg daily was superior to subcutaneous enoxaparin 40 mg daily for the prevention of VTE.[12,18–21] A meta-analysis of the major phase III trials demonstrated a highly significant relative risk reduction of 55% in the prevention of VTE with fondaparinux compared with enoxaparin (Figure 17.2).[23]

Phase II trials of fondaparinux

Based on the promising results of fondaparinux in trials of VTE, it was brought forward for evaluation in patients with acute coronary syndromes (ACS). There have been phase II dose-ranging studies performed in patients with non-ST-segment elevation (NSTE) ACS,[24] as well as in patients with ST-segment elevation myocardial infarction (STEMI)[25] and in those undergoing elective or urgent percutaneous coronary intervention (PCI).[26,27]

STEMI

In the PENTALYSE trial, 326 patients with STEMI presenting within 6 hours and treated with recombinant tissue-type plasminogen activator (rtPA) were randomized to

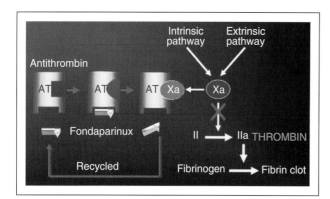

Figure 17.1
Mechanism of action fondaparinux. (Adapted from Turpie AG et al.[12]) (see color plate)

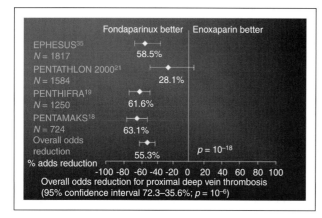

Figure 17.2
Overall efficacy of fondaparinux versus enoxaparin in prevention of versus thromboembolism: meta-analysis of trials in patients undergoing orthopedic surgery. (Adapted from Turpie AG et al.[23]) (see color plate)

receive either fondaparinux or UFH.[25] Fondaparinux was given in doses of either 4 mg (74 patients), 8 mg (74 patients) or 12 mg (79 patients) intravenously on day 1, then subcutaneously on days 2–5. UFH was given intravenously for 48–72 hours. Coronary angiography was performed at 90 minutes and at 6 days. At 90 minutes, there was little difference between fondaparinux compared with UFH in achieving Thrombolysis in Myocardial Infarction (TIMI) 2 or 3 flow (79% fondaparinux vs 82% UFH). At 6 days, rates of reocclusion were lower with fondaparinux compared with UFH (1/112 (0.9%) vs 3/43 (7%); $p=0.065$). There was no significant difference in the combined incidence of intracranial hemorrhage (ICH) or need for blood transfusion. There was only one non-fatal ICH, which occurred in a patient on the fondaparinux 4 mg dose. Excluding transfusions related to bypass surgery, there was no significant difference in the need for blood transfusions with fondaparinux: 3.3% versus 7.1% ($p=0.21$). TIMI major bleeding was 6.6% in the fondaparinux group and 4.7% in

the UFH group ($p=0.61$). TIMI minor bleeding was 6.2% in the fondaparinux group and 3.5% in the UFH group. Death was 2.5% in the fondaparinux group and 1.2% in the UFH group. Reinfarction was 3.8% and 3.6%, respectively. Revascularizations were lower in the fondaparinux group: 39% compared with 51% in the UFH group ($p=0.056$).

NSTE ACS

The dose of fondaparinux for the OASIS-5 UA/NSTEMI study (see below) was selected based on the results of the PENTUA trial.[24] In this trial, 1147 patients with symptoms of unstable angina/non-ST-segment-elevation myocardial infarction (UA/NSTEMI) presenting within 24 hours, with characteristic ECG changes and/or troponin I/T >0.1 ng/ml were enrolled. Of these patients, 1134 were randomized and treated with either one of four doses of fondaparinux sodium (2.5, 4, 8, or 12 mg once daily; intravenously on day 1, subcutaneously on days 2–7) or enoxaparin (1 mg/kg subcutaneously twice daily) for 3–7 days. The primary efficacy endpoint was the composite of death, MI, and recurrent ischemia (symptomatic or non-symptomatic, as measured on continuous 12-lead ECG monitoring) at day 9. This occured in 30.0%, 43.5%, 41.0% and 34.8% of patients treated with 2.5, 4, 8, and 12 mg fondaparinux, respectively, and in 40.2% of patients treated with enoxaparin 2.5 mg fondaparinux ($p = 0.04$). Death or myocardial infarction was observed in 1.4%, 4.3%, 3.3%, and 2.5% of patients in the fondaparinux groups and 1.9% in the enoxaparin group. At day 30, similar patterns were observed for both of these outcomes. Revascularization rates at day 9 were 16.7%, 22.2%, 20.2%, and 23.6% in the fondaparinux groups and 19.4% in the enoxaparin group. Major bleeding events occurred in none of the patients in the 2.5 mg fondaparinux and enoxaparin groups, and in 1.4%, 1.8% and 0.4% of patients treated with 4, 8, and 12 mg fondaparinux, respectively.

PCI

Fondaparinux (12 mg IV bolus) has been used in a series of 71 patients (11 patients receiving stents) undergoing coronary angioplasty. All patients received 500 mg intravenous aspirin. Acute thrombotic closure at a coronary dissection site occurred in one patient and distal embolization containing plaque in another patient. Flow was restored in both patients. At 24 hours, TIMI 3 flow was observed in all patients. Measurement of hematologic parameters showed no effect on activated clotting time (ACT), and significant drops in prothrombin fragment F1.2 and thrombin–antithrombin (TAT) levels after fondaparinux.

In the ASPIRE study, two doses of fondaparinux (2.5 and 5.0 mg intravenously) were compared with UFH in a randomized, double-blind trial in patients undergoing urgent or elective PCI.[26] There was a trend to a reduction in total bleeding with fondaparinux (combined doses) compared with UFH (7.7% vs 6.4%; hazard ratio (HR) 0.81, 95% confidence interval (CI) 0.35–1.84; $p=0.41$). Efficacy, as assessed by the composite of death, MI, urgent revascularization, or need for bailout glycoprotein GPIIb/IIIa (GPIIb/IIIa) antagonist was similar between fondaparinux and UFH (6.0% vs 6.0%). The lowest rates for both bleeding and efficacy were observed with the 2.5 mg dose of fondaparinux. Fondaparinux was superior to UFH in reducing F1.2, a marker of thrombin generation, without increasing the risk of bleeding. Vascular access site sheaths were removed within 6 hours of the PCI, with numerically fewer vascular access site complications occurring with fondaparinux (22 with UFH vs 16 with fondaparinux 2.5 mg and 10 with fondaparinux 5.0 mg). Thus, despite the longer half-life of fondaparinux, it was associated with less bleeding and fewer vascular access site complications compared with UFH in this pilot trial.

Phase III trials of fondaparinux

OASIS-5

OASIS-5 was a large, randomized, double-blind trial comparing fondaparinux with enoxaparin in 20 078 patients with UA or NSTE ACS.[28,29] Fondaparinux was administered in a dose of 1 mg/kg subcutaneously. The enoxaparin dosing was based upon renal function. Patients were treated for a mean of about 5 days, but in the large number of patients undergoing PCI, the treatment period was only 2 days. In those with a creatinine clearance >30 cm³/min, enoxaparin was dosed at 1 mg/kg twice daily and in those with creati-

nine clearance <30 cm³/min, the dose was reduced to 1 mg/kg once daily, as per FDA labelling.[28] Patients in the trial were eligible to be treated with aspirin, clopidogrel, or GPIIb/IIIa antagonists, and catheterization and PCI could be performed at any time after randomization. The hypothesis was that fondaparinux would be non-inferior to enoxaparin for efficacy, but superior to enoxaparin for safety, resulting in a superior net clinical benefit. The primary outcome was the composite of death, MI or refractory ischemia at 9 days.[28]

The results demonstrated definitively that fondaparinux was non-inferior to enoxaparin at 9 days on the primary outcome of death, MI, or refractory ischemia (5.8% fondaparinux vs 5.7% enoxaparin; HR 1.01, 95% CI 0.90–1.13; p for non-inferiority = 0.007). However, at 30 days, fondaparinux was superior to enoxaparin in reducing all-cause mortality (2.9% vs 3.5%; HR 0.83, 95% CI 0.71–0.97; $p=0.02$), the first time any antithrombotic agent in ACS has demonstrated a reduction in mortality (Figure 17.3). In addition, the composite outcome of death or MI trended in favour of fondaparinux compared with enoxaparin (6.2% vs 6.8%; HR 0.90, 95% CI 0.81–1.01; $p=0.07$), as did the composite of death, MI, or refractory ischemia (8.0% vs 8.6%; HR 0.93, 95% CI 0.84–1.02; $p=0.13$). At 6 months' follow-up, there was a clear superiority of fondaparinux over enoxaparin in preventing the hard, irreversible outcomes of death, MI, or stroke (11.3% vs 12.5%; HR 0.89, 95% CI 0.82–0.97; $p=0.007$), and the mortality benefit persisted out to this longer-term follow-up (5.8% vs 6.5%; HR 0.92, 95% CI 0.84–1.00; $p=0.05$). In addition, fondaparinux reduced stroke as a single outcome compared with enoxaparin (1.3% vs 1.7%; HR 0.78, 95% CI 0.62–0.99; $p=0.04$).

For safety, there was a large reduction in major bleeding with fondaparinux compared with enoxaparin at 9 days

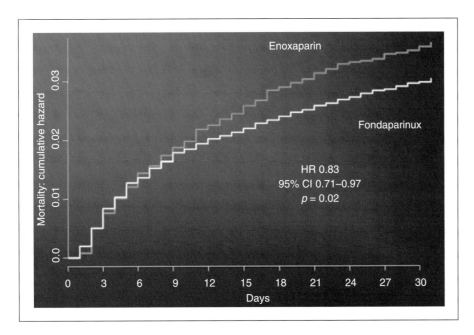

Figure 17.3
Fondaparinux reduces all-cause mortality compared with enoxaparin in patients with NSTE ACS.
(see color plate)

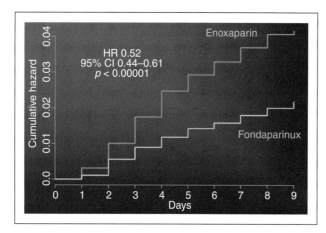

Figure 17.4
Fondaparinux reduces major bleeding substantially compared with enoxaparin in patients with NSTE ACS. (see color plate)

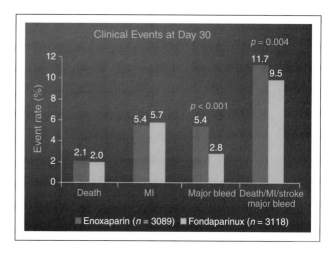

Figure 17.5
In patients undergoing PCI in OASIS-5, efficacy outcomes were similar between the enoxaparin and fondaparinux groups, but there was a large reduction in major bleeding in the latter, resulting in a significant net clinical benefit with fondaparinux. (see color plate)

(2.2% vs 4.1%; HR 0.52, 95% CI 0.44–0.61; $p<0.001$) (Figure 17.4). Bleeding was reduced as early as the first day after treatment, indicating that fondaparinux is safer than enoxaparin with even relatively short durations of treatment. In addition, fatal bleeding (i.e., a bleeding event that resulted in the death of the patient) was significantly reduced with fondaparinux compared with enoxaparin (7 fatal bleeds with fondaparinux vs 22 with enoxaparin $p=0.005$) and severe bleeding according to the TIMI scale (70 TIMI major bleeds with fondaparinux vs 126 with enoxaparin; HR 0.55, 95% CI 0.41–0.74; $p<0.001$). In addition, bleeding requiring surgical intervention to stop it was lower with fondaparinux compared with enoxaparin (41 vs 77), as were retroperitoneal bleeding (9 vs 37) and need for blood transfusion (164 vs 287) ($p<0.001$ for all comparisons).

In patients undergoing PCI, efficacy in terms of death, MI, or stroke was similar between the fondaparinux and enoxaparin groups at 9 days (6.3% vs 6.2%; HR 1.03, 95% CI 0.84–1.25; $p=0.79$).[30] However, there was a large and highly significant reduction in major bleeding with fondaparinux group compared with the enoxaparin group (2.3% vs 4.9%; HR 0.48, 95% CI 0.31–0.72; $p=0.0005$) (Figure 17.5).[30] Similarly, there were large and highly significant reductions in minor bleeding and total bleeding with fondaparinux. Major bleeding at 9 days was 5.1% in those patients where study drug was not restarted after PCI compared with 3.1% in patients where study drug was restarted (relative risk (RR) 0.61, 95% CI 0.47–0.80, $p<0.0001$). In addition, fondaparinux was superior to enoxaparin in reducing major bleeding irrespective of whether study drug was restarted after PCI (1.9% vs 4.4%; HR 0.42, 95% CI 0.29–0.60; $p<0.00001$) or whether it was not restarted after the procedure (3.7% vs 6.6%; HR 0.55, 95% CI 0.35–0.84; $p<0.00001$). Thus, restarting of study drug after PCI did not increase the rate of major bleeding in OASIS 5, and, regardless of whether study drug was restarted, fondaparinux was associated with lower rates of major

bleeding compared with enoxaparin. Patients undergoing PCI who experienced a major bleeding event during the initial hospitalization had substantially higher rates of death (10.1% vs 1.7%; HR 6.00, 95% CI 3.82–9.42; $p<0.00001$), MI (14.3% vs 5.3%; HR 2.77, 95% CI 1.93–3.99; $p<0.00001$), and stroke (3.1% vs 0.5%; HR 5.99, 95% CI 2.64–13.56; $p<0.00001$) at 30 days. The differences persisted at 6 months: death (HR 4.31, 95% CI 2.89–6.42; $p<0.00001$), MI (HR 2.47, 95% CI 1.76–3.47; $p<0.00001$), and stroke (HR 5.55, 95% CI 2.81–10.94; $p<0.00001$).[30]

Thus, in PCI patients, the net clinical composite of death, MI, stroke, or major bleeding was significantly lower with fondaparinux compared with enoxaparin at day 9 (8.2% vs 10.4%; HR 0.78, 95% CI 0.67–0.93; $p=0.004$) (Figure 17.5).[30] This net clinical benefit of fondaparinux was preserved at longer-term follow-up out to day 30 and to 6 months, highlighting the clinical superiority of fondaparinux over enoxaparin in PCI patients.

Outcomes in patients undergoing early PCI

In patients undergoing PCI within the first 24 hours, death, MI, or stroke occurred in 5.3% in the fondaparinux group and 5.4% in the enoxaparin group (HR 0.98, 95% CI 0.71–1.34), with a marked and highly significant reduction in major bleeding with fondaparinux compared with enoxaparin (2.3% vs 4.9%; HR 0.48; $p=0.0005$).[30] Major bleeding was reduced with fondaparinux compared with enoxaparin as early as the day of randomization (i.e., within hours after administration of the first dose of study drug). Similarly, major bleeding was lower with fondaparinux compared with enoxaparin on the first day and subsequent days after randomization. Thus, even with very short durations of therapy, major bleeding was lower with fondaparinux than with enoxaparin.

The net clinical benefit of death, MI, stroke, or major bleeding favored fondaparinux in those undergoing early PCI (7.3% vs 9.5%; HR 0.76; $p = 0.035$).[30]

Use of UFH

In the OASIS-5 trial, enoxaparin-treated patients undergoing PCI 6 hours after the last subcutaneous dose received guideline-recommended doses of UFH during PCI. Fondaparinux reduced major bleeding irrespective of whether PCI was performed within 6 hours of the last enoxaparin dose (1.5% vs 3.7%; HR 0.41; $p < 0.0001$) or later than 6 hours when UFH was given (1.4% vs 3.6%; HR 0.39; $p < 0.0001$).[30] Thus, the use of UFH did not increase the risk of bleeding in the enoxaparin group, and, both in those patients undergoing PCI with enoxaparin as the sole anticoagulant and in those receiving UFH, fondaparinux resulted in a marked reduction in major bleeding.

Catheter-related thrombus was observed more commonly when fondaparinux or enoxaparin was the sole anticoagulant (0.9% with fondaparinux alone, 0.4% with enoxaparin alone, and 0.2% when UFH was added to enoxaparin for PCI 6 hours after the last subcutaneous dose).[30] Importantly, catheter thrombus was virtually eliminated in the fondaparinux group with the use of conventional doses of UFH for the PCI procedure (mean dose 4000–5000 units with or without concurrent GPIIb/IIIa inhibitor.[30] In addition, the use of UFH for PCI in patients treated upstream with fondaparinux preserved the reduction in major bleeding with fondaparinux. Thus, in patients treated upstream with fondaparinux, it is recommended that standard UFH

with or without a GPIIb/IIIa antagonist be used for PCI anticoagulation. Bivalirudin was not used in the OASIS-5 trial, but previous randomized studies in patients undergoing elective or urgent PCI have demonstrated lower rates of bleeding with bivalirudin compared with UFH and a GPIIb/IIIa inhibitor. It follows that the use of bivalirudin during PCI in patients treated upstream with fondaparinux might be a very attractive option for the management of ACS patients. Such a strategy will be tested in future large-scale randomized controlled trials.

Mechanistic studies are attempting to address the issue of catheter-related thrombus with enoxaparin and with fondaparinux. In one trial of patients undergoing primary PCI with enoxaparin, catheter thrombus occurred in 3 patients out of 36 treated, requiring a change to the protocol.[31] Preliminary data with in situ models of thrombosis using angioplasty guiding catheters suggests that catheter thrombus is mediated by the extrinsic (or contact-mediated) coagulation pathway.[32] The use of agents with greater thrombin activity (such as UFH or direct thrombin inhibitors) appears to be the best way to avoid clotting due to this mechanism.[32] By contrast, thrombosis induced by spontaneous plaque rupture is mediated by tissue factor release, and agents with greater factor Xa activity (e.g., fondaparinux) may have a greater benefit. Thus, a combined approach of using a factor Xa inhibitor such as fondaparinux upstream with targeted therapy with a predominantly thrombin inhibitor (e.g., UFH or bivalirudin) may be an optimal approach for the management of ACS.

OASIS-6

The OASIS-6 trial evaluated the effects of fondaparinux in patients with STEMI.[33] Patients with ST-segment elevation

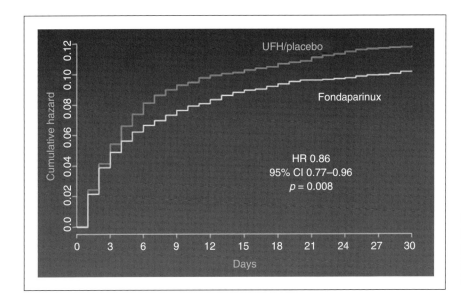

Figure 17.6
OASIS 6: fondaparinux reduces death or MI compared with standard care in STEMI. (Reproduced from Yusuf S et al.[33]) (see color plate)

Table 17.1   *OASIS-6: fondaparinux reduced mortality as well as MI in STEMI patients at study end without increasing major bleeding*

	Percentage of events				
	Control (6056 patients)	Fondaparinux (6036 patients)	Hazard ratio	95% confidence interval	*p*
Death or re-MI	14.8	13.4	0.88	0.79–0.97	0.008
Death	11.6	10.5	0.88	0.79–0.99	0.029
Reinfarction	4.6	3.8	0.81	0.67–0.97	0.026

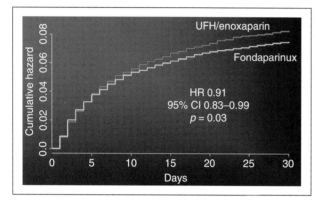

Figure 17.7
Combined analysis of OASIS-5 and -6 showing superiority of fondaparinux compared with UFH or enoxaparin. (see color plate)

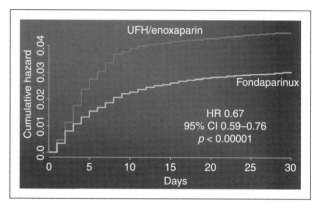

Figure 17.8
Combined analysis of OASIS-5 and -6 showing major bleeding at 30 days: fondaparinux versus UFH/enoxaparin. (see color plate)

presenting within 24 hours of onset of ischemic symptoms were eligible. Overall, 12 092 patients were randomized to receive fondaparinux 2.5 mg subcutaneously (with the first dose given intravenously) or control. Control therapy depended on whether, in the judgment of the principal investigator or treating physician, UFH was indicated (e.g., if a fibrin-specific thrombolytic or primary PCI was performed) or not (e.g., with non-fibrin-specific thrombolytic agents). Importantly, patients presenting late with STEMI were also eligible for this trial, as they represent up to 30% of patients presenting to hospital.

The results demonstrated that fondaparinux was superior to standard therapy in preventing death or myocardial infarction (9.7% vs 11.2%; HR 0.86; *p* = 0.008) (Figure 17.6). In addition, fondaparinux reduced all cause mortality at 30 days (7.8% vs 8.9%; HR 0.87; *p* = 0.03) as well as mortality and myocardial infarction alone at study end (Table 17.1). Major bleeding was not increased with fondaparinux (2.1% vs 1.8%; HR 0.83; *p* = 0.14). There were a significantly fewer pericardial bleeds and cardiac tamponade events in the fondaparinux group (0.5% vs 0.8%; HR 0.59; *p* = 0.02), perhaps due to lower infarct size or reinfarction in the fondaparinux group. The greatest benefit of fondaparinux was observed in those patients receiving either a fibrinolytic agent or no reperfusion treatment because of late presentation. In patients receiving a primary PCI, the results were neutral and there was an excess in catheter-related thrombosis when

fondaparinux was used alone (i.e., with no UFH) for the procedure. By contrast, patients who required rescue PCI, early PCI, or elective PCI, after the index event all received UFH in the trial, and there were no cases of catheter-related thrombus events and no increase in major bleeding in this group. Thus, UFH can be safely used with fondaparinux in STEMI if urgent or elective PCI is required after the index event. For primary PCI, standard UFH is still recommended as the standard therapy.

In summary, fondaparinux reduces mortality and reinfarction without an increase in bleeding in patients presenting with STEMI. There is a higher rate of catheter thrombosis if PCI is performed without UFH, but this is largely avoided if UFH is used during the procedure. There is a trend towards fewer severe bleeds with a significant reduction in cardiac tamponade with fondaparinux. The consistent results from OASIS 5 and OASIS 6 confirm the value of fondaparinux as a simple and widely applicable antithrombotic therapy in a broad group of patients with ACS.

Combined analysis of OASIS-5 and -6

A combined analysis of OASIS-5 and -6 demonstrated that, for efficacy, fondaparinux is superior to any control therapy in reducing mortality alone (4.8% vs 5.6%; HR 0.86;

$p=0.002$) as well as the composite of death, MI, or stroke at 30 days (8.0% vs 9.1%; HR 0.87; $p<0.0001$).[34] Compared with UFH or enoxaparin, fondaparinux reduced mortality (3.8% vs 4.3%; HR 0.89; $p=0.05$) (Figure 17.7) as well as the composite of death, MI, or stroke at 30 days (7.2% vs 8.0%; HR 0.91; $p=0.03$). Compared with placebo, fondaparinux also reduced mortality (9.1% vs 11.3%; HR 0.80; $p=0.006$) and the composite of death, MI or stroke (11.6% vs 14.6%; HR 0.78; $p=0.001$). For safety, fondaparinux reduced major bleeding by 41% compared with UFH or enoxaparin (2.1% vs 3.4%; HR 0.59; $p<0.00001$) (Figure 17.8), and compared with placebo did not increase bleeding (1.6% vs 2.3%; HR 0.69; $p=0.06$). In patients undergoing PCI, fondaparinux was similar to UFH or enoxaparin in reducing death, MI, or stroke (8.0% vs 8.0%) but reduced major bleeding (2.9% vs 5.5%; HR 0.52; $p<0.0001$), resulting in superior net clinical benefit as assessed by death, MI, stroke or major bleeding (9.0% vs 11.8%; HR 0.75; $p=0.01$). Thus, data in over 32 000 patients demonstrate that fondaparinux reduces all-cause mortality and ischemic events as well as major bleeding across the entire spectrum of acute coronary syndromes.

References

1. Weitz JI, Bates SM. New anticoagulants. J Thromb Haemost 2005;3:1843–53.
2. Walenga JM, Bara L, Petitou M et al. The inhibition of the generation of thrombin and the antithrombotic effect of a pentasaccharide with sole anti-factor Xa activity. Thromb Res 1988;51:23–33.
3. Turpie AG, Eriksson BI, Lassen MR, Bauer KA. Fondaparinux, the first selective factor Xa inhibitor. Curr Opin Hematol 2003;10:327–32.
4. Bauer KA, Hawkins DW, Peters PC et al. Fondaparinux, a synthetic pentasaccharide: the first in a new class of antithrombotic agents – the selective factor Xa inhibitors. Cardiovasc Drug Rev 2002;20:37–52.
5. Turpie AG. Fondaparinux: a Factor Xa inhibitor for antithrombotic therapy. Expert Opin Pharmacother 2004;5:1373–84.
6. Walenga JM, Petitou M, Lormeau JC et al. Antithrombotic activity of a synthetic heparin pentasaccharide in a rabbit stasis thrombosis model using different thrombogenic challenges. Thromb Res 1987;46:187–98.
7. Walenga JM, Jeske WP, Bara L et al. Biochemical and pharmacologic rationale for the development of a synthetic heparin pentasaccharide. Thromb Res 1997;86:1–36.
8. Walenga JM, Jeske WP, Samama MM et al. Fondaparinux: a synthetic heparin pentasaccharide as a new antithrombotic agent. Expert Opin Invest Drugs 2002;11:397–407.
9. Petitou M, Duchaussoy P, Driguez PA et al. New synthetic heparin mimetics able to inhibit thrombin and factor Xa. Bioorg Med Chem Lett 1999;9:1155–60.
10. Boneu B, Necciari J, Cariou R et al. Pharmacokinetics and tolerance of the natural pentasaccharide (SR90107/Org31540) with high affinity to antithrombin III in man. Thromb Haemost 1995;74:1468–73.
11. Petitou M, Duchaussoy P, Jaurand G et al. Synthesis and pharmacological properties of a close analogue of an antithrombotic pentasaccharide (SR 90107A/ORG 31540). J Med Chem 1997;40:1600–7.
12. Turpie AG, Gallus AS, Hoek JA. A synthetic pentasaccharide for the prevention of deep-vein thrombosis after total hip replacement. N Engl J Med 2001;344:619–25.
13. Turpie AG. Pentasaccharide Org31540/SR90107A clinical trials update: lessons for practice. Am Heart J 2001;142:S9–15.
14. Elalamy I, Lecrubier C, Potevin F et al. Absence of in vitro cross-reaction of pentasaccharide with the plasma heparin-dependent factor of twenty-five patients with heparin-associated thrombocytopenia. Thromb Haemost 1995;74:1384–5.
15. Bijsterveld NR, Moons AH, Boekholdt SM et al. Ability of recombinant factor VIIa to reverse the anticoagulant effect of the pentasaccharide fondaparinux in healthy volunteers. Circulation 2002;106:2550–4.
16. Bijsterveld NR, Vink R, van Aken BE et al. Recombinant factor VIIa reverses the anticoagulant effect of the long-acting pentasaccharide idraparinux in healthy volunteers. Br J Haematol 2004;124:653–8.
17. Weitz JI. Emerging anticoagulants for the treatment of venous thromboembolism. Thromb Haemost 2006;96:274–84.
18. Bauer KA, Eriksson BI, Lassen MR, Turpie AG. Fondaparinux compared with enoxaparin for the prevention of venous thromboembolism after elective major knee surgery. N Engl J Med 2001;345:1305–10.
19. Eriksson BI, Bauer KA, Lassen MR, Turpie AG. Fondaparinux compared with enoxaparin for the prevention of venous thromboembolism after hip-fracture surgery. N Engl J Med 2001;345:1298–304.
20. Eriksson BI, Lassen MR. Duration of prophylaxis against venous thromboembolism with fondaparinux after hip fracture surgery: a multicenter, randomized, placebo-controlled, double-blind study. Arch Intern Med 2003;163:1337–42.
21. Turpie AG, Bauer KA, Eriksson BI, Lassen MR. Postoperative fondaparinux versus postoperative enoxaparin for prevention of venous thromboembolism after elective hip-replacement surgery: a randomised double-blind trial. Lancet 2002;359:1721–6.
22. Cohen AT, Davidson BL, Gallus AS et al. Efficacy and safety of fondaparinux for the prevention of venous thromboembolism in older acute medical patients: randomised placebo controlled trial. BMJ 2006;332:325–9.
23. Turpie AG, Bauer KA, Eriksson BI, Lassen MR. Fondaparinux vs enoxaparin for the prevention of venous thromboembolism in major orthopedic surgery: a meta-analysis of 4 randomized double-blind studies. Arch Intern Med 2002;162:1833–40.
24. Simoons ML, Bobbink IW, Boland J et al. A dose-finding study of fondaparinux in patients with non-ST-segment elevation acute coronary syndromes: the Pentasaccharide in Unstable Angina (PENTUA) study. J Am Coll Cardiol 2004;43:2183–90.
25. Coussement PK, Bassand JP, Convens C et al. A synthetic factor-Xa inhibitor (ORG31540/SR9017A) as an adjunct to fibrinolysis in acute myocardial infarction. The PENTALYSE study. Eur Heart J 2001;22:1716–24.
26. Mehta SR, Steg PG, Granger CB et al. Randomized, blinded trial comparing fondaparinux with unfractionated heparin in patients undergoing contemporary percutaneous coronary intervention: Arixtra Study in Percutaneous Coronary Intervention: a Randomized Evaluation (ASPIRE) pilot trial. Circulation 2005;111:1390–7.
27. Vuillemenot A, Schiele F, Meneveau N et al. Efficacy of a synthetic pentasaccharide, a pure factor Xa inhibitor, as an antithrombotic agent – a pilot study in the setting of coronary angioplasty. Thromb Haemost 1999;81:214–20.
28. Mehta SR, Yusuf S, Granger CB et al. Design and rationale of the MICHELANGELO Organization to Assess Strategies in Acute Ischemic Syndromes (OASIS)-5 trial program evaluating fondaparinux, a synthetic factor Xa inhibitor, in patients with non-ST-segment elevation acute coronary syndromes. Am Heart J 2005;150:1107.
29. Yusuf S, Mehta SR, Chrolavicius S et al. Comparison of fondaparinux and enoxaparin in acute coronary syndromes. N Engl J Med 2006;354:1464–76.
30. Mehta SR, Granger CB, Bassand JP et al. Fondaparinux is associated with substantially less major bleeding and vascular access site complications compared with enoxaparin in patients with acute coronary

syndrome undergoing percutaneous coronary intervention: insights from the OASIS 5 trial. J Am Coll Cardiol 2006;47(4 Suppl A):205A (Abst 821-5).

31. Buller CE, Pate GE, Armstrong PW et al. Catheter thrombosis during primary percutaneous coronary intervention for acute ST elevation myocardial infarction despite subcutaneous low-molecular-weight heparin, acetylsalicylic acid, clopidogrel and abciximab pretreatment. Can J Cardiol 2006;22:511–15.

32. Weitz J. Anticoagulation during PCI: fondaparinux and catheter thrombosis. Accessed at http:/www.theheart.org (22 October 2006, 11 June 2007).

33. Yusuf S, Mehta SR, Chrolavicius S et al. Effects of fondaparinux on mortality and reinfarction in patients with acute ST-segment elevation myocardial infarction: the OASIS-6 randomized trial. JAMA 2006;295:1519–30.

34. Mehta SR, on behalf of the OASIS 6 and 6 Steering Committee. Benefit of fondaparinux on mortality, ischemic events and bleeding across the entire spectrum of acute coronary syndromes: results of the combined analysis of OASIS 5 and OASIS 6. Presented at the Europen Society of Cardiology and World Congress of Cardiology. Hotline Session, 2006.

35. Lasser MR, Bauer KA, Eriksson BI, Turpie AG. Postoperative fonda-parinux versus preoperative enoxaparin for prevention of venous thromboembolism in elective hip-replacement surgery: a randomised double-blind comparison. Lancet 2002;359:1715–20.

18

Tissue factor inhibitors

Christian T Ruff, David A Morrow, and Robert P Giugliano

Introduction

Anticoagulation is the cornerstone of therapy in the treatment of venous and arterial thromboembolism. Traditional anticoagulants – unfractionated heparin (UFH), low-molecular-weight heparin (LMWH), and warfarin – have many significant limitations. Both UFH and warfarin have narrow therapeutic windows of adequate anticoagulation without bleeding and a highly variable dose–response relation among individuals that requires frequent monitoring by laboratory testing.[1–3] UFH, and to a lesser extent LMWH, is associated with the occurrence of thrombocytopenia, a potentially fatal complication that may be associated with thrombosis.[4,5] Importantly, current antithrombotic strategies do not suppress generation of thrombin, the critical enzyme that generates fibrin and activates platelets.[6–9] An important aspect of this system is that at each branch in the pathway, one molecule of enzyme is able to activate many molecules of its substrate protein, thereby amplifying each step in the cascade. Given this cascade of interactions, an approach that intervenes at the earliest trigger to activation of the system has a potential for more effective inhibition of thrombin generation than strategies that rely upon inhibition of later steps.

Coagulation cascade and platelet activation

Endothelial injury or the rupture of vulnerable atherosclerotic plaque triggers the release of tissue factor (TF), a surface glycoprotein that is expressed by endothelial cells, monocytes, and smooth muscle cells and is upregulated in response to vascular endothelial injury (Figure 18.1). When exposed to circulating blood, TF binds to the serine protease factor (F) VII, forming a complex that activates FIX, which then activates FX; alternatively, TF:FVII can directly activate FX. It is at this step that tissue factor pathway inhibitor (TFPI) regulates the extrinsic coagulation pathway by forming a complex with FXa, which then forms an inhibitory quaternary complex with – TF:VIIa.[10,11] FXa forms a complex with FVa and calcium to catalyze the conversion of prothrombin to thrombin (FIIa), the critical enzyme that generates fibrin.[6,8,9] In addition to forming fibrin and activating FXIII, which crosslinks and stabilizes the fibrin network, thrombin activates platelet aggregation and plays a crucial role in the positive feedback mechanisms of the coagulation cascade by activating FV and FVIII as well as platelet-bound FXI.[7] TF also plays a role in platelet activation both through binding of fibrin to platelet integrins and through direct interaction via the G-protein-coupled receptor family known as protease-activated receptors (PARs).[12,13] The TF:FVIIa–FXa complex acts as a cofactor for activation of both PAR-2 (endothelial cells) and PAR-1 (platelets).[14] Moreover, the accumulation of TF in developing thrombus is believed to occur through a mechanism involving P-selectin on the platelet surface.[15,16]

This amplification is enhanced by the cooperative interaction between the coagulation and platelet pathways.[17] Given that TF serves as the gatekeeper to this amplification process, an agent that interferes with the ability of TF to initiate this process has a potential to be a more effective inhibitor of thrombin generation than strategies that inhibit downstream steps.

Role of tissue factor in thrombosis and cardiovascular disease

Experimental studies have established the presence of tissue factor within thrombus (Figure 18.2). For example, thrombus that precipitates on pig arterial media devoid of TF and thrombus that precipitates on collagen-coated glass slides (also devoid of TF) when exposed to flowing human blood both stain intensely for TF. Interestingly, antibodies against TF caused a 70% reduction in the amount of thrombus formed.[18] In hyperlipidemic mice, TF expression localizes in neointimal macrophages after arterial injury.[19] TF mRNA

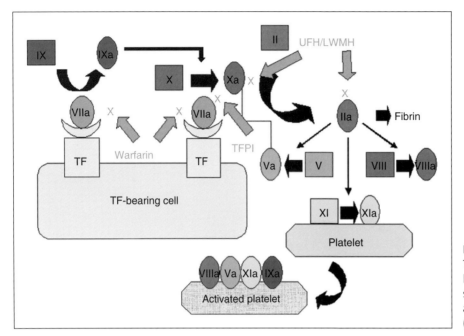

Figure 18.1
The role of the coagulation cascade leading to platelet activation and the sites of action of various anticoagulants. See text for details. (see color plate)

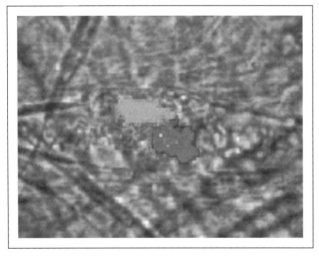

Figure 18.2
Tissue factor, platelet, and fibrin deposition during thrombus formation. Using color-coded antibodies during the experimental induction of thrombi in mice, the constituents of a growing thrombus (25% of maximum size) includes predominantly platelets (red), tissue factor (green), fibrin (blue), tissue factor + platelets (yellow), with lesser amounts of fibrin (turquoise) and platelets + fibrin (magenta). (Adapted with permission from Chou et al.[50]) (see color plate)

expression in human carotid and coronary atherosclerotic plaques is significantly increased in lipid-rich compared with fibrous plaque components.[19]

There is a substantial amount of data implicating high levels of circulating TF as possibly responsible for the increased thrombotic complications associated with certain cardiovascular risk factors such as hyperlipidemia, diabetes, hypertension, and smoking.[20,21] For example, patients with improvement in glycemic control show a reduction in circulating TF, whereas levels are increased in a dose-related fashion after smoking cigarettes.[20] Levels are elevated in hyperlipidemic subjects compared with healthy volunteers.[20] Statins have been shown to reduce TF expression in monocytes, endothelial cells, and vascular smooth muscle cells.[22–24] In mice they inhibit TF expression in advanced plaques independent of plasma lipid levels.[25] TF plasma antigen levels are elevated in hypertensive subjects and can be lowered by antihypertensive drugs, especially angiotensin-converting enzyme (ACE) inhibitors and angiotensin II type I receptor (AT-1) blockers.[21]

Although TF is primarily a membrane bound protein, it is detectable in circulating plasma at low concentrations (0.0067 nmol/l) in healthy individuals and at modestly but detectably higher concentrations in patients presenting with unstable angina (0.01 nmol/l),[9] as well as among patients with complications during angioplasty.[17] TF is also more abundant in atherosclerotic plaque from patients with unstable compared with stable angina, and there is a close correlation between the amount of TF antigen and TF activity.[18,26] In particular, TF expression is increased on macrophages in patients with unstable angina and myocardial infarction,[12,27,28] and this increase is associated with an adverse prognosis.

In addition to activation of the coagulation cascade, TF has been implicated in short- and long-term adverse effects mediated through inflammatory pathways. Almost all systemic inflammatory responses, ranging from coronary artery disease to sepsis,[26,29] lead to derangement of the coagulation system mediated by proinflammatory cytokines.[30,31] This observation suggests the potential for inhibition of TF to have not only anticoagulant actions but also anti-inflammatory effects.

Tissue factor inhibitors

There are many agents that interfere with TF expression, its activation of the coagulation cascade, and its role in platelet aggregation through non-specific anti-inflammatory or antiplatelet effects, but we will focus on agents developed specifically to interfere with TF and the TF–FVIIa complex (Table 18.1). At present, no drugs are clinically available for therapeutic use, but several are being evaluated in clinical studies in man.

Endogenous Inhibition – tissue factor pathway inhibitor

Tissue factor pathway inhibitor (TFPI) regulates the initial step of the extrinsic coagulation pathway mediated by TF.[32] TFPI is present on endothelium and circulates in association with plasma lipoproteins and platelets. It exerts its inhibitory action by forming a complex with FXa, which then forms an inhibitory quaternary complex with TF:FVIIa.[10,11]

Experimental data

Evaluation of recombinant TFPI in animal models has demonstrated promise for TFPI as an inhibitor of arterial

Table 18.1 *Tissue factor inhibitors*

Drug	Site of action	Mechanism	Preclinical data	Clinical data
Tissue factor pathway inhibitor (TFPI)	FXa	Forms a complex with FXa, which then forms an inhibitory complex with TF:FVIIa	Inhibition of arterial thrombosis in animals Decreased mortality in animal model of sepsis	Dose-dependent inhibition of coagulation cascade in human endotoxemia
Active site-blocked factor VIIa (FVIIai)	TF	Competitive inhibitor of FVIIa for TF binding	Inhibition of arterial thrombosis in animals	Negative phase II study comparing FVIIai + heparin vs heparin alone in patients undergoing PCI
Sunol cH-36: a mouse/human monoclonal antibody to TF	TF	Binds TF at the FX-binding site	Inhibition of thrombin generation in whole blood assay	No major bleeding but dose-dependent increase in minor bleeding in phase I study in patients with CAD
Recombinant nematode anticoagulant protein (rNAPc2)	FXa	Binds to the catalytic site of FXa	Inhibition of arterial and venous thrombosis in animals Attenuation of procoagulant response in animal model of peritonitis	Decreased DVT in patients undergoing elective, unilateral total knee replacement Decreased thrombin generation in dose-escalation trial in patients with CAD scheduled for elective PCI In patients with NSTE ACS, demonstrated a dose-dependent inhibition of thrombin generation, reduction in ischemia on continuous ECG, and similar rates of bleeding

TF, tissue factor; FXa (etc.), factor Xa (etc.); PCI, percutaneous coronary intervention; CAD, coronary artery disease; DVT, deep vein thrombosis; NSTE ACS, non-ST-elevation acute coronary syndromes.

thrombosis. An early study determined that reocclusion of electrically thrombosed dog femoral arteries after thrombolysis with tissue-type plasminogen activator (tPA) could be prevented by infusing recombinant TFPI.[33] Investigators using a rabbit model to examine the effect of recombinant TFPI infusion on restenosis rates after balloon angioplasty of femoral arteries demonstrated that TFPI reduced angiographic restenosis and decreased neointimal hyperplasia.[34] The results of a study of balloon-injured porcine carotid arteries treated locally with adenovirus encoding human TFPI demonstrated decreased cyclic flow variations after artery occlusion compared with controls.[15] Encouragingly, animal studies of infused anti-TF antibodies showed no increase in bleeding.[16]

In a study of baboons administered a lethal dose of *Escherichia coli*, infusion of recombinant TFPI resulted in survival of 5/5 baboons, while none (0/5) of controls survived.[35] Although a randomized controlled trial in humans evaluating the efficacy and safety of recombinant TFPI (Tifacogin) in severe sepsis found no effect on all-cause mortality and an increased risk of bleeding,[36] prior animal studies of infused anti-TF antibodies showed no increase in bleeding.[16]

Clinical studies

The number of clinical studies remains low. TFPI has been shown to dose-dependently inhibit coagulation activation in human endotoxemia without influencing the fibrinolytic and cytokine response. In a double-blind, randomized, placebo-controlled crossover study, subjects received bolus injections (4 ng/kg) of endotoxin followed by 6-hour continuous infusion of TFPI (both a high-dose (0.2 mg/kg) and a low-dose (0.05 mg/kg) group) or placebo. TFPI infusion demonstrated dose-dependent attenuation of thrombin generation as measured by plasma levels of the prothrombin fragment F1.2 and thrombin–antithrombin complexes, with complete blockade of coagulation after high-dose TFP.[37] Interestingly, TFPI did not influence the fibrinolytic and cytokine response to endotoxin.

Active site-blocked factor VIIa

FVIIai, an inactivated form of FVIIa that lacks catalytic activity, is a competitive inhibitor of FVIIa for TF binding. Blocking this complex prevents the activation of FX, which regulates the conversion of prothrombin to thrombin.

Experimental data

In rabbit models of arterial thrombosis, administration of FVIIai at arterial trauma sites improved vessel patency compared with controls.[38,39] A single 10-minute infusion exerted a complete antithrombotic effect for at least 6 hours, despite the fact that plasma FVIIai levels were well below threshold concentrations.[39]

Clinical studies

Based on promising preclinical studies, a phase II trial was performed comparing FVIIai plus heparin versus heparin alone in patients undergoing percutaneous coronary intervention (PCI).[40] A total of 491 patients undergoing elective or urgent coronary stenting or balloon angioplasty were randomized to receive either adjuvant heparin or adjuvant modified recombinant human activated factor VII (FFR–FVIIa) at one of six escalating dosage levels with supplemental heparin. There was no difference in the primary endpoint of death, myocardial infarction (MI), urgent revascularization, abrupt vessel closure or glycoprotein IIb/IIIa (GPIIb/IIIa) bailout (20% in the control group and 5.5–38.9% in the heparin–FFR–FVIIa groups; $p=$NS). No differences were observed in the rates of major or minor bleeding complications. Further clinical development of this compound has been placed on hold.

Antibodies to tissue factor

Antibodies directed against TF have been evaluated both in vivo and in preliminary clinical trials. There has been interest in a specific mouse/human monoclonal antibody to TF, Sunol-cH36, which specifically binds to human TF at the FX-binding site, preventing formation of the TF:VIIa–FX complex and thereby preventing thrombin formation by blocking the production of FXa and FXia. Sunol-cH36 has a long elimination half-life (about 70 hours) and requires recombinant FVIIa for reversal of its anticoagulant effects.

Experimental data

In a rabbit carotid artery thrombosis model, administration of an anti-TF monoclonal antibody (AP-1) reduced reocclusion rates and shortened tPA lysis time.[41] Another study performed in a rabbit coronary artery ligation model demonstrated a reduction in infarct size by up to 61% after administration of an anti-TF antibody, which correlated with a decrease in chemokine expression and leukocyte infiltration.[42] An experimental study of human atherosclerotic arterial segments in a coronary stenosis model observed that an anti-TF polyclonal antibody reduced thrombogenicity of disrupted atherosclerotic plaques by impairing platelet and fibrin deposition.[43]

The potency of Sunol-cH36 as an anticoagulant has been evaluated using a minimally altered whole blood assay. Clot formation initiated with 40 pmol/l of recombinant human TF was significantly delayed by the addition of Sunol-cH36, with evidence of inhibition of thrombin generation via measurement of fibrinopeptide A.[44]

Clinical studies

Sunol-cH36 has been studied in a phase I study of patients with coronary artery disease (CAD): PROXIMATE–TIMI 27. In this study, the tolerability and pharmacokinetics of Sunol-cH36 were evaluated in an open-label, dose-escalating design among 26 subjects with stable CAD.[44] Five separate doses of Sunol-cH36 (0.03, 0.06, 0.08, 0.1, and 0.3 mg/kg) were administered as a single intravenous bolus. No major bleeding (≥2 g/dl hemoglobin decline) occurred. Spontaneous minor bleeding occurred in a dose-related pattern, exhibiting an anticoagulant effect of this agent for the first time in humans. Interestingly, the majority of spontaneous bleeding episodes were clinically consistent with platelet-mediated bleeding without thrombocytopenia. This finding, along with concurrent in vitro studies, raised the hypothesis that the mucosal bleeding observed with this potent inhibitor of thrombin generation reflect antiplatelet effects resulting from interference of networking between the coagulation cascade and platelet pathways mediated by TF's binding of fibrin to platelet integrins and direct activation of PARs on platelets and endothelial cells (Figure 18.1). The median terminal half-life of the drug was 72.2 hours. The study was not designed to detect significant differences in ischemic event rates.

Nematode anticoagulant protein (NAPc2)

Nematode anticoagulant proteins (NAPs) are a family of small proteins (75–84 residues) that inhibit blood coagulation in picomolar concentrations and are found in hookworm parasites. The inhibition of thrombin formation occurs by direct binding to the catalytic site of FXa.[45] A novel recombinant analogue of nematode anticoagulant protein c2 (rNAPc2), initially isolated from the canine hookworm (*Ancylostoma caninum*), has been developed and shown to inhibit FVIIa bound to TF in a FX/Xa-dependent fashion. The agent is characterized by a long elimination half-life (about 60 hours). Reversal of anticoagulation with this agent requires recombinant FVIIa.

Experimental data

The antithrombotic activity of rNAPc2 has been assessed in preclinical studies in rats and pigs, where significant antithrombotic efficacy of rNAPc2 was demonstrated in models of both arterial and venous blood clot formation. rNAPc2 has also been studied in animal models of peritonitis, which is associated with an increase in TF levels and procoagulant effects as reflected by fibrinogen deposition. Mice given an intraperitoneal injection of live *E. coli* with concurrent treatment with rNAPc2 had a strongly attenuated procoagulant response compared with controls. However, there was no difference in dissemination of infection or survival.[46]

Clinical studies

rNAPc2 has been studied as an anticoagulant in both venous and arterial thrombosis. rNAPc2 was evaluated for the prevention of venous thromboembolism after elective unilateral total knee replacement.[47] Each enrolled patient received one of three dosages of rNAPC2: 1.5, 3.0, or 5.0 μg/kg. The first dose was administered initially within 6–12 hours or within 1 hour after surgery. Patients received a dose on days 1, 3, 5, and 7. Primary efficacy outcome was a composite of overall deep vein thrombosis (DVT) based on mandatory unilateral venography (day 7 ± 2) and confirmed symptomatic venous thromboembolism recorded ≤48 hours after the last dose. Observed rates of overall DVT were similar across the three regimens in which rNAPc2 was administered within 6–12 hours after surgery (mean 21.5%). When rNAPc2 was initiated within 1 hour after surgery, the overall DVT rate for the 3 μg/kg dosage group fell to 12.2% (95% confidence interval (CI) 5.7–21.8%). No substantial differences occurred in rates of minor bleeding among the five regimens, but there was increased major bleeding at the highest dosage of rNAPc2.

rNAPc2 has been studied in 154 patients with CAD scheduled for elective PCI in a multicenter, randomized, double blinded, dose-escalation trial.[48] In addition to aspirin and unfractionated heparin (UFH), participants received placebo or rNAPc2 at doses of 3.5, 5.0, 7.5, and 10.0 μg/kg as a single subcutaneous administration 2–6 hours before angioplasty. Clopidogrel was administered after the intervention if stent implantation was performed. The minor bleeding rate for the doses of 3.5–7.5 μg/kg was comparable to that of placebo (6.7%), but was significantly higher in the 10 μg/kg dose group (26.9%). Major bleeding (excessive drainage after emergency bypass grafting, sustained oral oozing after tracheal intubation, and a suspected cerebral vascular accident) occurred in the 5.0 μg/kg ($n = 3$) and 7.5 μg/kg ($n = 1$) dose groups. The three patients in the 5.0 μg/kg dose group who had major bleeding also received a GPIIb/IIa inhibitor. Systemic thrombin generation, as measured by prothrombin fragment F1.2, was suppressed in all rNAPc2 dose groups to levels below pretreatment values for at least 36 hours. In the placebo group, a significant increase in F1.2 levels was observed after cessation of heparin. Interestingly, although the patients in the study were not considered high risk, there was a sustained elevation of thrombin generation beyond 30 hours post PCI.

Following the above-described promising safety and anticoagulant effects of rNAPc2 in combination with aspirin, clopidogrel and UFH (but limited experience in combination with GPIIb/IIIa inhibitors), a trial in patients with non-ST-elevation a coronary syndromes (NSTE ACS) was undertaken. The ANTHEM (Anticoagulation with rNAPc2 To Help Eliminate Major adverse cardiac events) – TIMI 32 trial was designed to evaluate the safety and efficacy of a range of doses of the agent in patients with unstable angina/non-ST-elevation myocardial infarction (UA/NSTEMI) managed predominantly with invasive therapy, with a high proportion receiving GPIIb/IIIa antagonists.[49] In this study, 203 patients aged up to 75 years with moderate- to high-risk NSTE ACS <48 hours managed invasively on UFH or enoxaparin were randomized to double-blinded rNAPc2 (1.5–10 µg/kg) or placebo every 48 hours for one to three doses in dose-ranging. Another 52 patients receiving 10 µg/kg rNAPc2 were studied in an open-label UFH de-escalation phase (26 patients each with half-dose UFH and 26 patients with no UFH). All patients had 3-lead continuous ECG monitoring for 1 week, serial measurements of prothrombin time (PT) and F1.2, and assessment of clinical events to 6 months. rNAPc2 prolonged PT in a dose-related fashion, and this was strongly correlated with drug concentration. Higher-dose rNAPc2 ($\geq$7.5 µg/kg) suppressed F1.2 levels at 2–6 (trend p = 0.001)and 48 hours (trend p = 0.002). Overall, rates of clinically significant bleeding were similar between patients receiving rNAPc2 and placebo (3.7% vs. 2.5%; p = NS), although the risk of major bleeding was increased with rNAPc2 if coronary artery bypass graft (CABG) surgery was performed within 4 days of the last dose. Ischemia on continuous ECG was reduced by >50% with higher-dose rNAPc2. Some heparin appears to be necessary to prevent catheter-related thrombosis during intracoronary procedures, although the possibility remains that rNAPc2 could be used as the sole anticoagulant outside during the medical management phase. Larger studies will be needed to evaluate whether this will translate into a reduction in clinical events.

Summary

The clinical use of anticoagulants is central in our attempt to limit pathologic thrombus. Current agents have significant limitations and do not effectively suppress the generation of new thrombin, spurring interest in novel proximally acting anticoagulants with greater efficacy that maintain a favorable safety profile. The pathophysiologic rationale for inhibition of TF as a therapeutic target is compelling both because of the possibility of improved efficacy as an anticoagulant and because of the potential for interruption of other pathologic consequences of TF release, including its contribution to inflammatory activation. Accumulating findings from experimental studies provide strong support for dose-dependent anticoagulant actions of this class of agents. To date, clinical data are sparse; however, the findings thus far provide confirmation of the anticoagulant actions of the drugs in humans, with preliminary evidence suggesting an acceptable safety profile. Studies evaluating the effect of these agents with respect to cardiovascular outcomes have not yet been completed.

References

1. Hirsh J, Raschke R. Heparin and low-molecular-weight heparin: the Seventh ACCP Conference on Antithrombotic and Thrombolytic Therapy. Chest 2004;126:188S–203S.
2. Eitzman DT, Chi L, Saggin L et al. Heparin neutralization by platelet-rich thrombi. Role of platelet factor 4. Circulation 1994;89:1523–9.
3. Kucher N, Connolly S, Beckman JA et al. International Normalized Ratio increase before warfarin-associated hemorrhage: brief and subtle. Arch Intern Med 2004;164:2176–9.
4. Warkentin TE, Greinacher A. Heparin-induced thrombocytopenia: recognition, treatment, and prevention: the Seventh ACCP Conference on Antithrombotic and Thrombolytic Therapy. Chest 2004;126:311S–37S.
5. Prandoni P, Siragusa S, Girolami B, Fabris F; BELZONI Investigators Group. The incidence of heparin-induced thrombocytopenia in medical patients treated with low-molecular-weight heparin: a prospective cohort study. Blood 2005;106:3049–54.
6. Camerer E, Kolsto AB, Prydz H. Cell biology of tissue factor, the principal initiator of blood coagulation. Thromb Res 1996;81:1–41.
7. Dahlback B. Blood coagulation. Lancet 2000;355:1627–32.
8. Moreno PR, Bernardi VH, Lopez-Cuellar J et al. Macrophages, smooth muscle cells, and tissue factor in unstable angina. Implications for cell-mediated thrombogenicity in acute coronary syndromes. Circulation 1996;94:3090–7.
9. Mann KG. Biochemistry and physiology of blood coagulation. Thromb Haemost 1999;82:165–74.
10. Broze GJ Jr. The role of tissue factor pathway inhibitor in a revised coagulation cascade. Semin Hematol 1992;29:159–69.
11. Girard TJ, Warren LA, Novotny WF et al. Functional significance of the Kunitz-type inhibitory domains of lipoprotein-associated coagulation inhibitor. Nature 1989;338:518–20.
12. Misumi K, Ogawa H, Yasue H et al. Comparison of plasma tissue factor levels in unstable and stable angina pectoris. Am J Cardiol 1998;81:22–6.
13. Soejima H, Ogawa H, Yasue H et al. Heightened tissue factor associated with tissue factor pathway inhibitor and prognosis in patients with unstable angina. Circulation 1999;99:2908–13.
14. Ahamed J, Ruf W. Protease-activated receptor 2-dependent phosphorylation of the tissue factor cytoplasmic domain. J Biol Chem 2004;279:23038–44.
15. Zoldhelyi P, McNatt J, Shelat HS et al. Thromboresistance of balloon-injured porcine carotid arteries after local gene transfer of human tissue factor pathway inhibitor. Circulation 2000;101:289–95.
16. Harker LA, Hanson SR, Kelly AB. Antithrombotic strategies targeting thrombin activities, thrombin receptors and thrombin generation. Thromb Haemost 1997;78:736–41.
17. Byzova TV, Plow EF. Networking in the hemostatic system. Integrin $\alpha_{IIb}\beta_3$ binds prothrombin and influences its activation. J Biol Chem 1997;272:27183–8.
18. Giesen PL, Rauch U, Bohrmann B et al. Blood-borne tissue factor: another view of thrombosis. Proc Natl Acad Sci U S A 1999;96:2311–15.
19. Hutter R, Valdiviezo C, Sauter BV et al. Caspase-3 and tissue factor expression in lipid-rich plaque macrophages: evidence for apoptosis as link between inflammation and atherothrombosis. Circulation 2004;109:2001–8.

20. Sambola A, Osende J, Hathcock J et al. Role of risk factors in the modulation of tissue factor activity and blood thrombogenicity. Circulation 2003;107:973–7.

21. Felmeden DC, Spencer CG, Chung NA et al. Relation of thrombogenesis in systemic hypertension to angiogenesis and endothelial damage/dysfunction (a substudy of the Anglo-Scandinavian Cardiac Outcomes Trial [ASCOT]). Am J Cardiol 2003;92:400–5.

22. Steffel J, Luscher TF, Tanner FC. Tissue factor in cardiovascular diseases: molecular mechanisms and clinical implications. Circulation 2006;113:722–31.

23. Eto M, Kozai T, Cosentino F et al. Statin prevents tissue factor expression in human endothelial cells: role of Rho/Rho-kinase and Akt pathways. Circulation 2002;105:1756–9.

24. Brandes RP, Beer S, Ha T, Busse R. Withdrawal of cerivastatin induces monocyte chemoattractant protein 1 and tissue factor expression in cultured vascular smooth muscle cells. Arterioscler Thromb Vasc Biol 2003;23:1794–800.

25. Bea F, Blessing E, Shelley MI et al. Simvastatin inhibits expression of tissue factor in advanced atherosclerotic lesions of apolipoprotein E deficient mice independently of lipid lowering: potential role of simvastatin-mediated inhibition of Egr-1 expression and activation. Atherosclerosis 2003;167:187–94.

26. Ardissino D, Merlini PA, Ariens R et al. Tissue-factor antigen and activity in human coronary atherosclerotic plaques. Lancet 1997;349:769–71.

27. Kaikita K, Ogawa H, Yasue H et al. Tissue factor expression on macrophages in coronary plaques in patients with unstable angina. Arterioscler Thromb Vasc Biol 1997;17:2232–7.

28. Soejima H, Ogawa H, Yasue H et al. Effects of enalapril on tissue factor in patients with uncomplicated acute myocardial infarction. Am J Cardiol 1996;78:336–40.

29. Levi M, Ten Cate H. Disseminated intravascular coagulation. N Engl J Med 1999;341:586–92.

30. Levi M, van der Poll T, ten Cate H, van Deventer SJ. The cytokine-mediated imbalance between coagulant and anticoagulant mechanisms in sepsis and endotoxaemia. Eur J Clin Invest 1997;27:3–9.

31. van der Poll T, Buller HR, ten Cate H et al. Activation of coagulation after administration of tumor necrosis factor to normal subjects. N Engl J Med 1990;322:1622–7.

32. Rao LV, Rapaport SI. Studies of a mechanism inhibiting the initiation of the extrinsic pathway of coagulation. Blood 1987;69:645–51.

33. Haskel EJ, Torr SR, Day KC et al. Prevention of arterial reocclusion after thrombolysis with recombinant lipoprotein-associated coagulation inhibitor. Circulation 1991;84:821–7.

34. Jang Y, Guzman LA, Lincoff AM et al. Influence of blockade at specific levels of the coagulation cascade on restenosis in a rabbit atherosclerotic femoral artery injury model. Circulation 1995;92:3041–50.

35. Creasey AA, Chang AC, Feigen L et al. Tissue factor pathway inhibitor reduces mortality from *Escherichia coli* septic shock. J Clin Invest 1993;91:2850–60.

36. Abraham E, Reinhart K, Opal S et al. OPTIMIST Trial Study Group. Efficacy and safety of tifacogin (recombinant tissue factor pathway inhibitor) in severe sepsis: a randomized controlled trial. JAMA 2003;290:238–47.

37. de Jonge E, Dekkers PE, Creasey AA et al. Tissue factor pathway inhibitor dose-dependently inhibits coagulation activation without influencing the fibrinolytic and cytokine response during human endotoxemia. Blood 2000;95:1124–9.

38. Arnljots B, Ezban M, Hedner U. Prevention of experimental arterial thrombosis by topical administration of active site-inactivated factor VIIa. J Vasc Surg 1997;25:341–6.

39. Golino P, Ragni M, Cirillo P et al. Antithrombotic effects of recombinant human, active site-blocked factor VIIa in a rabbit model of recurrent arterial thrombosis. Circ Res 1998;82:39–46.

40. Lincoff AM. First clinical investigation of a tissue-factor inhibitor administered during a percutaneous coronary revascularization: a randomized, double-blinded, dose-escalation trial assessing safety and efficacy of FFR–FVIIa in percutaneous transluminal coronary angioplasty (ASIS) trial. J Am Coll Cardiol 2000;36(1):312–3(abstr.)

41. Ragni M, Cirillo P, Pascucci I et al. Monoclonal antibody against tissue factor shortens tissue plasminogen activator lysis time and prevents reocclusion in a rabbit model of carotid artery thrombosis. Circulation 1996;93:1913–18.

42. Erlich JH, Boyle EM, Labriola J et al. Inhibition of the tissue factor–thrombin pathway limits infarct size after myocardial ischemia–reperfusion injury by reducing inflammation. Am J Pathol 2000;157:1849–62.

43. Badimon JJ, Lettino M, Toschi V et al. Local inhibition of tissue factor reduces the thrombogenicity of disrupted human atherosclerotic plaques: effects of tissue factor pathway inhibitor on plaque thrombogenicity under flow conditions. Circulation 1999;99:1780–7.

44. Morrow DA, Murphy SA, McCabe CH et al. Potent inhibition of thrombin with a monoclonal antibody against tissue factor (Sunol-cH36): results of the PROXIMATE-TIMI 27 trial. Eur Heart J 2005;26:682–8.

45. Duggan BM, Dyson HJ, Wright PE. Inherent flexibility in a potent inhibitor of blood coagulation, recombinant nematode anticoagulant protein c2. Eur J Biochem 1999;265:539–48.

46. Weijer S, Schoenmakers SH, Florquin S et al. Inhibition of the tissue factor/factor VIIa pathway does not influence the inflammatory or antibacterial response to abdominal sepsis induced by *Escherichia coli* in mice. J Infect Dis 2004;189:2308–17.

47. Lee A, Agnelli G, Buller H et al. Dose–response study of recombinant factor VIIa/tissue factor inhibitor recombinant nematode anticoagulant protein c2 in prevention of postoperative venous thromboembolism in patients undergoing total knee replacement. Circulation 2001;104:74–8.

48. Moons AH, Peters RJ, Bijsterveld NR et al. Recombinant nematode anticoagulant protein c2, an inhibitor of the tissue factor/factor VIIa complex, in patients undergoing elective coronary angioplasty. J Am Coll Cardiol 2003;41:2147–53.

49. Giugliano RP, Wiviott SD, Stone PH et al. Recombinant nematode anticoagulant protein c2 in patients with non-ST-segment elevation acute coronary syndrome: the ANTEM-TIMI 32 trial. J Am Coll Cardiol 2007;49:2398–2407.

50. Chou J, Mackman N, Merrill-Skoloff G et al. Hematopoietic cell-derived microparticle tissue factor contributes to fibrin formation during thrombus propagation. Blood 2004;104:3190–7.

Section II.D

Antithrombotic drugs: fibrinolytic therapy

19

Fibrinolytics: current indications and treatment modalities in the absence of mechanical reperfusion

Peter R Sinnaeve and Frans J Van de Werf

Introduction

Acute myocardial infarction (MI) remains the leading cause of death in industrialized countries. Numerous studies during the past decades have firmly established the paradigm of achieving early, complete, and sustained infarct-related artery patency in patients with an MI, resulting in a reduction in an average 30-day mortality of 18% in the pre-fibrinolytic era to less than 6% in the context of contemporary clinical trials. In general, reperfusion can be attained by mechanical reperfusion using primary percutaneous coronary intervention (PCI) or pharmacological reperfusion using fibrinolytic agents. Because primary PCI achieves higher patency rates and is associated with fewer intracranial bleeding complications than fibrinolysis, current guidelines recommend primary PCI if the procedure can be performed by an experienced team within 90 minutes after initial medical contact. Fibrinolysis, however, is more widely available and requires less logistics, and therefore remains a valuable alternative. Indeed, lytic therapy is still used for the treatment of acute MI in the majority of centers worldwide.

Fibrinolytic therapy and reperfusion

Acute MI is generally caused by rupture of an atherosclerotic plaque, triggering the formation of an occlusive coronary thrombus. Coronary artery occlusion sets off a wave front of myocardial necrosis spreading from endocardium to epicardium, with an inverse relation between the time to perfusion and the ultimate size and extent of transmurality of the infarct. To rescue myocardial muscle at risk from undergoing necrosis, rapid restoration of coronary blood flow is essential. In the absence of access to immediate primary PCI, clot lysis can be achieved by activating the endogenous fibrinolytic system using plasminogen-activating agents. These agents convert plasminogen to plasmin, which then degrades fibrin, a major constituent of clots (Figure 19.1).

The advantages conferred by lytic therapy are clearly time-dependent. Although administering fibrinolytics up to 12 hours after the onset of symptoms may be beneficial in terms of outcome, every minute that reperfusion is postponed will unavoidably result in more extensive necrosis and a worse outcome. In a meta-analysis, the mortality reduction following fibrinolytic therapy was calculated to be 44% in patients treated within 2 hours versus 20% in those treated later.[1] Early in the course of ST-segment-elevation MI (STEMI), the thrombus may be smaller and easier to lyse, which might in part explain the more prominent benefit of lytics in the first hours after symptom onset.

Angiographically documented acute coronary reocclusion occurs in 5–15% of patients after lytic-induced reperfusion, resulting in a significant further worsening of left ventricular function and a steep increase in in-hospital mortality.[2,3] Rethrombosis may be mediated by the interaction of vasospasm, aggregating platelets, clot-bound thrombin, the thrombogenicity of partially lysed clot and ruptured atheroma, or the persistence of a flow-limiting stenosis in the absence of a PCI. Paradoxical procoagulant and platelet-activating side effects of fibrinolytic agents might also trigger reocclusion, especially with fibrin-specific drugs.[4] In a pooled analysis of 15 trials, alteplase, for instance, was associated with higher rates of reocclusion compared with streptokinase, underscoring the importance of antithrombotic co-therapy with fibrin-selective fibrinolytics.[5]

Indications for fibrinolytic therapy

Patients younger than 76 years with typical chest pain of less than 12 hours duration presenting with ECG ST-segment

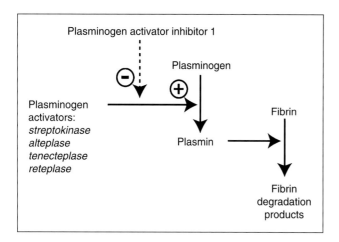

Figure 19.1
Mechanism of plasminogen activators.

elevations or new bundle branch block are eligible for fibrinolytic therapy.[6] Patients presenting later are generally not considered good candidates for fibrinolysis (class III). Likewise, patients older than 75 years of age have often been excluded from randomized trials, mainly because of an increased risk of bleeding complications. Nevertheless, elderly patients may benefit from fibrinolytic therapy, provided that they do not present with contraindications.

The usual ECG criterion for administration of fibrinolytic therapy is at least 0.1 mV of ST-segment elevation in two or more contiguous leads. Since mortality is significantly higher in patients with complete bundle branch block, administration of a fibrinolytic agent is also recommended in this population.[7] Indeed, fibrinolysis in patients presenting with a new bundle branch block, obscuring ST-segment analysis, reduces mortality by 25%. There is no evidence of benefit, however, of lytic therapy in patients presenting with non-ST-segment-elevation acute coronary syndromes.

Universally established contraindications to fibrinolysis are in essence precautions to avoid excessive hemorrhage in patients with comorbidities that increase the risk of bleeding complications (Table 19.1). In these patients, including those with a previous history of stroke or recent major surgery, primary PCI should be considered. Since arterial hypertension increases the risk of intracranial hemorrhage, patients presenting with hypertension are usually not eligible for lytic therapy, although a history of systemic hypertension in itself does not predispose to intracranial hemorrhage after lytic therapy. Fibrinolytic trials have adopted different approaches with regard to patients presenting with hypertension. In the ASSENT-3 trial, patients were only excluded if they had a diastolic blood pressure >110 mmHg and/or systolic blood pressure >180 mmHg on repeated measurements.[8] Accordingly, in this trial, patients could still receive fibrinolysis after successful treatment of

their high initial blood pressure on admission. In contrast, patients were excluded after a single reading of diastolic blood pressure >110 mmHg and/or systolic blood pressure >180 mmHg in many other trials, including GUSTO-V and most TIMI trials.[9] Nevertheless, because there is a substantial mortality benefit with lytics in patients even presenting with hypertension, lytics should still be considered in patients with high blood pressure on admission after initiation of antihypertensive treatment, when primary PCI is not available.

Fibrinolytic agents

Fibrinolytic agents are generally divided into fibrin-specific and non-fibrin-specific agents (Table 19.2). Fibrin-specific drugs are more efficient in dissolving thrombi and do not deplete systemic coagulation factors, in contrast with non-fibrin-specific agents. First-generation fibrinolytic regimens including streptokinase and recombinant tissue-type plasminogen activator (rtPA: alteplase) required continuous intravenous infusion. Contemporary lytic strategies, however, consist of intravenous bolus administration of second and third generation fibrinolytics.

Unfortunately, fibrinolytic regimens suffer from several limitations. Fibrinolytics need 30–45 minutes on average to recanalize the infarct-related artery, and complete patency is only achieved in 60–80% of patients. Also, reocclusion due to prothrombotic side effects is common, occurring in 5–15% of previously recanalized arteries.[10] Furthermore, even when blood flow to the infarct-related artery is restored, microcirculatory reperfusion can still be absent (the 'no-reflow' phenomenon).[11] Finally, bleeding complications, especially intracranial hemorrhage (ICH), continue to be a concern. Although contemporary pharmacological reperfusion strategies (see Table 19.3) now focus on antithrombotic co-therapies and improved strategies such as pre-hospital treatment and facilitated PCI, the search for the ideal fibrinolytic agent continues.

Streptokinase

Streptokinase is a non-fibrin-specific fibrinolytic agent that indirectly activates plasminogen. Because of its lack of fibrin specificity, streptokinase induces a systemic lytic state. Since a benefit of heparin with streptokinase has not been convincingly demonstrated in clinical trials, its use is optional. Although newer fibrin-specific fibrinolytics have theoretical and clinical advantages, streptokinase remains widely used in part because of its low cost. Preexisting anti-streptokinase antibodies may impede reperfusion after treatment with streptokinase.[12] Administration of streptokinase also invariably induces anti-streptokinase antibodies, precluding re-administration.

Table 19.1 *Contraindications to fibrinolysis*

Absolute	Relative
• Previous hemorrhagic stroke at any time • Non-hemorrhagic (ischemic) stroke <6 months • Intracranial neoplasm or damage • Recent surgery or trauma (including head trauma) within 2–4 weeks • Active internal bleeding • Gastrointestinal bleeding within last month • Known bleeding diatheses • Suspected aortic dissection	• Transient ischemic attack <6 months • Uncontrolled or refractory hypertension on presentation (blood pressure >180/100 mmHg) • Traumatic cardiopulmonary resuscitation • Current use of anticoagulant • Recent internal bleeding (2–4 weeks) • Non-compressible vascular punctures • Pregnancy • Active peptic ulcer • Previous use of streptokinase, anistreplase (APSAC),or staphylokinase

Table 19.2 *Fibrinolytic agents*

	Streptokinase	Alteplase	Reteplase	Tenecteplase
Fibrin-specificity	–	++	+	+++
Half-life (min)	18–23	3–4	18	20
Administration	1-hour infusion	90-minute infusion	Double bolus	Single bolus
Antigenicity	+++	–	–	–

The first large trial to show a significant reduction in mortality with a fibrinolytic agent was the landmark GISSI-1 trial.[13] In this study, 11 806 patients with acute MI presenting within 12 hours of symptom onset were randomized to either reperfusion therapy with streptokinase or standard non-fibrinolytic therapy. The in-hospital mortality rate was 10.7% in patients treated with intravenous streptokinase versus 13.1% in controls, resulting in 23 lives saved per 1000 patients treated. This benefit in mortality was preserved at 1-year and 10-year follow-up.[14] Another landmark trial, ISIS-2, corroborated these results.[15] In this trial, 17 187 patients received streptokinase, aspirin daily for 1 month, both treatments, or neither. Treatment with aspirin or streptokinase alone resulted in a significant reduction in mortality (23% and 24%, respectively), an effect that was additive, as witnessed by a 43% reduction in the combination group.

Alteplase

Alteplase is a single-chain tissue-type plasminogen activator molecule. It has considerably greater fibrin-specificity than streptokinase, but nevertheless induces mild systemic fibrinogen depletion. Because of its short half-life, alteplase requires a continuous infusion.

In two mortality trials, ISIS-3 and GISSI-2, alteplase, given as a 3-hour continuous infusion, was not superior to streptokinase.[16,17] The question which of the two fibrinolytic drugs is the most effective in terms of mortality reduction was nevertheless answered in the first GUSTO trial.[18] In this trial, a 'front-loaded' 90-minute dosing regimen of alteplase was used, which had earlier been shown to achieve higher patency rates than the 3-hour scheme. The 30-day mortality rate was 6.3% in patients receiving alteplase, compared with 7.4% in patients treated with streptokinase ($p=0.001$). The 1% lower mortality rate at 30 days with front-loaded alteplase corresponded to a significantly higher Thrombolysis in Myocardial Infarction (TIMI) flow grade 3 rate at 90 minutes: 54% versus only 32% with streptokinase.[19]

Reteplase

Reteplase, a second-generation fibrinolytic agent, was a first attempt to improve on the shortcomings of alteplase. It is a mutant of alteplase in which the finger, the kringle-1 domain, and epidermal growth factor domains are removed. This results in a decreased plasma clearance, allowing double-bolus administration. The removal of the finger domain diminishes fibrin specificity, whereas inactivation by plasminogen activator inhibitor (PAI-1; Figure 19.1) remains similar to that with alteplase.

In two pilot trials, different doses of reteplase were evaluated in STEMI patients.[20,21] In RAPID-I, patients treated with two boluses of 10 MU reteplase given 30 minutes apart had a significantly higher rate of TIMI flow grade 3 (63%) compared with patients treated with a 3-hour infusion of alteplase (49%). Reteplase also achieved significantly higher TIMI flow grade 3 rates than 90-minute front-loaded alteplase (60% vs 45%) in RAPID-II (Figure 19.2).

In the GUSTO-III trial, which was designed as a superiority trial, 15 059 patients were randomized to double-bolus reteplase, given 30 minutes apart, or front-loaded alteplase.[22] Mortality at 30 days was similar in both treatment arms (7.47% vs 7.24%, respectively), as was the incidence of hemorrhagic stroke or other major bleeding complications (Figures 19.2 and 19.3). Similar mortality rates were maintained for both treatment groups at 1-year follow-up.[23] Thus, higher TIMI flow grade 3 rates at 90 minutes with reteplase, as seen in the two pilot studies, did not translate into lower short- or long-term mortality rates. The reason for this incongruity remains unclear, but might be explained in part by increased platelet activation and surface receptor expression with reteplase compared with alteplase.

Tenecteplase

Tenecteplase (TNK-tPA) is derived from alteplase after mutations at three places (T103, N117, KHRR296–299), increasing fibrin binding and specificity, plasma half-life, and resistance to PAI-1. Its slower clearance allows convenient single-bolus administration. Tenecteplase leads to faster recanalization compared with alteplase, and also has higher fibrinolytic potency on platelet-rich clots than its parent molecule.

Efficacy of clot lysis was evaluated in the TIMI-10A and -10B trials.[24,25] In the TIMI-10A trial, the rate of TIMI flow grade 3 was 59% and 64% with 30 and 50 mg tenecteplase, respectively. In the TIMI-10B trial, 837 patients were randomized to single-bolus tenecteplase (30, 40, or 50 mg), or

front-loaded alteplase. TIMI flow grade 3 rates were identical after single-bolus administration of 40 mg tenecteplase compared with alteplase (63%) (Figure 19.2). The 50 mg dose of tenecteplase, however, was discontinued early because of an excess of intracranial hemorrhages.

In the double-blind ASSENT-2 trial, 16 949 patients were randomized to weight-adjusted single-bolus tenecteplase or standard front-loaded alteplase.[26] Specifically designed as an equivalence trial, this study showed that tenecteplase and alteplase had equivalent 30-day mortality rates (6.18% vs 6.15%) (Figure 19.2). Mortality rates remained similar at 1-year follow-up.[27] Although the rates of ICH were similar for tenecteplase (0.93%) and alteplase (0.94%) (Figure 19.3), female patients, elderly (>75 years), and patients weighing <67 kg tended to have lower rates of ICH after treatment with tenecteplase.[28] Non-cerebral bleeding complications occurred less frequently in the tenecteplase group, and, as a consequence, there was also less need for blood transfusion after tenecteplase, especially in high-risk patients.

Adjunctive antithrombotic therapy with lytics
Antiplatelet therapy
Aspirin

In ISIS-2, low-dose aspirin was associated with improved outcome in STEMI patients receiving fibrinolysis.[15] Aspirin also significantly reduced non-fatal re-infarction (1.0% vs 2.0%) and was not associated with any significant increase in intracranial hemorrhages. In the most recent meta-analysis of the Antithrombotic Trialists' Collaboration including

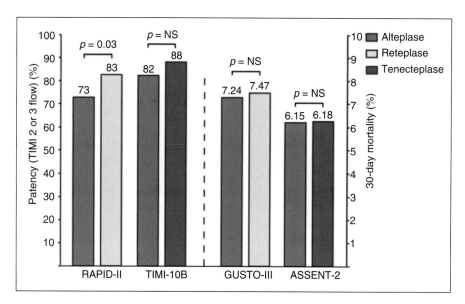

Figure 19.2
Patency rates (TIMI flow grade 2 or 3) and mortality rates with reteplase or tenecteplase versus alteplase.
(see color plate)

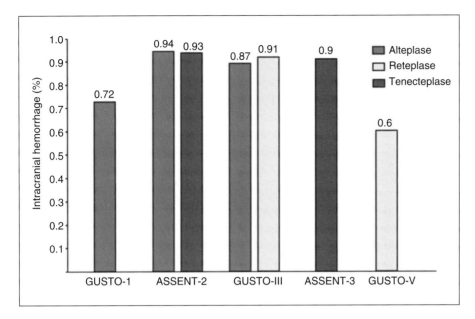

Figure 19.3
Rates of intracranial hemorrhage after alteplase, reteplase or tenecteplase (UFH groups only). (see color plate)

19 288 patients from 15 STEMI trials, aspirin use was associated with a significant reduction in cardiovascular death (23 lives saved per 1000 patients treated) and non-fatal reinfarction (13 events prevented per 1000 patients treated).[29] Overall, a small increase in ICH (1–2 per 1000) was seen in patients taking low-dose aspirin.

The benefit of aspirin in the setting of lytic therapy appears to be time-dependent. In a small trial, patients who received aspirin before fibrinolysis had a lower 7-day mortality rate than patients who received the first dose of aspirin after administration of the fibrinolytic agent (2.5% vs 6.0%; $p = 0.01$).[30] Similarly, patients with a STEMI had a better survival rate at 30 days when they received aspirin before hospital admission compared with in-hospital initiation.[31]

Clopidogrel

Even after aspirin became standard therapy for all STEMI patients, reocclusion and reinfarction after successful pharmacological reperfusion continued to be a problem. The CLARITY trial examined whether addition of the platelet adenosine diphosphate (ADP) receptor inhibitor clopidogrel (300 mg bolus followed by 75 mg daily) to aspirin was associated with higher rates of infarct-related artery patency in patients treated with a fibrinolytic agent.[32] At angiographic follow-up at least 2 days after fibrinolytic therapy, patients treated with clopidogrel had significantly lower TIMI flow grade 0 or 1 rates (11.7% vs 18.4% with placebo). Clopidogrel appeared to improve patency rates by preventing reocclusion rather than through facilitating early reperfusion.[33] No increased risk of bleeding complications was observed with clopidogrel. Since no patients >75 years of age were included, however, it remains uncertain whether dual antiplatelet therapy is safe in the elderly treated with lytic therapy. Clopidogrel also significantly reduced the risk

of in-hospital death after STEMI in the large COMMIT trial (−7%, 95% CI −1% to −13%); in this trial, however, no loading dose was used and only half of the patients received fibrinolysis.[34]

Clopidogrel also improved outcome after PCI in CLARITY, regardless of the duration of pretreatment or whether patients received additional glycoprotein (GP) IIb/IIIa inhibitors.[35] These results also suggest that starting clopidogrel at the time of fibrinolysis could obviate the need for additional GPIIb/IIIa inhibitors if a rescue PCI became necessary.

GPIIb/IIIa inhibitors

The addition of GPIIb/IIIa inhibitors such as abciximab, eptifibatide, and tirofiban to fibrinolytic regimens is useful in reducing the risk of recurrent ischemia and reocclusion due to the prothrombotic side-effects of fibrinolytic drugs. Several trials indeed indicate that abciximab with a half-dose fibrinolytic not only modestly enhances recanalization of the culprit epicardial vessel but also improves tissue reperfusion.[36] The effect of improved epicardial patency rates on outcome with combination therapy using abciximab was tested in the GUSTO-V and ASSENT-3 trials. In the GUSTO-V trial, an open-label non-inferiority trial, 16 588 patients were randomized to either reteplase or half-dose reteplase with weight-adjusted abciximab.[9] The 30-day mortality rates were 5.9% for reteplase and 5.6% for the combined reteplase–abciximab group. Unsurprisingly, the 1-year follow-up mortality rates were identical.[37] Combination therapy with reteplase and abciximab resulted in a significant reduction of ischemic complications after acute MI. ICH rates were equal (0.6%) in the overall study population for both treatment arms (Figure 19.3), although in patients >75 years of age, the rate of intracranial bleeding was almost twice as high in the combination-treatment arm. Similarly, in the ASSENT-3 study, a significant decrease in ischemic complications with abciximab plus half-dose tenecteplase was observed, without significant differences in 30-day and 1-year mortality rates.[8,38] Although ICH rates were comparable between treatment arms (Figure 19.3), major and minor bleeding complications, thrombocytopenia, and transfusion rates were more frequent in the half-dose tenecteplase plus abciximab arm. As in the GUSTO-V trial, patients aged >75 years experienced significantly more bleeding complications.[39] Taken together, combination therapy with fibrinolysis and abciximab results in a significant reduction in ischemic complications after acute MI, but this benefit is offset by an increased risk of bleeding complications, particularly in elderly patients. Nevertheless, the combination of half-dose lytic and full-dose abciximab might be an attractive approach in combined pharmacological and mechanical reperfusion strategies, as currently being tested in the CARESS and FINESSE studies.[40,41]

Anticoagulant therapy

Unfractionated heparin and low-molecular-weight heparin

Unfractionated heparin (UFH) has been standard adjunctive antithrombotic therapy with fibrin-specific fibrinolytics since GUSTO-I, although early studies were unconvincing. Low-molecular-weight heparin (LMWH) offers several advantages over conventional UFH. It has a more stable and predictable anticoagulant response that eliminates the need for activated partial thromboplastin time (aPTT) monitoring. Also, a better anti-factor Xa:factor IIa ratio than that of UFH more efficiently enhances the inhibition of thrombin generation. In addition, subcutaneous administration and a longer half-life greatly facilitate administration when compared to UFH.

Studies showed improved patency rates and less reocclusion with LMWH.[42,43] In contrast, in the ENTIRE–TIMI-23 trial, enoxaparin achieved similar complete reperfusion (TIMI flow grade 3) rates compared with UFH at 60 minutes.[44] Nevertheless, although this study was relatively small, a significant reduction in the composite endpoint of death and reinfarction at 30 days was seen with full-dose tenecteplase and enoxaparin (4.4%) compared with UFH (15.9%), largely due a reduction in reinfarction rates. Major hemorrhages were less frequent in the tenecteplase and enoxaparin group. In the ASSENT-3 study, a significant improvement in the primary combined efficacy and safety endpoint was seen with tenecteplase and enoxaparin when compared with standard tenecteplase and UFH, although no difference in 30-day and 1-year mortality was seen.[8,38] Using an age-adjusted dose, enoxaparin was also associated with fewer ischemic complications

than UFH in STEMI patients receiving fibrinolytic therapy in the ExTRACT–TIMI-25 study.[45] Major bleeding complications, but not ICH, were more frequent in the enoxaparin group (2.1% vs 1.4% for UFH). A recent meta-analysis of trials comparing LMWH, given for 4–8 days, with UFH as an adjunct to fibrinolysis clearly demonstrated that LMWH reduces the risk of reinfarction but not death, and is associated with a higher risk of minor but not major bleeding complications.[46]

Another LMWH, reviparin, was tested in the CREATE study. In this, 15 570 patients with a STEMI, of whom over 70% received lytic therapy, were randomized to either placebo or reviparin subcutaneously twice daily for 7 days.[47] Reviparin significantly reduced 30-day mortality with 13% and reinfarction with 23%. However, bleeding complications were more frequent with reviparin, especially in patients receiving reperfusion therapy.

Fondaprinux

Fondaparinux, a synthetic pentasaccharide, is a factor Xa inhibitor that selectively binds antithrombin. As with LMWH, fondaparinux does not need monitoring of its anticoagulant effect. In the PENTALYSE pilot trial, fondaparinux was compared with UFH in 333 patients with STEMI.[48] Epicardial patency rates at 90 minutes and at 5 days were similar for both groups, but there was a trend towards less reocclusion of the infarct-related artery and fewer revascularizations during the 30-day follow-up in patients receiving fondaparinux. In the OASIS-6 trial, fondaparinux was compared with UFH in 12 092 patients with STEMI.[49] In the 45% patients ($n = 5436$) who were treated with lytic therapy, fondaparinux was associated with a significant 21% lower risk of death or MI when compared with standard heparin or placebo. Unfortunately, no direct efficacy and safety comparison between fondaparinux and UFH in lytic-treated patients was provided.

Bivalirudin

In contrast with UFH, which only inhibits fluid-phase thrombin, bivalirudin is a direct thrombin-specific anticoagulant that inhibits both fibrin-bound and fluid-phase thrombin. Because inadequately inactivated thrombin at the site of thrombus is in part responsible for the procoagulant side-effect of thrombolysis, direct inhibition of thrombin might thus reduce the occurrence of ischemic complications after reperfusion.

In the HERO-1 study, reperfusion rates were assessed in 412 patients receiving streptokinase with bivalirudin or UFH.[50] TIMI flow grade 3 rates were higher in the bivalirudin group (48%) than in the UFH group (35%), while no increase in bleeding complications in patients receiving bivalirudin was observed. In the HERO-2 trial, 17 073 patients were then randomized to streptokinase and UFH or streptokinase and bivalirudin.[51] Mortality at 30 days was not different for the two regimens, but the reinfarction rate was significantly lower in the bivalirudin group (1.6% vs 2.3% for UFH), suggesting that early and more efficient inhibition of thrombin can inhibit reocclusion. Mild to moderate bleeding complications were higher in the bivalirudin group, possibly due to higher aPTT values observed in that group, although ICH occurred infrequently in both groups (0.6% and 0.4% for bivalirudin and UFH, respectively).

Current fibrinolytic strategies in STEMI (Table 19.3)

Fibrinolysis or transport for primary PCI?

Current guidelines unequivocally recommend primary PCI in patients presenting with STEMI.[6,52] They require that an experienced team start the intervention within 90 minutes after initial presentation. Patients presenting at a hospital without interventional facilities need to be transported to the nearest PCI center, requiring established communication and transportation routines between the referring and receiving hospitals. In a real-world setting, however, door-to-balloon times are often longer than 90 minutes: in the National Registry of Myocardial Infarction (NRMI)

3 and 4 cohorts, for instance, the median door-to-balloon delay was 180 minutes, with only 4% of patients being treated within 90 minutes.[53] In the recent second Euro Heart Survey, median door-to-balloon time has nevertheless decreased to 70 minutes, which is 23 minutes less than the first survey 4 years earlier.[54]

Uncertainties about delays associated with communicating with the receiving catheterization laboratory, arranging patient transfer, and mobilizing an interventional team within a 90-minute interval often confuse physicians referring patients for primary PCI. Results from studies comparing on-site fibrinolysis with primary PCI led to the impression that the superiority of primary PCI in terms of ischemic complications justifies long treatment delays caused by transportation. Meta-analyses pooling these studies, however, suggested that the mortality benefit of primary PCI over fibrinolysis disappears with door-to-balloon delays of 1 hour or more.[55,56] In contrast, a more recent pooled analysis showed that the mortality benefit of primary PCI over fibrinolysis was independent of treatment delays of up to 2 hours.[57] Nevertheless, as with fibrinolysis, mortality rates do increase with longer treatment delays or interhospital delays in patients undergoing primary PCI, indicating that the total ischemic time needs to be as short as possible, regardless of reperfusion strategy.[57,58]

A recent analysis of the NRMI databases shed more light on how to triage patients to fibrinolysis or transport for primary PCI (Figure 19.4).[59] Increasing delay (door-to-balloon time minus door-to-needle time) was found to be associated with impaired outcome: a 10% increased risk of in-hospital mortality for every 30 minutes delay. When the

Table 19.3 *Fibrinolytic strategies*			
Antiplatelet therapy	• Loading dose: **Aspirin** (150–325) mg chewable, non-enteric-coated (≤100 mg daily lifelong) • Loading dose: **Clopidogrel** 300 mg (75 mg daily for 1 month)		
Fibrinolysis	**Tenecteplase** Single bolus according to weight: <60 kg: 30 mg 60–69.9 kg: 35 mg 70–79.9 kg: 40 mg 80–89.9 kg: 45 mg >90 kg: 50 mg	**Reteplase** Double bolus: 10 + 10 MU (30 min apart)	**Streptokinase** 1.5 MU in 1-hour infusion
Anticoagulation	**Enoxaparin** Bolus 30 mg IV 1 mg/kg SC (age >75: no bolus) 1 mg/kg per 12 h (max. 100 mg for first 2 doses) (0.75 mg/kg if age >75) *or* **UFH** 60 U/kg (max. 4000 U) 12 U/kg/h (max. 1000 U/h) Age 50–70: first measurement at 3 h		

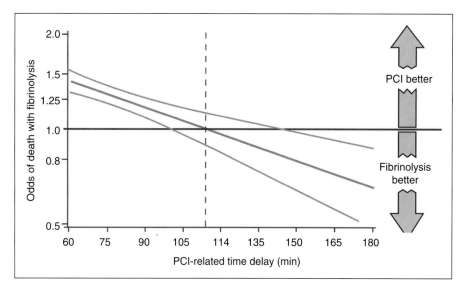

Figure 19.4
Odds of death with fibrinolysis versus primary PCI per PCI-related treatment delay (door-to-balloon minus door-to-needle). Data from Pinto et al[82] suggest that fibrinolysis might be superior to primary PCI with PCI-related treatment delays longer than 114 minutes.

PCI-related delay reaches 114 minutes, the benefit of primary PCI over fibrinolysis disappears in the overall population. The advantage of primary PCI over fibrinolysis in terms of outcome is lost even at much shorter PCI-related delays in younger patients (<65 years) presenting with an anterior infarction within 2 hours of symptom onset (Figure 19.5). The benefit of lytic therapy might indeed be more pronounced in fresh occlusive clots jeopardizing a large myocardial area at risk, while younger patients are less at risk for bleeding complications. Furthermore, in a general acute coronary syndrome population including 34% STEMI patients, in-hospital outcome was comparable regardless whether patients first presented to a hospital with or without a catheterization laboratory.[60] On aggregate, when primary PCI is not available within 90 minutes or when there is doubt about transportation delays, STEMI patients should receive lytic therapy in the absence of contraindications, especially with a large amount of ischemic myocardium at risk.

Pre-hospital fibrinolysis

As stated before, the benefits conferred by fibrinolytic therapy are clearly time-dependent. Although administering fibrinolytic agents up to 12 hours after the onset of symptoms may be beneficial in terms of outcome,[61] every minute that reperfusion is postponed will inevitably result in more extensive necrosis. Since GUSTO-I, however, it has proven difficult to decrease treatment delays using conventional in-hospital strategies.[62] Time lost between symptom onset and hospitalization indeed remains a crucial contributor to treatment delay in STEMI. In this respect, bolus fibrinolytic agents undoubtedly facilitate pre-hospital reperfusion protocols. Less complicated fibrinolytic regimens might also facilitate initiation of pre-hospital fibrinolytic treatment by trained paramedical staff. Indeed, the administration of a bolus fibrinolytic by paramedical ambulance staff does not appear to influence efficacy and safety.[63]

Several trials and registries have compared pre-hospital fibrinolysis with in-hospital fibrinolysis. A meta-analysis of six trials including 6434 patients clearly demonstrates that the time gained with pre-hospital treatment resulted in a significant 17% mortality reduction compared with in-hospital fibrinolysis.[64] In a more recent cohort study, time to fibrinolysis was almost 1 hour shorter with pre-hospital diagnosis and lytics administered by trained paramedics in the ambulance, when compared with regular in-hospital lytic therapy.[65] The significant amount of time gained by administrating fibrinolytics in the pre-hospital setting resulted in a reduction of adjusted 1-year mortality by almost 30%. In the French USIC registry, the risk of death at 1 year was even >50% lower after pre-hospital fibrinolysis, compared with other treatment strategies (relative risk (RR) 0.49, 95% confidence interval (CI) 0.24–1.00; $p < 0.05$) (Figure 19.6).[66] In patients treated pre-hospitally within 3.5 hours of symptom onset, the 1-year survival rate was close to 99%.

The combination of single-bolus tenecteplase plus enoxaparin, which emerged as a convenient and attractive therapy in the ASSENT-3 study, has also been investigated in the pre-hospital setting in the ASSENT-3 PLUS trial. In this trial, 1639 patients with acute MI received pre-hospital tenecteplase and were randomized to either enoxaparin or UFH.[67] A time gain of 47 minutes was observed, increasing the fraction of patients treated within 2 hours of symptom onset from 29% in ASSENT-3 to 52% in ASSENT-3 PLUS. Early treatment (<2 hours) was associated with a lower 30-day mortality rate (4.4% vs 6.2 (2–4 hours) and 10.4% (4–6 hours)), but no significant difference in outcome was observed between enoxaparin and heparin.

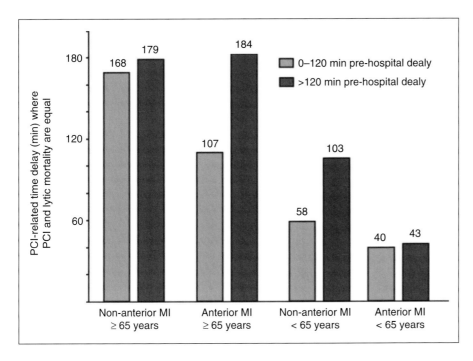

Figure 19.5
PCI-related treatment delays (door-to-balloon minus door-to-needle) where mortality after fibrinolysis is equal to that after primary PCI, categorized according to age, infarct localization, and time to treatment. Data are from Pinto et al.[82]

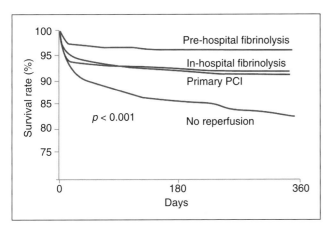

Figure 19.6
Age-adjusted 1-year survival rate after pre-hospital fibrinolysis versus in-hospital fibrinolysis, primary PCI, or no reperfusion; data from the French USIC registry (n=1922). Reproduced form Danchin N et al.[66]

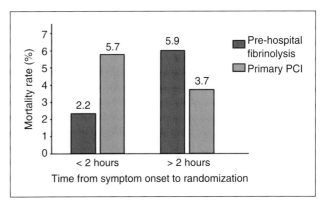

Figure 19.7
Mortality rates in patients randomized within or after 2 hours of symptom onset, to pre-hospital fibrinolysis or transport for primary PCI in the French CAPTIM study.

Studies comparing on-site fibrinolysis with transport for primary PCI in low-risk patients suggest that, even with transport-related time delays up to 90 minutes, primary PCI is superior to fibrinolysis. Nevertheless, time gained with pre-hospital administration might level this difference in outcome. In the CAPTIM trial, patients were randomized to either pre-hospital fibrinolysis with accelerated alteplase or primary PCI after transport to a center with interventional facilities (Figure 19.7).[68] In essence, CAPTIM compared two reperfusion *strategies*, because >30% of patient in the pre-hospital lytic arm underwent urgent (rescue) angiography. Unfortunately, the trial was stopped prematurely because of low enrolment. Nevertheless, results from

CAPTIM suggest that outcome after pre-hospital fibrinolysis is at least comparable to that with primary PCI, especially in patients presenting very early after symptom onset.[68,69] Similarly, tenecteplase followed by mandatory PCI within 24 hours or rescue PCI when necessary was as effective as primary PCI in the recent WEST trial, in which almost 40% of the 304 patients were randomized pre-hospitally.

As a MI is often the cause of sudden death, bolus fibrinolytics have also been studied in refractory cardiopulmonary resuscitation. Earlier pilot trials using infusional fibrinolytics in this setting showed promising results.[70,71] More recently, however, a large international trial examining the safety and efficacy of a bolus fibrinolytic given during CPR for cardiac arrest has been halted prematurely because of futility.[72]

Fibrinolysis in the elderly

Fibrinolytic therapy for acute MI in the elderly remains controversial. Elderly patients with STEMI are often less intensively treated and investigated than their younger counterparts, as indicated by the second Euro Heart Survey.[73] Registries suggest an excess mortality in lytic-treated patients aged over 75 years compared with those treated with primary PCI, possibly due to an excess of major bleeding complications.[74,75] This excessive mortality might also be explained in part by negative selection, as fitter elderly patients might have been more likely amenable for primary PCI. Also, a significant portion of elderly patients receiving fibrinolysis actually might have had one or more contraindications. Conversely, elderly patients with contraindications to fibrinolysis often do receive lytic therapy.[76] This is apparently not without risk, as demonstrated by the higher mortality in patients older than 80 years receiving fibrinolysis versus those who did not. Mortality rates in observational studies, however, are in contrast with findings from large randomized trials. In the SENIOR PAMI trial, primary PCI was not found to be superior to primary PCI in 481 elderly patients (≥70 years). Also, data from the Fibrinolytic Therapy Trialists (FTT) group in 3300 patients over the age of 75 presenting within 12 hours of symptom onset with ST-segment elevation or bundle branch block revealed a significant 15% relative mortality reduction by fibrinolytic therapy.[77] This represents an absolute mortality reduction of 34 patients per 1000 randomized, in contrast with 16 per 1000 in those younger than 55 years. Furthermore, data from the GISSI-1 study suggest that the greatest absolute benefit of fibrinolysis occurs in elderly patients, due to their higher baseline risk.[78] Interestingly, lower ICH rates with tenecteplase as compared with alteplase in older patients in the ASSENT-2 study indicate that the timely use of a more fibrin-specific agent might be preferable in older patients without contraindications to fibrinolytic therapy.[28]

Concomitant antithrombotic therapy also appears to influence outcome in elderly patients receiving fibrinolysis. As in non-ST-segment elevation MI treatment combinations, elderly patients might receive inappropriately high doses of antiplatelet and anticoagulant agents, which might impact on outcome.[79] Indeed, in ASSENT-3 and ASSENT-3 PLUS, the combined safety–efficacy endpoint was considerably higher in patients above 75 years of age treated with enoxaparin or abciximab versus unfractionated heparin (Figure 19.8).[39] In order to reduce bleeding complications in the elderly, patients older than 75 years treated with lytics received a reduced dose of enoxaparin (0.75 mg/kg subcutaneously and no bolus) in the ExTRACT-TIMI-25 trial.

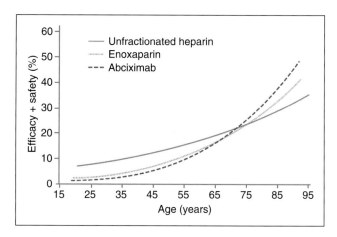

Figure 19.8
Combined efficacy plus safety endpoint according to age and antithrombotic regimen in ASSENT-3 and ASSENT-3 PLUS.[39]

Although enoxaparin was associated with a 50% increase in major bleeding complications in the overall populations, there was no excess of major bleedings in the elderly compared with younger patients.[45] On aggregate, elderly patients receiving fibrinolysis preferably should be treated with either UFH or reduced-dose enoxaparin.

Conclusion: Is there a future for fibrinolytic therapy?

For many STEMI patients worldwide, fibrinolysis remains the best and often only option for reperfusion treatment. When given early after symptom onset, fibrinolysis can match primary PCI in terms of outcome, especially when expected transport delays to the catheterization laboratory are long. In recent years, much effort has been put into the development of a combined pharmacological and mechanical reperfusion strategy (see Chapter X). The hypothesis behind combining both reperfusion options is that early administration of a lytic agent limits myocardial damage and prevents evolution to cardiogenic shock, while an early planned PCI prevents acute or subacute reocclusion. Unfortunately, a recent large international trial comparing fibrinolysis followed by early mandatory PCI versus primary PCI alone (ASSENT-4 PCI) was stopped prematurely because of a significant lower in-hospital mortality rate in the PCI-alone arm.[80] This was explained in part by a conservative concomitant antithrombotic regimen in the combined arm, leading to a higher risk of early reocclusion. The results might also indicate that an early PCI is perhaps not indicated in all patients receiving lytic therapy. Further randomized clinical trials will have to determine which subsets of patients really benefit from fibrinolysis with adequate upfront antithrombotic therapy when anticipated transport delays are long, and whether very early PCI might need to be reserved only for patients in whom fibrinolysis fails. Also, since fibrinolysis works at its best when time to treatment is relatively short, and because pre-hospital initiation of lytic therapy consistently decreases total ischemic time in clinical studies, all effort should be made to initiate lytic therapy in the pre-hospital setting. In this respect, pre-hospital triage and treatment of STEMI patients is strongly advocated by the European Society of Cardiology.[81]

References

1. Boersma E, Maas AC, Deckers JW, Simoons ML. Early thrombolytic treatment in acute myocardial infarction: reappraisal of the golden hour. Lancet 1996;348:771.
2. Hudson MP, Granger CB, Topol EJ et al. Early reinfarction after fibrinolysis: experience from the Global Utilization of Streptokinase and Tissue Plasminogen Activator (Alteplase) for Occluded Coronary Arteries (GUSTO I) and Global Use of Strategies to Open Occluded Coronary Arteries (GUSTO III) trials. Circulation 2001;104:1229.
3. Ohman EM, Califf RM, Topol EJ et al. Consequences of reocclusion after successful reperfusion therapy in acute myocardial infarction. TAMI Study Group. Circulation 1990;82:781.
4. Hoffmeister HM, Kastner C, Szabo S et al. Fibrin specificity and procoagulant effect related to the kallikrein- contact phase system and to plasmin generation with double-bolus reteplase and front-loaded alteplase thrombolysis in acute myocardial infarction. Am J Cardiol 2000;86:263.
5. Barbagelata NA, Granger CB, Oqueli E et al. TIMI grade 3 flow and reocclusion after intravenous thrombolytic therapy: a pooled analysis. Am Heart J 1997;133:273.
6. van de Werf FJ, Ardissino D, Betriu A et al. Management of acute myocardial infarction in patients presenting with ST-segment elevation. The Task Force on the Management of Acute Myocardial Infarction of the European Society of Cardiology. Eur Heart J 2003;24:28.
7. Al-Faleh H, Fu Y, Wagner G et al. Unraveling the spectrum of left bundle branch block in acute myocardial infarction: insights from the Assessment of the Safety and Efficacy of a New Thrombolytic (ASSENT 2 and 3) trials. Am Heart J 2006;151:10–15.
8. Efficacy and safety of tenecteplase in combination with enoxaparin, abciximab, or unfractionated heparin: the ASSENT-3 randomised trial in acute myocardial infarction. Lancet 2001;358:605.
9. Topol EJ. Reperfusion therapy for acute myocardial infarction with fibrinolytic therapy or combination reduced fibrinolytic therapy and platelet glycoprotein IIb/IIIa inhibition: the GUSTO V randomised trial. Lancet 2001;357:1905.
10. Topol EJ. Acute myocardial infarction: thrombolysis. Heart 2000;83:122.
11. Ito H, Maruyama A, Iwakura K et al. Clinical implications of the 'no reflow' phenomenon. A predictor of complications and left ventricular remodeling in reperfused anterior wall myocardial infarction. Circulation 1996;93:223.
12. Juhlin P, Bostrom PA, Torp A, Bredberg A. Streptokinase antibodies inhibit reperfusion during thrombolytic therapy with streptokinase in acute myocardial infarction. J Intern Med 1999;245:483.
13. Effectiveness of intravenous thrombolytic treatment in acute myocardial infarction. Gruppo Italiano per lo Studio della Streptochinasi nell'Infarto Miocardico (GISSI). Lancet 1986;i:397.
14. Franzosi MG, Santoro E, De Vita C et al. Ten-year follow-up of the first megatrial testing thrombolytic therapy in patients with acute myocardial infarction: results of the Gruppo Italiano per lo Studio della Sopravvivenza nell'Infarto-1 study. The GISSI Investigators. Circulation 1998;98:2659.
15. ISIS-2 (Second International Study of Infarct Survival) Collaborative Group. Randomised trial of intravenous streptokinase, oral aspirin, both, or neither among 17,187 cases of suspected acute myocardial infarction: ISIS-2. Lancet 1988;ii:349.
16. Gruppo Italiano per lo Studio della Sopravvivenza nell'Infarto Miocardico. GISSI-2: a factorial randomised trial of alteplase versus streptokinase and heparin versus no heparin among 12,490 patients with acute myocardial infarction. Lancet 1990;336:65.
17. ISIS-3 (Third International Study of Infarct Survival) Collaborative Group. ISIS-3: a randomised comparison of streptokinase vs tissue plasminogen activator vs anistreplase and of aspirin plus heparin vs aspirin alone among 41,299 cases of suspected acute myocardial infarction. Lancet 1992;339:753.
18. The GUSTO investigators. An international randomized trial comparing four thrombolytic strategies for acute myocardial infarction. N Engl J Med 1993;329:673.
19. Simes RJ, Topol EJ, Holmes DR Jr et al. Link between the angiographic substudy and mortality outcomes in a large randomized trial of myocardial reperfusion. Importance of early and complete infarct artery reperfusion. GUSTO-I Investigators. Circulation 1995;91:1923.
20. Smalling RW, Bode C, Kalbfleisch J et al. More rapid, complete, and stable coronary thrombolysis with bolus administration of reteplase compared with alteplase infusion in acute myocardial infarction. RAPID Investigators. Circulation 1995;91:2725.
21. Bode C, Smalling RW, Berg G et al. Randomized comparison of coronary thrombolysis achieved with double-bolus reteplase (recombinant plasminogen activator) and front-loaded, accelerated alteplase (recombinant tissue plasminogen activator) in patients with acute myocardial infarction. The RAPID II Investigators. Circulation 1996;94:891.
22. The Global Use of Strategies to Open Occluded Coronary Arteries (GUSTO III) Investigators. A comparison of reteplase with alteplase for acute myocardial infarction. N Engl J Med 1997;337:1118.
23. Topol EJ, Ohman EM, Armstrong PW et al. Survival outcomes 1 year after reperfusion therapy with either alteplase or reteplase for acute myocardial infarction: results from the Global Utilization of Streptokinase and t-PA for Occluded Coronary Arteries (GUSTO) III trial. Circulation 2000;102:1761.
24. Cannon CP, McCabe CH, Gibson CM et al. TNK-tissue plasminogen activator in acute myocardial infarction. Results of the Thrombolysis in Myocardial Infarction (TIMI) 10A dose-ranging trial. Circulation 1997;95:351.
25. Cannon CP, Gibson CM, McCabe CH et al. TNK-tissue plasminogen activator compared with front-loaded alteplase in acute myocardial infarction: results of the TIMI 10B trial. Thrombolysis in Myocardial Infarction (TIMI) 10B Investigators. Circulation 1998;98:2805.
26. Assessment of the Safety and Efficacy of a New Thrombolytic Investigators. Single-bolus tenecteplase compared with front-loaded alteplase in acute myocardial infarction: the ASSENT-2 double-blind randomised trial. Lancet 1999;354:716.
27. Sinnaeve P, Alexander J, Belmans A et al. One-year follow-up of the ASSENT-2 trial: a double-blind, randomized comparison of single-bolus tenecteplase and front-loaded alteplase in 16,949 patients with ST-elevation acute myocardial infarction. Am Heart J 2003;146:27.
28. van de Werf FJ, Barron HV, Armstrong PW et al. Incidence and predictors of bleeding events after fibrinolytic therapy with fibrin-specific agents: a comparison of TNK-tPA and rt-PA. Eur Heart J 2001;22:2253.
29. Antithrombotic Trialists' Collaboration. Collaborative meta-analysis of randomised trials of antiplatelet therapy for prevention of death, myocardial infarction, and stroke in high risk patients. BMJ 2002;324:71–86.
30. Freimark D, Matetzky S, Leor J et al. Timing of aspirin administration as a determinant of survival of patients with acute myocardial infarction treated with thrombolysis. Am J Cardiol 2002;89:381.

31. Barbash IM, Freimark D, Gottlieb S et al. Outcome of myocardial infarction in patients treated with aspirin is enhanced by pre-hospital administration. Cardiology 2002;98:141.

32. Sabatine MS, Cannon CP, Gibson CM et al. Addition of clopidogrel to aspirin and fibrinolytic therapy for myocardial infarction with ST-segment elevation. N Engl J Med 2005;352:1179–89.

33. Scirica BM, Sabatine MS, Morrow DA et al. The role of clopidogrel in early and sustained arterial patency after fibrinolysis for ST-segment elevation myocardial infarction: the ECG CLARITY-TIMI 28 Study. J Am Coll Cardiol 2006;48:37–42.

34. Chen ZM, Jiang LX, Chen YP et al. Addition of clopidogrel to aspirin in 45,852 patients with acute myocardial infarction: randomised placebo-controlled trial. Lancet 2005;366:1607–21.

35. Sabatine MS, Cannon CP, Gibson CM et al. Effect of clopidogrel pretreatment before percutaneous coronary intervention in patients with ST-elevation myocardial infarction treated with fibrinolytics: the PCI-CLARITY study. JAMA 2005;294:1224–32.

36. Rebeiz AG, Johanson P, Green CL et al. Comparison of ST-segment resolution with combined fibrinolytic and glycoprotein IIb/IIIa inhibitor therapy versus fibrinolytic alone (data from four clinical trials). Am J Cardiol 2005;95:611–14.

37. Lincoff AM, Califf RM, van de Werf FJ et al. Mortality at 1 year with combination platelet glycoprotein IIb/IIIa inhibition and reduced-dose fibrinolytic therapy vs conventional fibrinolytic therapy for acute myocardial infarction: GUSTO V randomized trial. JAMA 2002;288:2130.

38. Sinnaeve PR, Alexander JH, Bogaerts K et al. Efficacy of tenecteplase in combination with enoxaparin, abciximab, or unfractionated heparin: one-year follow-up results of the Assessment of the Safety of a New Thrombolytic-3 (ASSENT-3) randomized trial in acute myocardial infarction. Am Heart J 2004;147:993.

39. Sinnaeve PR, Huang Y, Bogaerts K et al. Age, outcomes, and treatment effects of fibrinolytic and antithrombotic combinations: findings from Assessment of the Safety and Efficacy of a New Thrombolytic (ASSENT)-3 and ASSENT-3 PLUS. Am Heart J 2006;152:e1–9.

40. Di Mario C, Bolognese L, Maillard L et al. Combined Abciximab REteplase Stent Study in acute myocardial infarction (CARESS in AMI). Am Heart J 2004;148:378–85.

41. Ellis SG, Armstrong P, Betriu A et al. Facilitated percutaneous coronary intervention versus primary percutaneous coronary intervention: design and rationale of the Facilitated Intervention with Enhanced Reperfusion Speed to Stop Events (FINESSE) trial. Am Heart J 2004;147:E16.

42. Wallentin L, Dellborg DM, Lindahl B et al. The low-molecular-weight heparin dalteparin as adjuvant therapy in acute myocardial infarction: the ASSENT PLUS study. Clin Cardiol 2001;24:I12.

43. Ross AM, Molhoek P, Lundergan C et al. Randomized comparison of enoxaparin, a low-molecular-weight heparin, with unfractionated heparin adjunctive to recombinant tissue plasminogen activator thrombolysis and aspirin: second trial of Heparin and Aspirin Reperfusion Therapy (HART II). Circulation 2001;104:648.

44. Antman EM, Louwerenburg HW, Baars HF et al. Enoxaparin as adjunctive antithrombin therapy for ST-elevation myocardial infarction: results of the ENTIRE-Thrombolysis in Myocardial Infarction (TIMI) 23 Trial. Circulation 2002;105:1642.

45. Antman EM, Morrow DA, McCabe CH et al. Enoxaparin versus unfractionated heparin with fibrinolysis for ST-elevation myocardial infarction. N Engl J Med 2006;354:1477–88.

46. Eikelboom JW, Quinlan DJ, Mehta SR et al. Unfractionated and low-molecular-weight heparin as adjuncts to thrombolysis in aspirin-treated patients with ST-elevation acute myocardial infarction: a meta-analysis of the randomized trials. Circulation 2005;112:3855–67.

47. Yusuf S, Mehta SR, Xie C et al. Effects of reviparin, a low-molecular-weight heparin, on mortality, reinfarction, and strokes in patients with acute myocardial infarction presenting with ST-segment elevation. JAMA 2005;293:427–35.

48. Coussement PK, Bassand JP, Convens C et al. A synthetic factor-Xa inhibitor (ORG31540/SR9017A) as an adjunct to fibrinolysis in acute myocardial infarction. The PENTALYSE study. Eur Heart J 2001;22:1716.

49. Yusuf S, Mehta SR, Chrolavicius S et al. Effects of fondaparinux on mortality and reinfarction in patients with acute ST-segment elevation myocardial infarction: the OASIS-6 randomized trial. JAMA 2006;295:1519–30.

50. White HD, Aylward PE, Frey MJ et al. Randomized, double-blind comparison of hirulog versus heparin in patients receiving streptokinase and aspirin for acute myocardial infarction (HERO). Hirulog Early Reperfusion/Occlusion (HERO) Trial Investigators. Circulation 1997;96:2155.

51. White H. Thrombin-specific anticoagulation with bivalirudin versus heparin in patients receiving fibrinolytic therapy for acute myocardial infarction: the HERO-2 randomised trial. Lancet 2001;358:1855.

52. Antman EM, Anbe DT, Armstrong PW et al. ACC/AHA guidelines for the management of patients with ST-elevation myocardial infarction – executive summary: a report of the American College of Cardiology/American Heart Association Task Force on Practice Guidelines (Writing Committee to Revise the 1999 Guidelines for the Management of Patients With Acute Myocardial Infarction). Circulation 2004;110:588.

53. Nallamothu BK, Bates ER, Herrin J et al. Times to treatment in transfer patients undergoing primary percutaneous coronary intervention in the United States: National Registry of Myocardial Infarction (NRMI)-3/4 analysis. Circulation 2005;111:761–7.

54. Mandelzweig L, Battler A, Boyko V et al. The second Euro Heart Survey on acute coronary syndromes: characteristics, treatment, and outcome of patients with ACS in Europe and the Mediterranean Basin in 2004. Eur Heart J 2006;27:2285–93.

55. Kent DM, Lau J, Selker HP. Balancing the benefits of primary angioplasty against the benefits of thrombolytic therapy for acute myocardial infarction: the importance of timing. Eff Clin Pract 2001;4:214–20.

56. Nallamothu BK, Bates ER. Percutaneous coronary intervention versus fibrinolytic therapy in acute myocardial infarction: Is timing (almost) everything? Am J Cardiol 2003;92:824–6.

57. Boersma E. Does time matter? A pooled analysis of randomized clinical trials comparing primary percutaneous coronary intervention and in-hospital fibrinolysis in acute myocardial infarction patients. Eur Heart J 2006;27:779–88.

58. De Luca G, Suryapranata H, Ottervanger JP, Antman EM. Time delay to treatment and mortality in primary angioplasty for acute myocardial infarction: every minute of delay counts. Circulation 2004;109:1223–5.

59. Pinto DS, Kirtane AJ, Nallamothu BK et al. Hospital delays in reperfusion for ST-elevation myocardial infarction: implications when selecting a reperfusion strategy. Circulation 2006;114:2019–25.

60. Van de Werf F, Gore JM, Avezum A et al. Access to catheterisation facilities in patients admitted with acute coronary syndrome: multinational registry study. BMJ 2005;330:441.

61. Fibrinolytic Therapy Trialists' (FTT) Collaborative Group. Indications for fibrinolytic therapy in suspected acute myocardial infarction: collaborative overview of early mortality and major morbidity results from all randomised trials of more than 1000 patients. Lancet 1994;343:311.

62. Gibler WB, Armstrong PW, Ohman EM et al. Persistence of delays in presentation and treatment for patients with acute myocardial infarction: The GUSTO-I and GUSTO-III experience. Ann Emerg Med 2002;39:123.

63. Welsh RC, Goldstein P, Adgey J et al. Variations in pre-hospital fibrinolysis process of care: insights from the Assessment of the Safety

and Efficacy of a New Thrombolytic 3 Plus international acute myocardial infarction pre-hospital care survey. Eur J Emerg Med 2004;11:134.

64. Morrison LJ, Verbeek PR, McDonald AC et al. Mortality and prehospital thrombolysis for acute myocardial infarction: a meta-analysis. JAMA 2000;283:2686.

65. Bjorklund E, Stenestrand U, Lindback J et al. Pre-hospital thrombolysis delivered by paramedics is associated with reduced time delay and mortality in ambulance-transported real-life patients with ST-elevation myocardial infarction. Eur Heart J 2006;27:1146–52.

66. Danchin N, Blanchard D, Steg PG et al. Impact of prehospital thrombolysis for acute myocardial infarction on 1-year outcome: results from the French Nationwide USIC 2000 Registry. Circulation 2004;110:1909.

67. Wallentin L, Goldstein P, Armstrong PW et al. Efficacy and safety of tenecteplase in combination with the low-molecular-weight heparin enoxaparin or unfractionated heparin in the prehospital setting: the Assessment of the Safety and Efficacy of a New Thrombolytic Regimen (ASSENT)-3 PLUS randomized trial in acute myocardial infarction. Circulation 2003;108:135.

68. Bonnefoy E, Lapostolle F, Leizorovicz A et al. Primary angioplasty versus prehospital fibrinolysis in acute myocardial infarction: a randomised study. Lancet 2002;360:825.

69. Steg G, Bonnefoy E, Chabaud S et al. Impact of time to treatment on mortality after prehospital fibrinolysis or primary angioplasty – data from the CAPTIM randomized clinical trial. Circulation 2003;108:2851.

70. Bottiger BW, Bode C, Kern S et al. Efficacy and safety of thrombolytic therapy after initially unsuccessful cardiopulmonary resuscitation: a prospective clinical trial. Lancet 2001;19:1583.

71. Lederer W, Lichtenberger C, Pechlaner C et al. Recombinant tissue plasminogen activator during cardiopulmonary resuscitation in 108 patients with out-of-hospital cardiac arrest. Resuscitation 2001;50:71.

72. Spohr F, Arntz HR, Bluhmki E et al. International multicentre trial protocol to assess the efficacy and safety of tenecteplase during cardiopulmonary resuscitation in patients with out-of-hospital cardiac arrest: the Thrombolysis in Cardiac Arrest (TROICA) study. Eur J Clin Invest 2005;35:315–23.

73. Rosengren A, Wallentin L, Simoons M et al. Age, clinical presentation, and outcome of acute coronary syndromes in the Euroheart acute coronary syndrome survey. Eur Heart J 2006;27:789–95.

74. Berger AK, Radford MJ, Wang Y, Krumholz HM. Thrombolytic therapy in older patients. J Am Coll Cardiol 2000;36:366.

75. Thiemann DR, Coresh J, Schulman SP et al. Lack of benefit for intravenous thrombolysis in patients with myocardial infarction who are older than 75 years. Circulation 2000;101:2239.

76. Soumerai SB, McLaughlin TJ, Ross-Degnan D et al. Effectiveness of thrombolytic therapy for acute myocardial infarction in the elderly: cause for concern in the old-old. Arch Intern Med 2002;162:561.

77. White HD. Debate: Should the elderly receive thrombolytic therapy or primary angioplasty? Curr Control Trials Cardiovasc Med 2000;1:150.

78. Maggioni AP, Maseri A, Fresco C et al. Age-related increase in mortality among patients with first myocardial infarctions treated with thrombolysis. The Investigators of the Gruppo Italiano per lo Studio della Sopravvivenza nell'Infarto Miocardico (GISSI-2). N Engl J Med 1993;329:1442.

79. Alexander KP, Chen AY, Roe MT et al. Excess dosing of antiplatelet and antithrombin agents in the treatment of non-ST-segment elevation acute coronary syndromes. JAMA 2005;294:3108–16.

80. Primary versus tenecteplase-facilitated percutaneous coronary intervention in patients with ST-segment elevation acute myocardial infarction (ASSENT-4 PCI): randomised trial. Lancet 2006;367: 569–78.

81. Huber K, De Caterina R, Kristensen SD et al. Pre-hospital reperfusion therapy: a strategy to improve therapeutic outcome in patients with ST-elevation myocardial infarction. Eur Heart J 2005;26:2063–74.

82. Pinto DS, Southard M, Ciaglo L, Gibson CM. Door-to-balloon delays with percutaneous coronary intervention in ST-elevation myocardial infarction. Am Heart J 2006;151:S24–9.

20

Fibrinolytics and percutaneous coronary intervention

Pedro L Sánchez and Francisco Fernández-Avilés

Introduction

Cardiovascular disease continues to be the leading cause of death in developed countries – in particular, ischemic heart disease is responsible for more than 50% of cardiovascular deaths.[1] Prevention, rapid diagnosis and appropriate early treatment improve survival and reduce the risk of developing heart failure[2,3] Nonetheless, more than one-third of patients with ST-elevation myocardial infarction (STEMI) who are candidates for reperfusion therapy never actually receive this therapy.[4-7]

It is important to remember that reperfusion therapy should be administered as early as possible, given that any delay in its provision is related to worse clinical evolution, increase in infarct size, and higher mortality in the short and long term.[8] Therefore, in patients presenting with chest pain, over a period of less than 12 hours and with evidence of persistent ST elevation or left bundle branch block (LBBB), we should aim to give the patient urgent reperfusion therapy in an attempt to reopen the occluded coronary artery as quickly, effectively, and permanently as possible, and to re-establish epicardial and microvascular blood flow.[9-11] Furthermore, myocardial necrosis can even be aborted if this therapy is administered within the first hours of symptoms onset.[12]

Reperfusion therapies: fibrinolysis and primary PCI

For early, fast, complete and lasting restoration of epicardial and myocardial flow in patients with ST-elevation myocardial infarction (STEMI), there are two well-established therapies: fibrinolysis and primary percutaneous coronary intervention (PCI).

Primary PCI is considered the gold standard of myocardial reperfusion when promptly performed by skilled teams;[9-11] however, as the efficacy of this therapy is time-dependent, logistical barriers and other constraints limit its use to no more than 30% of STEMI patients worldwide.[4-7] Moreover, although it has been documented that a door-to-balloon time exceeding 120 minutes is associated with a 41–62% increase in mortality, even in well-developed countries the vast majority of patients with STEMI who undergo primary PCI achieve mechanical reopening of the infarct-related artery beyond the established time limit from which left ventricular preservation and clinical benefit are less probable.[13-15] In contrast, intravenous fibrinolysis is widely applicable, and has been shown to reduce mortality unequivocally when given within 12 hours of symptoms.[9-11] Furthermore, early administration of newer fibrin-specific thrombolytics is at least as effective as primary PCI, and can abort infarction and dramatically reduce mortality when given during the first 1–2 hours of onset.[16-18] Consequently, key elements from the current guidelines in Europe and in the USA recommend that patients with ST elevation or LBBB should be reperfused either by PCI performed 90 minutes after the first medical contact or by fibrinolysis within 30 minutes of presentation to hospital.[9,11] Thus, the choice of one or other therapy will depend basically on the medical service who attempt first patient contact, on how much time has elapsed since onset of symptoms, and on whether or not there is immediate access to perform primary PCI.[19]

Fibrinolytics and PCI: a crossroad in clinical practice

The advantages and disadvantages of these therapies generated two distinct viewpoints on reperfusion strategies in patients with infarction, denying the existence of alternatives that lay between one option and the other. However, this is not true in daily clinical practice. Furthermore, these two therapies of reperfusion are crossed in three clearly representative strategies: fibrinolytics-facilitated angioplasty, rescue PCI after failed fibrinolysis, and post-fibrinolysis PCI.

Time delay from first medical contact to balloon inflation constitutes overall the Achilles heel of primary PCI. This has led researchers to question whether administrating fibrinolytics to bridge the delay between first medical contact and primary PCI would improve outcomes. Thus, the concept of *fibrinolytic-facilitated angioplasty* came into being. Therefore, in randomized studies testing the concept of facilitated PCI, all patients (with or without fibrinolytics) should undergo planned primary PCI.

Rescue PCI is defined as PCI in a coronary artery that remains occluded despite thrombolytic therapy. Because fibrinolysis requires, on average, 45–60 minutes before reperfusion occurs, failed fibrinolysis should be suspected when persistent chest pain and non-resolution of ST elevation are evident 60–90 minutes after starting the administration.

Post-fibrinolysis PCI is defined as early percutaneous repair of the culprit artery in routine (i.e., not rescue), planned (i.e., not urgent) procedures, in patients with STEMI treated initially with fibrinolytics to open the artery.

The evidence available of these three different reperfusion strategies, where fibrinolytics and PCI coexist, could be identified in four recent meta-analysis.[20–23]

Fibrinolytic-facilitated angioplasty

In order to reduce the effects caused by delay in transferring the patient to perform primary angioplasty, many authors have advocated the initiation of intensive antithrombotic therapy at low or full doses of fibrinolytics to enhance the results of primary angioplasty and in some cases open the artery before the patient gets to the catheterization laboratory. Therefore, fibrinolytic-facilitated angioplasty is a variation of primary angioplasty whereby the patient receives fibrinolysis prior to the percutaneous intervention without entailing any additional delay to that due to the patient's transfer.

The rationale behind this approach is, on the one hand, the fact that the prognosis of patients referred for primary angioplasty substantially improves if the artery involved in infarction has normal epicardial flow on initial coronary arteriography and, on the other, that in the context of STEMI the thrombus is rich not only in fibrin but also in platelets. For this reason, the proposal is that therapy combining powerful antiagregants (such as glycoprotein (GP) IIb/IIIa inhibitors) and low or full doses of fibrinolytics might help to better dissolve the thrombus and thus improve

the epicardial flow index and the prognosis of patients who undergo primary angioplasty.

To this end, several different pre-primary angioplasty antithrombotic and firbinolytic strategies have been put to the test. As this is discussed in detail in other chapters of this book, we will summarize the principal studies where fibrinolytics in half or full doses have been used.

Facilitated angioplasty with full dose of fibrinolytics

The principal clinical trials conducted on the potential benefits of administration of fibrinolytics prior to urgent coronary angioplasty in STEMI patients are the PACT trial,[24] a subgroup analysis of the PRAGUE-1 trial,[25] and the ASSENT-4 PCI trial.[26]

Overall, 2474 patients were randomized, and although the coronary angiography showed better patency of the infarct-related artery in patients who received fibrinolytics, this epicardial benefit did not translate into clinical outcomes. Nonetheless, considering the rather discouraging results of ASSENT-4 PCI, caution must be exercised when recommending fibrinolytic-facilitated angioplasty.

The first study to consider the modern concept of fibrinolytic-facilitated angioplasty was the PACT trial ($N = 606$) published in 1999.[24] Patients initially received half the dose of alteplase followed by immediate coronary arteriography and angioplasty if Thrombolyis in Myocardial Infarction (TIMI) flow grade was less than 3 or alternatively fibrinolysis was completed if TIMI flow was normal. Arterial patency in this study was greater in patients randomised to fibrinolytic-facilitated angioplasty compared with controls (TIMI flow 2 or 3; 61% vs 34%; $p < 0.001$). Patients with optimal TIMI flow at catheterization also showed a better left ventricular function and clinical evolution at follow up. Overall for both strategies, mortality, reinfarction, and bleeding complications were similar at 30 days.

The PRAGUE-1 trial[25] compared three reperfusion strategies: isolated fibrinolysis ($N = 99$), fibrinolytic-facilitated angioplasty ($N = 100$), and primary angioplasty ($N = 101$). Comparative analysis of the last two groups showed that patients randomized to primary angioplasty presented a lower incidence in the primary endpoints of death, reinfarction, or cerebrovascular accident and in the incidence of bleeding complications at 30 days' follow-up as compared with the facilitated angioplasty group.

Anticipating the results of the FINESSE trial,[27] the ASSENT-4 PCI trial[26] discouraged the use of fibrinolytic-facilitated angioplasty. STEMI patients in ASSENT-4 were randomized to primary angioplasty ($N = 838$) versus fibrinolytic-facilitated angioplasty ($N = 828$) using full doses of tenecteplase. The trial had to be stopped prematurely due to a higher hospitalization death rate in the facilitated group (6% vs 3%). The final analysis showed a higher rate in the primary endpoint of death, heart failure, or cardiogenic shock at 90 days in the facilitated arm (19% vs 13%; p=0.004). The higher incidence of early ischemic coronary events should alert us or the pro-thrombotic effect of fibrinolytics during early-stage angioplasty.

Facilitated angioplasty with reduced dose of fibrinolytics and combination of GPIIb/IIIa inhibitors

The principal clinical trials aimed at studying the potential benefits of administering the combination of fibrinolytics and GPIIb/IIIa inhibitors prior to urgent coronary angioplasty in STEMI patients are the BRAVE[28] and ADVANCE MI[29] trials. The rationale for using this combination was that reducing the dose of fibrinolytic might lower the incidence of bleeding complications and that simultaneous administration of GPIIb/IIIa inhibitors might to counteract the prothrombotic effect of fibrinolytics.

Overall, 401 patients were randomized. The design of both studies compared two facilitated angioplasty strategies: combined fibrinolytics and GPIIb/IIIa inhibitors versus GPIIb/IIIa inhibitors alone. In a similar manner to full-dose fibrinolytic-facilitated angioplasty, although the combined treatment improved coronary patency, a higher incidence of clinical outcomes and bleeding complications was observed. Thus, facilitated interventions with fibrinolytic and GPIIb/IIIa inhibitors regimens should be avoided.

The BRAVE trial[28] (N=253) randomized patients to half doses of reteplase and abciximab (N=125) or abciximab alone (N=125). The principal endpoint was surrogate, based on the infaction size determined by single photon emission computed tomography (SPECT). No differences were observed in both groups: However, the rate of bleeding was higher in the combination-treatment group.

The ADVANCE MI trial[29] was designed with the intention to randomize 5640 patients; however, the study was stopped prematurely because of the very low recruitment rate. The two facilitated strategies consisted in the combination of half doses of tenecteplase and eptifibatide (N=69) versus eptifibatide alone (N=77). Although patients in the combination-treatment are showed better epicardial perfusion (TIMI flow 3; 40% vs 20%), the mortality (7% vs 0%) and bleeding (25% vs 10%) rates were also higher.

Figures 20.1–20.3 summarize the odds ratios for death, reinfarction, and bleeding complications in studies where the fibrinolytic-facilitated PCI strategy has been tested. These endpoints have been evaluated separately because the combined endpoint was not available in all studies.

Rescue angioplasty after failed fibrinolysis

In about 45–50% of patients who receive fibrinolytics, adequate coronary reperfusion (epicardial TIMI 3 flow) is not achieved.[19] Therefore, it is important to be aware of the

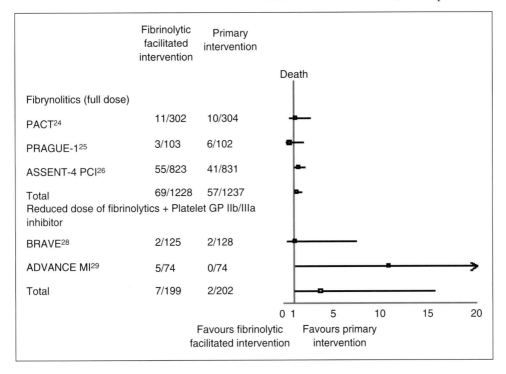

Figure 20.1
Odds ratio for death with fibrinolytic-facilitated PCI versus primary PCI.

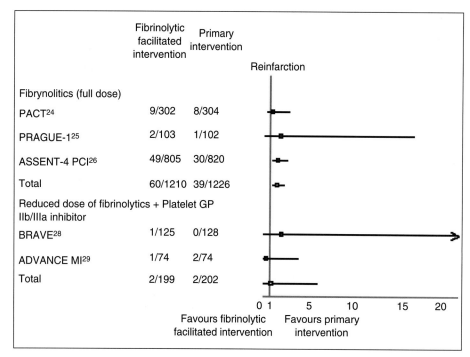

Figure 20.2
Odds ratio for reinfarction with fibrinolytic-facilitated PCI versus primary PCI.

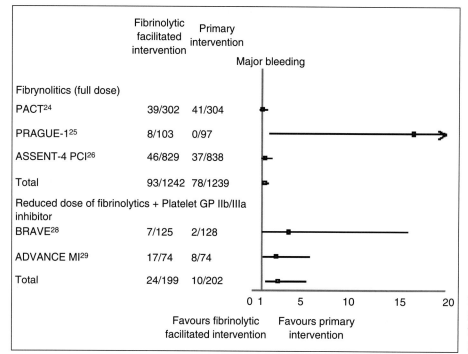

Figure 20.3
Odds ratio for major bleeding with fibrinolytic-facilitated PCI versus primary PCI.

signs of adequate reperfusion in terms of clinical parameters (relief of pain), electrocardiography (ST resolution >50%), enzymatic signs (rapid elevation of myocardial damage markers), and tissue perfusion. The combination of clinical data, electrocardiography (ECG), and measurement of enzyme activity helps to better evaluate whether or not adequate reperfusion has been achieved, although in the majority of cases, clinical and ECG assessments guided us in estimating the probability of adequate reperfusion. In fact, complete ST resolution is an excellent predictive factor of recovery of coronary patency, with a predictive value of >90% for an epicardial flow of TIMI 2 or 3 and 70–80% for TIMI 3.[30,31] On the contrary, its negative predictive value is very low (about 50%) – mainly due to the fact that ST resolution depends not only on epicardial perfusion but also on microvascular perfusion.[31] In any event, in the absence of clear reperfusion criteria 90 minutes after the administration of fibrinolytics, failure to restore patency must be ruled out by emergency catheterization and PCI. This procedure, known as rescue angioplasty, has been compared with a conservative strategy and readministration of fibrinolytics.

Rescue angioplasty versus a conservative strategy after failed fibrinolysis

Results of rescue PCI with balloon angioplasty alone were initially conflicting, taking into consideration that there were obviously biases due to a high recurrent reocclusion. The use of stents and concomitant administration of GPIIb/IIIa inhibitors have changed the thrombotic scenario, and therefore only studies from the 'stent era' are considered in this section. Studies aimed at analyzing the potential benefits of rescue angioplasty versus a conservative strategy including no reperfusion therapies of any kind are the MERLIN[32] and REACT[33] studies.

A total of 592 patients were randomized. Overall, there was a non-significant reduction in mortality in favor of rescue PCI. There was also a significant reduction of reinfarction in the rescue PCI group, especially at short-term follow-up. On the contrary, rescue PCI is associated with major bleeding as compared with a conservative treatment.

The MERLIN study[32] involved 307 patients with STEMI in whom reperfusion failed to occur (<50% ST resolution in the lead with maximal ST elevation) 60 minutes after the onset of fibrinolysis. The patients were randomly assigned to conservative treatment or rescue PCI. Stents were used in 50% of cases and GPIIb/IIIa inhibitors in 3%. Although 30-day mortality was similar in the two groups, the composite secondary endpoint of death, reinfarction, stroke, subsequent revascularization, or heart failure occurred less frequently in the rescue group (37% vs 50%; $p=0.02$). Strokes and transfusions were more common in the rescue group. The long-term follow-up results of the trial did not show any late survival advantage to rescue PCI, with only fewer unplanned revascularization procedures in the early phase of follow-up.[34]

The REACT trial[33] compared three different managements of failed fibrinolysis (using the same criteria as the MERLIN study, but at 90 minutes): repeated fibrinolysis ($N=142$), convervative treatment ($N=141$), and rescue PCI ($N=144$). Stents were used in approximately 90% of patients and GPIIb/IIIa inhibitors in 55%, thus reflecting current interventional practice. The comparative analysis of rescue angioplasty versus conservative treatment showed that patients randomized to rescue angioplasty presented a significant higher rate of event-free survival (85%) than patients receiving conservative therapy (70%). Bleeding, mostly at the sheath insertion site, was more common with rescue PCI.

Rescue angioplasty versus repeated fibrinolysis

Although the REACT trial[33] analyzed three different strategies of treatment in patients with failed fibrinolysis, it is the only clinical trial in which rescue PCI and repeated fibrinolysis have been compared. The agent used for repeat fibrinolytic therapy was tissue-type plasminogen activator (PA). Comparative analysis of these two groups showed that patients randomized to rescue PCI presented a lower incidence in the primary endpoint of death, reinfarction, stroke, or severe heart failure at 6 months' follow-up, as compared with the repeated fibrinolysis group (hazard ratio (HR) 0.47; 95% confidence interval (CI) 0.28–0.79; $p=0.004$).

Figure 20.4–20.6 summarize the odds ratios for death, reinfarction, and bleeding complications in studies where rescue PCI has been tested. These endpoints have been evaluated separately because a combined endpoint was not similar and available in all studies.

Routine angioplasty early post fibrinolysis

The standard treatment of a patient who has received fibrinolytics and presents signs of reperfusion was to assess the risk of future cardiac adverse events before discharge. The two most important parameters used to evaluate long- and short-term risk following myocardial infarction are left ventricular function and the extent and grade of myocardial ischemia. Thus, patients with spontaneous or induced severe ischemia or left ventricular dysfunction are candidates for angiography and revascularization. Beyond these circumstances, coronary arteriography was not recommended, as there was no evidence for any benefit to the patient if residual ischemia or left ventricular dysfunction was not observed.

Cardiac catheterization and systematized percutaneous procedures in patients with STEMI treated with fibrinolytic agents have been studied and discussed since the late 1980s. At that time, prior to the use of stents and GPIIb/IIIa inhibitors, or thienopyridines, results were disappointing.[35] However, current interventional practice, including the use of stents, thienopyridines, and GPIIb/IIIa inhibitors, has motivated different studies that have again revealed the role of early routine angioplasty in the management of STEMI patients treated with fibrinolysis.

Early and systematic post-fibrinolysis angioplasty versus guided or delayed angioplasty

Five randomized studies have contributed to the decision to recommend routine coronary angiography and, if applicable,

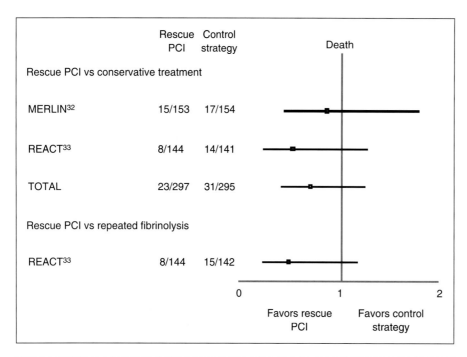

Figure 20.4
Odds ratio for death with rescue PCI versus a conservative approach or readministration of fibrinolysis.

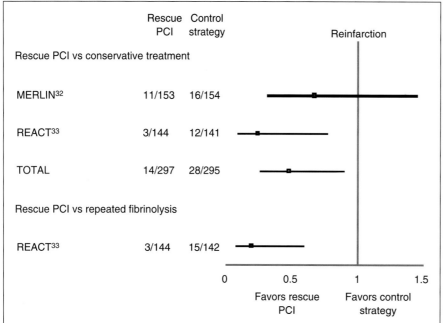

Figure 20.5
Odds ratio for reinfarction with rescue PCI versus a conservative approach or readministration of fibrinolysis.

PCI early post fibrinolysis compared with a guided or delayed angioplasty strategy: SIAM III,[36] GRACIA-1,[37] CAPITAL-AMI,[38] the Leipzig Prehospital Fibrinolysis Study,[39] and WEST.[40]

Overall, 1235 patients have been randomized. In the era of stents and GPIIb/IIIa inhibitors, early elective stenting following fibrinolysis is feasible and safe. Moreover, it permits rapid patient risk stratification, substantially reduces hospitalization, improves left ventricular evolution, and apparently reduces the incidence of adverse coronary events at 1 year. The clinical implications of these studies are

important, as they suggest that fibrinolysis, even if successful, should not be considered as the final treatment.

The SIAM III study[36] randomized 197 patients with STEMI treated with reteplase to two strategies: early and systematic angioplasty within 6 hours of fibrinolytic treatment or elective delayed angioplasty at 2 weeks post fibrinolysis. All patients received stents, and a GPIIb/IIIa inhibitor was administered to 10% of patients in the immediate stenting group and 16% of those in the delayed-stenting group. Immediate stenting was associated with a reduction in the primary composite endpoint (death,

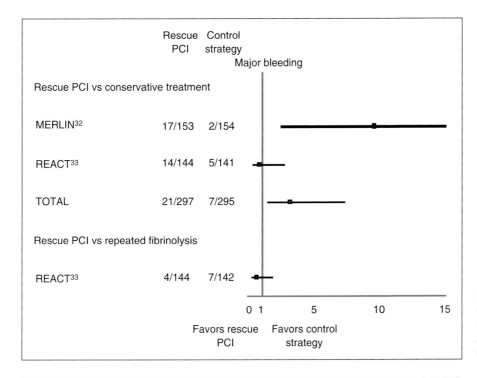

Figure 20.6
Odds ratio for major bleeding with rescue PCI versus a conservative approach or readministration of fibrinolysis.

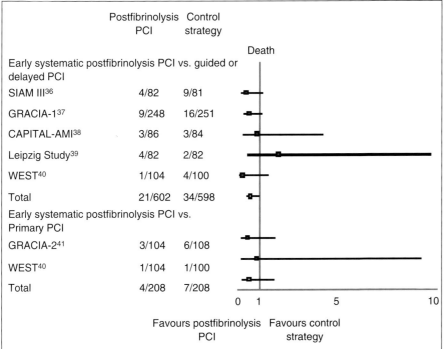

Figure 20.7
Odds ratio for death with early and systematic post-fibrinolysis PCI versus guided, delayed, or primary PCI.

reinfarction, unstable angina, or revascularization) compared with delayed stenting (26% vs 51%; $p = 0.001$).

The GRACIA-1 study[37] was a randomized multicenter clinical trial of 500 patients with STEMI and fibrinolytic treatment assigned either to coronary angiography within 24 hours of fibrinolysis followed by complete revascularization with stent or surgery or to conservative management guided by detection of spontaneous or provoked ischemia in post-infarction evaluation. The primary composite

endpoint was 1-year incidence of mortality, reinfarction, stroke, or ischemia-induced revascularization. In-hospital revascularization guided by detection of spontaneous or provoked ischemia in the conservative group was not considered an event, as it is standard in these patients. At 30 days, the primary endpoint was similar in both intervention and conservative groups (4.8% and 6%, respectively) with no differences in major bleeding or vascular complications. Hospitalization was significantly shorter in patients

Interventions of the European Society of Cardiology. Eur Heart J 2005;26:804–47.

12. Gersh BJ, Stone GW, White HD, Holmes DR Jr. Pharmacological facilitation of primary percutaneous coronary intervention for acute myocardial infarction: is the slope of the curve the shape of the future? JAMA 2005;293:979–86.

13. De Luca G, Suryapranata H, Ottervanger JP, Antman EM. Time delay to treatment and mortality in primary angioplasty for acute myocardial infarction: every minute of delay counts. Circulation 2004;109:1223–5.

14. Nallamothu BK, Bates ER, Herrin J et al. Times to treatment in transfer patients undergoing primary percutaneous coronary intervention in the United States: National Registry of Myocardial Infarction (NRMI)-3/4 analysis. Circulation 2005;111:761–7.

15. Nallamothu BK, Bates ER, Wang Y et al. Driving times and distances to hospitals with percutaneous coronary intervention in the United States: implications for prehospital triage of patients with ST-elevation myocardial infarction. Circulation 2006;113:1189–95.

16. Lamfers EJ, Hooghoudt TE, Hertzberger DP et al. Abortion of acute ST segment elevation myocardial infarction after reperfusion: incidence, patients' characteristics, and prognosis. Heart 2003;89:496–501.

17. Taher T, Fu Y, Wagner GS, Goodman SG et al. Aborted myocardial infarction in patients with ST-segment elevation: insights from the Assessment of the Safety and Efficacy of a New Thrombolytic Regimen-3 Trial Electrocardiographic Substudy. J Am Coll Cardiol 2004;44:38–43.

18. Lamfers EJ, Schut A, Hertzberger DP et al. Prehospital versus hospital fibrinolytic therapy using automated versus cardiologist electrocardiographic diagnosis of myocardial infarction: abortion of myocardial infarction and unjustified fibrinolytic therapy. Am Heart J 2004;147:509–15.

19. Sanchez PL, Fernandez-Aviles F. Appropriate invasive and conservative treatment strategies for patients with ST elevation myocardial infarction. Curr Opin Cardiol 2005;20:530–5.

20. Keeley EC, Boura JA, Grines CL. Comparison of primary and facilitated percutaneous coronary interventions for ST-elevation myocardial infarction: quantitative review of randomised trials. Lancet 2006;367:579–88.

21. Wijeysundera HC, Vijayaraghavan R, Nallamothu BK et al. Rescue angioplasty or repeat fibrinolysis after failed fibrinolytic therapy for ST-segment myocardial infarction: a meta-analysis of randomized trials. J Am Coll Cardiol 2007;49:422–30.

22. Collet JP, Montalescot G, Le May M et al. Percutaneous coronary intervention after fibrinolysis: a multiple meta-analyses approach according to the type of strategy. J Am Coll Cardiol 2006;48:1326–35.

23. Patel TN, Bavry AA, Kumbhani DJ, Ellis SG. A meta-analysis of randomized trials of rescue percutaneous coronary intervention after failed fibrinolysis. Am J Cardiol 2006;97:1685–90.

24. Ross AM, Coyne KS, Reiner JS et al. A randomized trial comparing primary angioplasty with a strategy of short-acting thrombolysis and immediate planned rescue angioplasty in acute myocardial infarction: the PACT trial. PACT investigators. Plasminogen-activator Angioplasty Compatibility Trial. J Am Coll Cardiol 1999;34:1954–62.

25. Widimsky P, Groch L, Zelizko M et al. Multicentre randomized trial comparing transport to primary angioplasty vs immediate thrombolysis vs combined strategy for patients with acute myocardial infarction presenting to a community hospital without a catheterization laboratory. The PRAGUE study. Eur Heart J 2000;21:823–31.

26. Assessment of Safety and Efficacy of a New Treatment Strategy with Percutaneous Coronary Intervention (ASSENT-4 PCI) Investigators. Primary versus tenecteplase-facilitated percutaneous coronary intervention in patients with ST-segment elevation acute myocardial infarction (ASSENT-4 PCI): randomised trial. Lancet 2006;367:569–78.

27. Ellis SG, Armstrong P, Betriu A et al. Facilitated percutaneous coronary intervention versus primary percutaneous coronary intervention: design and rationale of the Facilitated Intervention with Enhanced Reperfusion Speed to Stop Events (FINESSE) trial. Am Heart J 2004;147:E16.

28. Kastrati A, Mehilli J, Schlotterbeck K et al. Early administration of reteplase plus abciximab vs abciximab alone in patients with acute myocardial infarction referred for percutaneous coronary intervention: a randomized controlled trial. JAMA 2004;291:947–54.

29. The ADVANCE MI Investigators. Facilitated percutaneous coronary intervention for acute ST-segment elevation myocardial infarction: results from the prematurely terminated ADdressing the Value of facilitated ANgioplasty after Combination therapy or Eptifibatide monotherapy in acute Myocardial Infarction (ADVANCE MI) trial. Am Heart J 2005;150:116–22.

30. de Lemos JA, Morrow DA, Gibson CM et al. Early noninvasive detection of failed epicardial reperfusion after fibrinolytic therapy. Am J Cardiol 2001;88:353–8.

31. de Lemos JA, Braunwald E. ST segment resolution as a tool for assessing the efficacy of reperfusion therapy. J Am Coll Cardiol 2001;38:1283–94.

32. Sutton AG, Campbell PG, Graham R et al. A randomized trial of rescue angioplasty versus a conservative approach for failed fibrinolysis in ST-segment elevation myocardial infarction: the Middlesbrough Early Revascularization to Limit INfarction (MERLIN) trial. J Am Coll Cardiol 2004;44:287–96.

33. Gershlick AH, Stephens-Lloyd A, Hughes S et al. Rescue angioplasty after failed thrombolytic therapy for acute myocardial infarction. N Engl J Med 2005;353:2758–68.

34. Kunadian B, Sutton AG, Vijayalakshmi K et al. Early invasive versus conservative treatment in patients with failed fibrinolysis – no late survival benefit: the final analysis of the Middlesbrough Early Revascularisation to Limit Infarction (MERLIN) randomized trial. Am Heart J 2007;153:763–71.

35. Sanchez PL, Fernandez-Aviles F. [Facilitated angioplasty: neither black nor white]. Rev Esp Cardiol 2005;58:111–8.

36. Scheller B, Hennen B, Hammer B et al. Beneficial effects of immediate stenting after thrombolysis in acute myocardial infarction. J Am Coll Cardiol 2003;42:634–41.

37. Fernandez-Aviles F, Alonso JJ, Castro-Beiras A et al. Routine invasive strategy within 24 hours of thrombolysis versus ischaemia-guided conservative approach for acute myocardial infarction with ST-segment elevation (GRACIA-1): a randomised controlled trial. Lancet 2004;364:1045–53.

38. Le May MR, Wells GA, Labinaz M et al. Combined angioplasty and pharmacological intervention versus thrombolysis alone in acute myocardial infarction (CAPITAL AMI study). J Am Coll Cardiol 2005;46:417–24.

39. Thiele H, Engelmann L, Elsner K et al. Comparison of pre-hospital combination-fibrinolysis plus conventional care with pre-hospital combination-fibrinolysis plus facilitated percutaneous coronary intervention in acute myocardial infarction. Eur Heart J 2005;26:1956–63.

40. Armstrong PW. A comparison of pharmacologic therapy with/without timely coronary intervention vs. primary percutaneous intervention early after ST-elevation myocardial infarction: the WEST (Which Early ST-elevation myocardial infarction Therapy) study. Eur Heart J 2006;27:1530–8.

41. Fernandez-Aviles F, Alonso JJ, Pena G et al. Primary angioplasty vs. early routine post-fibrinolysis angioplasty for acute myocardial infarction with ST-segment elevation: the GRACIA-2 non-inferiority, randomized, controlled trial. Eur Heart J 2007;28:949–60

Section III

Special situations

21

Role of facilitated percutaneous coronary intervention in ST-elevation myocardial infarction

Karthik Reddy and Howard C Herrmann

Introduction

In the mid-1970s, Davies et al[1] demonstrated that the mechanism of acute myocardial infarction (AMI) in most cases results from rupture of an atherosclerotic plaque leading to thrombosis and occlusion of the coronary artery. The recognition that the prompt restoration of flow salvages myocardium, reduces infarct size, and prolongs life has been the driving force behind a large number of clinical trials assessing reperfusion therapy for AMI. The goal of reperfusion therapy in ST-elevation myocardial infarction (STEMI) is to achieve early, full, and sustained coronary blood flow in the culprit vessel. Both primary percutaneous coronary intervention (PPCI) and fibrinolytic therapy fulfill some but not all of these goals.

Fibrinolytic therapy can rapidly be initiated, but normal Thrombolysis in Myocardial Infarction (TIMI) grade 3 flow is restored in only 50–60% of arteries,[2,3] and 29% of patients are prone to recurrent ischemia before hospital discharge.[4] Furthermore, prediction of successful infarct-related artery thrombolysis by electrocardiogram (ECG) or other noninvasive markers of reperfusion is limited. Nonetheless, major advantages of fibrinolytic therapy are its ease of administration, consistent performance, and widespread availability.

PPCI is more effective than thrombolytic therapy for the treatment of STEMI when delivered soon after the onset of symptoms by an experienced team. This benefit was nicely summarized in a pooled analysis by Keeley et al[5] from 23 randomized trials in which 7739 patients were enrolled. PPCI, as compared with fibrinolysis, achieves higher recanalization rates as well as direct and immediate verification of procedural success. However, performance of PPCI in a timely fashion can be logistically challenging. Time to reperfusion with PPCI is a critical determinant of outcome,[6] and few hospitals consistently perform PPCI rapidly on a full-time, emergency basis. Most studies demonstrate that a longer door-to-balloon time worsens outcome as assessed by myocardial infarct size as well as mortality.[7] Despite the apparent limitation of PPCI if not performed rapidly, five randomized trials comparing fibrinolysis with transfer to another hospital for primary angioplasty summarized in two meta-analyses have been interpreted to demonstrate that transfer for primary angioplasty is a better treatment than fibrinolysis at the presenting hospital.[7]

Transfer times in the real world greatly exceed those evaluated in randomized trials, which likely reduces the benefit that PPCI can offer compared with fibrinolytic therapy.[8] Nallamothu et al[9] demonstrated from a large registry of MI in the USA that the 'total' door-to-balloon time in 4278 transfer patients was a median of 180 minutes, with only 4% of patients having a door-to-balloon time of less than 90 minutes and 15% are less than or equal to 120 minutes. These values contrast with the current American College of Cardiology/American Heart Association guidelines, which recommend a goal of less than 90 minutes for total door-to-balloon time.[10] The longest delay occurred in patients with comorbid conditions, a delayed presentation after symptom onset, non-specific ECG findings, and presentation during off hours and to non-teaching hospitals in rural areas.[9]

The benefits of earlier reperfusion with fibrinolytics coupled with the more complete and sustained coronary blood flow achievable with PPCI gave rise to the concept of facilitated percutaneous intervention (facilitated PCI), a strategy of administration of a pharmacological agent or combination of agents before planned immediate percutaneous intervention (Figure 21.1).[11] Some of the potential benefits of facilitated PCI are recanalization of the occluded coronary artery as soon as possible, improved patient stability during the intervention; greater technical success, and the potential to fuse the best aspects of fibrinolytic therapy and primary angioplasty.[12] The time window during which reperfusion exerts maximum benefit on myocardial salvage and mortality is fairly brief: within 3 hours of symptom onset.[13] The average patient with AMI presents about 2 hours after symptom onset, and receives thrombolytic therapy about 30 minutes later, and another 60 minutes is

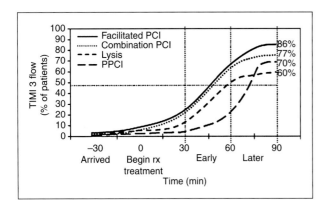

Figure 21.1
Hypothetical proportions of patients who achieve TIMI grade 3 flow with current STEMI treatment strategies. The patterns are based on clinical trial data for full-dose fibrinolysis (Lysis), PPCI, combination therapy with a reduced-dose lytic agent and GPIIb/IIIa inhibitor, and facilitated PCI utilizing a combination of pharmacologic therapy and planned PCI. (Reprinted with permission from Herrmann HC.[36])

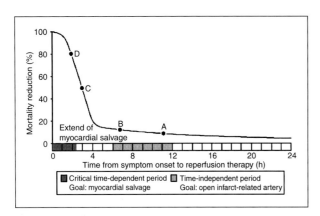

Figure 21.2
The mortality reduction in STEMI with fibrinolytic therapy is greatest in the first few hours after the onset of symptoms. (Reproduced with permission from Gersh BJ et al.[13])

required on average before reperfusion is established. Thus, unless the patient presents very early (within 60–90 minutes of symptom onset), the time window to salvage the majority of myocardium is lost (Figure 21.2). In this regard, the concept of pre-hospital initiation of a reperfusion strategy is appealing. Thiele et al[14] showed in the Leipzig Prehospital Fibrinolysis Study that when combination fibrinolysis was administered in the field, pre-hospital initiated facilitated PCI resulted in the highest percentage of complete ST-segment recovery compared with pre-hospital combination fibrinolysis or PPCI.

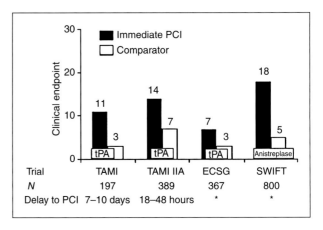

Figure 21.3
Early trials of facilitated PCI examined whether an invasive strategy was better than a conservative strategy after the administration of a thrombolytic agent. These studies did not show any significant benefit of an early invasive strategy. See the text for study details tPA, alteplase. (Reproduced with permission from Herrmann HC.[36])

Early studies of facilitated PCI

Some of the early studies exploring the facilitated PCI concept focused on determining whether an invasive strategy was better than a conservative strategy after the administration of a thrombolytic agent and the timing of the invasive strategy (Figure 21.3). The Thrombolysis and Angioplasty in Myocardial Infarction (TAMI) trial was a randomized multicenter study performed to determine whether immediate or elective (7-day) coronary angioplasty was preferable once infarct vessel recanalization had been confirmed.[15] With the exception of a higher rate of emergent PCI in the deferred PCI group, there were no differences in outcomes between the two groups.

In the ECSG (European Cooperative Study Group) trial, 367 patients treated with alteplase were randomized to immediate angiography with angioplasty or to non-invasive management.[16] Although, on follow-up angiography, immediate angioplasty did result in a lower residual stenosis in the infarct-related artery compared with conservative management, early intervention was associated with more recurrent ischemia, bleeding, hypotension, and higher mortality.

The SWIFT (Should We Intervene Following Thrombolysis?) trial compared routine angiography and revascularization versus conservative treatment after thrombolysis with anistreplase in acute myocardial infarction.[17] A total of 397 patients were randomized to early angiography, and 1 year infarction-free survival did not differ between treatment strategies ($p = 0.32$).

The TIMI 3B (Thrombolysis in Myocardial Ischemia phase IIIB) trial compared the effects of thrombolytic therapy and of an early invasive strategy on clinical outcome after unstable angina or non-Q-wave MI in 1473 patients.[18]

At 6 weeks, the principal endpoint for comparison of the two strategies (death, myocardial infarction, or an unsatisfactory symptom-limited exercise stress test at 6 weeks) occurred in 16.2% of the patients randomized to the early invasive strategy versus 18.1% of those assigned to the early conservative strategy ($p = NS$). At 1 year, the incidence of death or non-fatal infarction was also similar for the early invasive and early conservative strategies (10.8% vs 12.2% $p = 0.42$).

In a meta-analysis of randomized controlled trials published in 1995, Michels et al[19] showed that PCI used as an adjunct to thrombolytic therapy provided little benefit. When mortality at 6 weeks was analyzed, four of the five different approaches to angioplasty (immediate PCI compared with no PCI, early PCI compared with no PCI, delayed PCI versus no PCI, and immediate PCI compared with delayed PCI) showed trends toward increased risk in the more aggressively treated group. In none of these categories were these differences significant – nor were they significant when the categories were combined.

These early trials did not show any significant benefit of an early invasive strategy compared with a conservative strategy following the administration of a thrombolytic. However, these trials were performed before stents were available, and before the routine use of glycoprotein (GP) IIb/IIIa inhibitors and thienopyridines.

Recent studies with fibrinolysis

Some of the more recent trials using fibrinolytics compared these agents with the combination approach of facilitated PCI and with PPCI alone (Figure 21.4). With realistic concerns about the increased bleeding complications seen with facilitated PCI, some of the trials attempted to decrease that risk by varying the dosage of thrombolytics. Therefore, some studies examined full-dose thrombolytics while others examined reduced-dose thrombolytics in conjunction with PCI or compared with PCI alone.

SIAM III (the Southwest German Interventional Study in Acute Myocardial Infarction) investigated the efficacy of immediate stenting after thrombolysis versus a more conservative treatment regimen in patients with AMI.[20] All patients were enrolled at community hospitals without on-site catheterization laboratories. Patients received reteplase (two boluses of 10 U 30 minutes apart) and were randomized to immediate transfer (within 6 hours of thrombolysis) to a central facility for coronary angiography, including stenting of the infarct-related artery (IRA) ($n = 82$) or delayed coronary angiography and intervention 2 weeks after thrombolysis ($n = 81$). TIMI grade 3 flow rates at 2-week angiography were 98% in the immediate-stenting arm versus 59% in the delayed-stenting arm ($p < 0.001$).

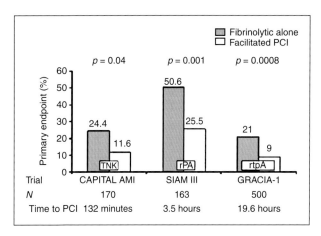

Figure 21.4
More recent trials using fibrinolytics compared these agents with the combination approach of facilitated PCI and primary PCI alone. See the text for study details. TNK, tenecteplase; rPA, reteplase; rtpA, alteplase. (Reproduced with permission from Herrmann HC.[36])

The primary composite endpoint of ischemic events, death, reinfarction, and target lesion revascularization (TLR) was significantly lower in the immediate-stenting arm compared with the delayed-stenting arm (25.6% vs 50.6%; $p = 0.001$). The reduction was driven primarily by a reduction in ischemic events (4.9% vs 28.4%, $p = 0.01$). There was no difference in rates of reinfarction (2.4% vs 2.5%, $p = 0.685$) or TLR (19.5% vs 23.5%; $p = 0.336$), but mortality was non-significantly lower in the immediate-stenting arm (4.9% vs 11.1%; $p = 0.119$). There was no difference in major bleeding between the immediate-stenting and delayed-stenting arms (9.8% vs 7.4%; $p = 0.400$).

The BRAVE (Bavarian Reperfusion Alternatives Evaluation) trial was a randomized controlled trial of 253 patients to assess whether early administration of reteplase plus abciximab produces better results compared with abciximab alone in patients with AMI referred for PCI.[21] The majority of patients (76%) in this study were transferred following randomization from treatment centers without PCI to centers with PCI. The median time from treatment to angiography was 2 hours. Pre PCI, TIMI grade 3 flow was present more frequently in the combination-therapy arm versus the abciximab-alone arm (40% vs 18%), and TIMI grade 0 flow was present less frequently (25% vs 50%; $p < 0.001$). However, there was no difference in post-PCI TIMI grade 3 flow (87% each; $p = 0.73$), and the primary endpoint of final infarct size did not differ between the treatment arms (13% in the combination arm vs 11.5% in the abciximab-alone arm; $p = 0.81$). Major bleeding occurred in 5.6% of patients in the combination arm versus 1.6% of patients in the abciximab-alone arm ($p = 0.16$). While the results of the trial were negative, it should be noted that the sample size was relatively small and the duration from diagnosis to angiography was short.

In addition, this trial compared two facilitated PCI pharmacological regimes, not the concept itself, since there was no placebo arm of PPCI alone.

In the ADVANCE MI (Addressing the Value of Facilitated Angioplasty after Combination Therapy or Eptifibatide Monotherapy in Acute Myocardial Infarction) trial, patients with STEMI with planned PPCI were randomly assigned to receive eptifibatide plus half the standard-dose tenecteplase or eptifibatide plus placebo before PCI.[22] The trial was terminated prematurely after only 148 patients were randomized due to slow recruitment. Among both populations, epicardial infarct artery patency and myocardial tissue perfusion on pre-PCI angiography were improved in the tenecteplase group, but ST-segment resolution at 60 minutes was similar.

In a randomized trial comparing stenting within 24 hours of thrombolysis ($n = 248$) versus an ischemia-guided conservative approach ($n = 252$) (GRACIA-1: Grappo de Análisis de la Cardiopatia Isquémica Aguda 1), the primary endpoint (combined rate of death, reinfarction, or revascularization at 12 months) was lower in the interventional arm (9% vs 21%; risk ratio (RR) 0.44; $p = 0.0008$).[23] The reduction in events was driven by a lower revascularization rate in the intervention arm (4% vs 12%; RR 0.30; $p = 0.001$).[23] There were trends to reduction of death (4% vs 6%; RR 0.55; $p = 0.16$) and MI (4% vs 6%; RR 0.60; $p = 0.22$).

The CAPITAL AMI (Combined Angioplasty and Pharmacological Intervention Versus Thrombolytics Alone in Acute Myocardial Infarction) trial evaluated the safety and efficacy of treatment with thrombolytic therapy alone (tenecteplase) compared with thrombolytic therapy followed by transfer and subsequent PCI.[24] Patients were randomized to full-dose tenecteplase alone ($n = 84$) or full-dose tenecteplase followed by immediate transfer for PCI ($n = 86$). Patients who failed medical therapy alone were subsequently transferred for PCI, which was performed in 91% of patients in the combination-therapy arm. In the tenecteplase alone arm, 50% of patients underwent PCI during the index hospitalization. The composite 6-month event rate of death, reinfarction, recurrent unstable ischemia, or stroke was lower in the combination-therapy arm compared with the tenecteplase-alone arm (11.6% vs 24.4%; $p = 0.04$), driven by a reduction in recurrent unstable ischemia (8.1% vs 20.7%; $p = 0.03$) and a trend toward less reinfarction (5.8% vs 14.6%; $p = 0.07$). There was no difference in death (3.5% vs 3.7%) or stroke (1.2% each).

The GRACIA-2 trial compared optimal primary PCI (within 3 hours with or without abciximab; $n = 108$) with facilitated PCI ($n = 104$).[25] Facilitated PCI patients were treated with tenecteplase bolus and enoxaparin immediately and stent or coronary artery bypass graft (CABG) within 3–12 hours. The median time from randomization to catheterization was 1.1 hours in the primary PCI arm and 5.9 hours in the facilitated PCI arm. Coronary flow at angiography was better in the facilitated PCI arm, with higher rates of TIMI flow

grade 3 (67.0% vs 13.7%; $p < 0.001$) and lower TIMI frame counts (20.9 frames vs 30.6 frames; $p = 0.034$). Infarct size assessed by creatine kinese MB isoenzyne and troponin were similar in the two arms. There were no differences between treatment arms in the composite endpoint of death/MI/ disabling stroke/ischemic-driven revascularization (9.6% vs 12.0%; $p = NS$) and major bleeding events (1.9% vs 2.8%; $p = NS$).

Definitive conclusions cannot be drawn from these trials as a result of the small sample sizes and the wide range of results. For this reason, ASSENT-4 PCI (Assessment of the Safety and Efficacy of a New Treatment Strategy with Percutaneous Coronary Intervention) was widely anticipated as the largest contemporary trial to evaluate the safety and efficacy of full-dose thrombolysis immediately prior to PPCI compared with PPCI alone.[26] Patients with STEMI were randomized to full-dose tenecteplase followed by primary PCI ($n = 829$) or PPCI alone ($n = 838$). Glycoprotein (GP) IIb/IIIa inhibitors were allowed in the PPCI arm at the discretion of the physician; however, GPIIb/IIIa inhibitors were only allowed for bailout use in the tenecteplase plus PCI group. The trial had a planned enrollment of 4000 patients, but was discontinued early by the Data Safety Monitoring Board after enrollment of 1667 patients due to worse outcomes in the facilitated PCI arm. The median time from symptom onset to randomization was 140 minutes in the tenecteplase PCI group and 135 minutes in the PCI-alone group; 20% of patients were randomized in the ambulance. PCI was performed in 91.1% of the primary PCI group and 87.1% of the tenecteplase plus PCI group ($p = 0.01$), at a median of 104 minutes following tenecteplase bolus administration. GPIIb/IIIa inhibitors were used more frequently in the PCI-alone group both prior to the PCI (3.0% vs 0.2%; $p < 0.001$) and during the PCI (50% vs 10%; $p < 0.001$). Clopidogrel/ticlopidine was used in 63% of patients, while additional unfractionated heparin (UFH) was given in 70% of the PPCI arm and 67% of the tenecteplase plus PCI arm.

TIMI grade 3 flow prior to PCI was present more frequently in the tenecteplase PCI arm (43% vs 15%; $p < 0.001$). Post-PCI patency (TIMI grade 2 or 3 flow) was slightly higher in the PCI-alone group (98% vs 95%). At 90 days, the primary composite endpoint of death, congestive heart failure (CHF), or shock was higher in the tenecteplase plus PCI group (19% vs 13%; $p = 0.0055$) (Figure 21.5). There were no significant differences in the individual components of the composite endpoint, including death (7% vs 5%; $p = 0.141$), shock (6% vs 5%; $p = 0.19$), or CHF (12% vs 9%; $p = 0.064$). Total stroke in-hospital occurred more often in the tenecteplase plus PCI group (1.8% vs 0%; $p < 0.0001$), as did intracranial hemorrhage (1.0% vs 0%; $p = 0.0037$).

Limitations of ASSENT-4 PCI include that the randomization-to-balloon times were similar in the two groups, at less than 120 minutes. Potentially, the rapid timing from tenecteplase to balloon of 104 minutes played a role in the

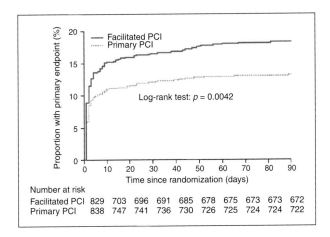

Figure 21.5
Kaplan–Meier curves for the primary endpoint (death, congestive heart failure, or shock) in the ASSENT-4 PCI trial. (Reproduced with permission ASSENT-4 PCI Investigators.[26])

worse outcomes, whereas benefit might be seen if there were a longer delay between thrombolytic and PCI, as seen in SIAM III. Another major potential confounder of the strategy of full-dose tenecteplase followed by immediate PCI in this study may be the lack of adequate antiplatelet therapy to counteract the activation produced by fibrinolysis. Less than 10% of patients received a GPIIb/IIIa inhibitor and only 63% received clopidogrel or ticlopidine. While TIMI grade 3 flow was present more frequently in the tenecteplase plus PCI group than the PPCI-alone group, the rate of grade 3 flow (44%) was lower than in most contemporary fibrinolytic trials 90 minutes post lytic administration. Similarly, the mortality achieved with PPCI was very low at 3.8%, as compared with 7.0% in a recent meta-analysis.[5] Despite these limitations, the ASSENT-4 trial raises sufficient concerns that a routine strategy of fibrinolysis before PPCI can no longer be advocated.

More recent studies with GPIIb/IIIa inhibitors

With the development of GPIIb/IIIa inhibitors, there has been renewed interest in the potential role of these agents to facilitate PPCI. One of the first trials to examine this concept was the pilot trial (SPEED) to GUSTO-5.[11] A total of 528 patients with AMI participated in dose-finding or confirmation phases of varying doses of reteplase with abciximab. Angiograms were performed between 60 and 90 minutes in 424 patients, and immediate PCI was performed in 76%. Although the decision to perform PCI was not random, baseline characteristics were similar among patients who received and those who did not receive PCI. Patients

receiving PCI had significantly less recurrent MI, transfusions, and urgent revascularizations by 30 days. Clinical success, defined as freedom from death, MI, and urgent revascularization at 30 days, was 94% in those receiving early PCI versus 84% in those who did not.[11]

The ADMIRAL (Abciximab before Direct Angioplasty and Stenting in Myocardial Infarction Regarding Acute and Long-Term Follow-up) trial compared primary stenting plus platelet GPIIb/IIIa receptor inhibition with primary stenting alone in 300 patients with AMI.[27] TIMI grade 3 flow rates at 24 hours were higher in the abciximab group (85.6% vs 78.4%; $p < 0.05$), and the combined endpoint of death, reinfarction, and urgent revascularization at 30 days was significantly reduced with abciximab compared with placebo (10.7% vs 20.0%; $p < 0.03$). Of the 300 patients, 78 (26%) were randomly assigned to one of the two study groups early (in the mobile intensive care unit or emergency department), and the remaining were assigned on admission to the intensive care unit or in the catheterization laboratory. The patients who received their randomly assigned treatment with abciximab early had a greater benefit with respect to the primary endpoint at both 30 days and 6 months than did those treated with abciximab in the intensive care unit or catheterization laboratory, thereby demonstrating the potential benefit of a facilitated strategy.

The INTAMI (Integrilin in Acute Myocardial Infarction) trial evaluated adjunctive therapy with the GPIIb/IIIa inhibitor eptifibatide administered early in the emergency department ($n = 53$) compared with late, optional administration in the catheterization laboratory ($n = 49$).[28] TIMI grade 3 flow at the time of angiography was higher in the early-eptifibatide group compared with the late/no-eptifibatide group (34.0% vs. 10.2%; $p = 0.01$). The presence of visible thrombus also trended lower in the early group (57.7% vs 70.8%; $p = 0.1$). However, there was no difference in post-PCI TIMI flow grade 3, TIMI myocardial perfusion grade 3, ST resolution, and clinical events or bleeding by 30 days.

The TITAN (Time to Integrilin Therapy in Acute Myocardial Infarction) – (TIMI 34) trial compared a strategy of early initiation of eptifibatide in the emergency department ($n = 174$) with that of initiating eptifibatide in the cardiac catheterization laboratory ($n = 142$).[29] The primary endpoint of corrected TIMI frame count on diagnostic angiography was lower (i.e., faster) in the emergency department group (77.5 frames vs 84.3 frames; $p = 0.049$). TIMI myocardial perfusion grade 3 was present more frequently in the emergency department group (24.3% vs 14.2%; $p = 0.026$). By 30 days, there was no difference in mortality (4.0% for the emergency department group vs 2.8% for the catheterization laboratory group) and there were two cases of reinfarction in each group.

These small studies seem to favor the use of platelet GPIIb/IIIa inhibition early in the emergency department before planned PCI for STEMI patients with a minimal risk for increased bleeding. Larger studies are needed to confirm these results as well as to explore the combination of novel antithrombotic agents and GPIIb/IIIa inhibitors in conjunction with PCI.

Trials in progress

Several ongoing trials, including CARESS in AMI,[30] TRANSFER-AMI[31] and FINESSE,[32] will help clarify the safety and efficacy of different regimens of facilitated PCI. CARESS in AMI (Combined Abciximab Reteplase Stent Study in AMI) is a trial comparing emergent PCI versus conservative management of STEMI patients treated with abciximab and half-dose reteplase. The study plans to enroll 1800 high-risk STEMI patients within 12 hours of symptom onset. The primary endpoint is the 30-day combined incidence of mortality, reinfarction, and refractory ischemia. Secondary endpoints include the 1-year composite endpoint of mortality, reinfarction, refractory ischemia, and hospital readmission because of heart failure; resource use at 30 days and 1 year; and the incidence of in-hospital stroke and bleeding complications in the two groups.

TRANSFER-AMI (Trial of Routine Angioplasty and Stenting after Fibrinolysis to Enhance Reperfusion in Acute Myocardial Infarction) is comparing standard treatment after thrombolysis with transfer for urgent PCI within 6 hours after thrombolysis. This is a Canadian multicenter trial enrolling 1200 patients with anterior or high-risk inferior STEMI. The primary endpoint is death, reinfarction, recurrent unstable angina, CHF, or shock at 30 days.

Finally, the FINESSE (Facilitated Intervention with Enhanced Reperfusion Speed to Stop Events) trial is an ongoing 3000-patient, randomized, double-blind, placebo-controlled, double-dummy trial in patients with STEMI that will examine the efficacy and safety of facilitated PCI with reduced-dose reteplase plus abciximab, and compare this strategy with facilitated PCI using early abciximab alone, or PPCI with abciximab just before the procedure. The study will determine whether facilitated PCI is superior to PPCI in patients when the door-to-balloon time is between 1 and 4 hours after initial presentation. Study enrollment in this trial was recently completed, and the results are expected by the end of 2007.

Favorable characteristics for facilitated PCI

Delays in the delivery of both fibrinolytic therapy and PPCI are associated with increased mortality rates. An additional delay of 60 minutes for PPCI compared with fibrinolytic therapy is considered acceptable, because this reperfusion treatment is associated with higher patency rates of the infarct vessel and better survival. This PCI-related delay may be presented as the door-to-balloon (DB) time minus the door-to-needle (DN) time.

Two recent meta-analyses assessed the relation between PCI-related time delay and the effectiveness of this intervention in decreasing death compared with fibrinolysis. Betriu and Masotti[33] analyzed data from 21 randomized controlled trials. After adjustment for patient-level data, they demonstrated that the loss of mortality advantage with PPCI occurred at a DB–DN time of 110 minutes.[33] In another pooled analysis by the PCAT-2 (Primary Coronary Angioplasty versus Thrombolysis 2) investigators of the delay times in 22 randomized studies, suggested that a survival benefit of PPCI could still be present with PCI-related delays of up to 2 hours.[34]

Pinto et al[35] analyzed data from the large NRMI (National Registries of Myocardial Infarction) 2, 3, and 4, and reported that while selecting a reperfusion strategy for patients presenting with STEMI, apart from time delays (presentation delay and PCI-related delay), baseline characteristics of the patient and the infarct should be also taken into account when choosing a reperfusion strategy (Figure 21.6). In this study, data from 192 509 patients, treated between June 1994 and August 2003 at 645 hospitals in the USA, was included. Hospitals were divided into four categories of increasing PCI-related delays: <60, 60–89, 90–120, and >120 minutes. For each of the four categories, hospital and patient characteristics were analyzed. The effect of the PCI-related delay in specific subgroups of patients were stratified by risk factors, including age (<65 years vs >65 years), infarct location (anterior versus non-anterior), and time from symptom onset to hospital arrival (2 hours vs >2 hours). In the total study population, there was a 10% increase in the relative risk of in-hospital death with every 30-minute increase in the

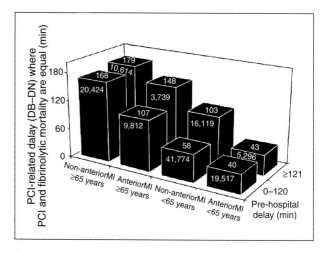

Figure 21.6
The PCI-related delay (door-to-balloon minus door-to-needle time: DB–DN that results in equal mortality for fibrinolysis and primary PCI. See the text for details. (Reproduced with permission from Pinto DS et al.[35])

PCI-related delay. The survival benefit of PPCI over fibrinolytic therapy was lost when the PCI-related delay was 114 minutes, a time delay very similar to the 30-day mortality survival advantage of 110 minutes calculated from the randomized trials.[33]

Importantly, the PCI-related delay beyond which the survival benefit of PPCI was lost varied considerably and depended on patient characteristics. The shortest permissible time delay associated with a survival benefit for PCI (<1 hour) was found in patients <65 years of age presenting with an anterior infarction within 2 hours after symptom onset. A longer time delay for PCI of almost 3 hours was acceptable without an increase in mortality in patients >65 years of age with a non-anterior infarction presenting more than 2 hours after symptom onset. For example, a patient who is <65 years old and presents with an anterior MI within 2 hours of symptom onset only gains a mortality advantage from PPCI if the DB–DN time is short (<40 minutes). This finding is likely due to the fact that thromboresistance has not emerged (better fibrinolytic efficacy), the risk of intracranial hemorrhage is low due to a younger age (improved fibrinolytic safety), and there are advantages of more rapid restoration of flow as a larger amount of ischemic myocardium is at risk (an advantage of fibrinolytic therapy). In contrast, a patient who is >65 years of age with a non-anterior infarction presenting more than 2 hours after symptom onset may have a greater tendency toward thromboresistance (reduced fibrinolytic efficacy), an increased risk of intracranial hemorrhage due to age (reduced fibrinolytic safety), and a relatively good prognosis with either therapy due to the smaller amount of myocardium at risk. Thus, a reperfusion strategy for STEMI should be selected based not only on the benefits and limitations of the reperfusion strategy and time delays (presentation delay and PCI-related delay), but must also consider patient characteristics.

Conclusions

PPCI is more effective than thrombolytic therapy for the treatment of STEMI when delivered soon after the onset of symptoms by an experienced team. However, time to reperfusion is a critical determinant of outcome with both fibrinolysis and PPCI. As the PCI-related delay to reperfusion increases, it dilutes or negates the benefit that PPCI can offer compared with fibrinolytic therapy. Registries have shown that only a small percentage of patients in the real world meet the current guidelines of a door-to-balloon time of less than 90 minutes. Facilitated PCI offers both theoretical and practical appeal to overcome some of these issues. To date, trials that have compared PPCI with facilitated PCI with full-dose fibrinolytics have failed to show a clinical benefit, although infarct artery patency rates before the PCI were significantly higher in the facilitated PCI arm.

Ongoing trials will provide important insight into the potential benefits of a facilitated PCI strategy with GPIIb/IIIa inhibitors, or combination therapy with a reduced-dose fibrinolytic plus a GPIIb/IIIa inhibitor. In this regard, it is likely that, apart from the benefits and limitations of the reperfusion strategy and time delays, patient characteristics will also be important considerations for optimal outcomes.

References

1. Davies MJ, Woolf N, Robertson WB. Pathology of acute myocardial infarction with particular reference to occlusive coronary thrombi. Br Heart J 1976;38:659–64.
2. The GUSTO Angiographic Investigators. The effects of tissue plasminogen activator, streptokinase, or both on coronary artery patency, ventricular function, and survival after acute myocardial infarction. N Engl J Med 1993;329:1615–22.
3. Granger CB, White HD, Bates ER et al. A pooled analysis of coronary arterial patency and left ventricular function after intravenous thrombolysis for acute myocardial infarction. Am J Cardiol 1994;74:1220–28
4. Pilote L, Miller DP, Califf RM, Topol EJ; Global Utilization of Streptokinase and Tisssue Plasminogen Activator for Occluded Coronary Arteries (GUSTO-I) Investigators. Recurrent ischemia after thrombolysis for acute myocardial infarction. Am Heart J 2001;141:559–65.
5. Keeley EC, Boura JA, Grines CL. Primary angioplasty versus intravenous thrombolytic therapy for acute myocardial infaction: a quantitative review of 23 randomized trials. Lancet 2003;361:13–20.
6. De Luca G, Suryapranata H, Ottervanger JP, Antman EM. Time delay to treatment and mortality in primary angioplasty for acute myocardial infarction: every minute of delay counts. Circulation 2004;109:1223–5.
7. Herrmann HC. Transfer for primary angioplasty: the importance of time. Circulation 2005;111:718–20.
8. Pinto DS, Kirtane AJ, Nallamothu BK et al. Hospital delays in reperfusion for ST-elevation myocardial infarction: implications when selecting a reperfusion strategy. Circulation 2006;114:2019–25.
9. Nallamothu BK, Bates ER, Herrin J. Times-to-treatment in transfer patients undergoing primary percutaneous coronary intervention in the United States: a National Registry of Myocardial Infarction-3/4 analysis. Circulation 2005;111:761–7.
10. Antman EM, Anbe DT, Armstrong PW et al. ACC/AHA guidelines for the management of patients with ST-elevation myocardial infarction: executive summary. J Am Coll Cardiol 2004;44:671–719.
11. Herrmann HC, Moliterno DJ, Ohman EM et al. Facilitation of early percutaneous coronary intervention after reteplase with or without abciximab in acute myocardial infarction: results from the SPEED (GUSTO-4 pilot) trial. J Am Coll Cardiol 2000;36:1489–96.
12. Herrmann HC. Triple therapy for acute myocardial infarction: combining fibrinolysis, platelet IIb/IIIa inhibition, and percutaneous coronary intervention. Am J Cardiol 2000;85(8 Suppl 1):10–16.
13. Gersh BJ, Stone GW, White HD, Holmes DR Jr. Pharmacological facilitation of primary percutaneous coronary intervention for acute myocardial infarction: Is the slope of the curve the shape of the future? JAMA 2005;293:979–86.
14. Thiele H, Scholz M, Engelmann L et al. ST-segment recovery and prognosis in patients with ST-elevation myocardial infarction reperfused by prehospital combination fibrinolysis, prehospital initiated facilitated percutaneous coronary intervention, or primary percutaneous coronary intervention. Am J Cardiol 2006;98:1132–9.

15. Topol EJ, Califf RM, Kereiakes DJ, George BS. Thrombolysis and Angioplasty in Myocardial Infarction (TAMI) trial. J Am Coll Cardiol 1987;10(5 Suppl B):65B–74B.

16. Simoons ML, Betriu A, Col J et al. European Cooperative Study Group for Recombinant Tissue-type Plasminogen Activator (rTPA). Thrombolysis with tissue plasminogen activator in acute myocardial infarction: no additional benefit from immediate percutaneous coronary angioplasty. Lancet 1988;331:197–203.

17. SWIFT (Should We Intervene Following Thrombolysis?) Trial Study Group. SWIFT trial of delayed elective intervention v conservative treatment after thrombolysis with anistreplase in acute myocardial infarction. BMJ 1991;302:555–60.

18. Thrombolysis in Myocardial Ischemia. Effects of tissue plasminogen activator and a comparison of early invasive and conservative strategies in unstable angina and non-Q-wave myocardial infarction. Results of the TIMI IIIB trial. Circulation 1994;89:1545–56.

19. Michels KB, Yusuf S. Does PTCA in acute myocardial infarction affect mortality and reinfarction rates? A quantitative overview (meta-analysis) of the randomized clinical trials. Circulation 1995;91:476–85.

20. Scheller B, Hennen B, Hammer B et al. Beneficial effects of immediate stenting after thrombolysis in acute myocardial infarction. J Am Coll Cardiol 2003;42:634–41.

21. Kastrati A, Mehilli J, Schlotterbeck K et al. Early administration of reteplase plus abciximab vs abciximab alone in patients with acute myocardial infarction referred for percutaneous coronary intervention: a randomized controlled trial. JAMA 2004;291:947–54.

22. The ADVANCE MI Investigators. Facilitated percutaneous coronary intervention for acute ST-segment elevation myocardial infarction: results from the prematurely terminated ADdressing the Value of facilitated ANgioplasty after Combination therapy or Eptifibatide monotherapy in acute Myocardial Infarction (ADVANCE MI) trial. Am Heart J 2005;150:116–22.

23. Fernandez-Aviles F, Alonso JJ, Castro-Beiras A et al. Routine invasive strategy within 24 hours of thrombolysis versus ischaemia-guided conservative approach for acute myocardial infarction with ST-segment elevation (GRACIA-1): a randomised controlled trial. Lancet 2004;364:1045–53.

24. Le May MR, Wells GA, Labinaz M et al. Combined Angioplasty and Pharmacological Intervention Versus Thrombolysis Alone in Acute Myocardial Infarction (CAPITAL AMI Study). J Am Coll Cardiol 2005;46:417–24.

25. Fernandez-Aviles F, Alonso JJ, Pena G et al. Primary angioplasty vs. early routine post-fibrinolysis angioplasty for acute myocardial infarction with ST-segment elevation: the GRACIA-2 non-inferiority, randomized, controlled trial. Eur Heart J 2007;28:949–60.

26. Assessment of the Safety and Efficacy of a New Treatment Srategy with Percutaneous Coronary Intervention (ASSENT T-4 PCI) Investigators. Primary versus tenecteplase-facilitated percutaneous coronary intervention in patients with ST-segment elevation acute myocardial infarction (ASSENT-4 PCI): randomized trial. Lancet 2006;367:569–78.

27. Montalescot G, Barragan P, Wittenberg O et al. ADMIRAL Investigators. Platelet glycoprotein IIb/IIIa inhibition with coronary stenting for acute myocardial infarction. N Engl J Med 2001;344:1895–903.

28. Zeymer U, Zahn R, Schiele R et al. Early eptifibatide improves TIMI 3 patency before primary percutaneous coronary intervention for acute ST elevation myocardial infarction: results of the randomized Integrilin in Acute Myocardial Infarction (INTAMI) pilot trial. Eur Heart J 2005;26:1971–7.

29. Gibson CM, Kirtane AJ, Murphy SA et al. Early initiation of eptifibatide in the emergency department before primary percutaneous coronary intervention for ST-segment elevation myocardial infarction: results of the Time to Integrilin Therapy in Acute Myocardial Infarction (TITAN)-TIMI 34 trial. Am Heart J 2006;152:668–75.

30. Di Mario C, Bolognese L, Maillard L et al. Combined Abciximab REteplase Stent Study in acute myocardial infarction (CARESS in AMI). Am Heart J 2004;148:378–85.

31. Cantor WJ, Burnstein J, Choi R et al. Transfer for urgent percutaneous coronary intervention early after thrombolysis for ST-elevation myocardial infarction: the TRANSFER-AMI pilot feasibility study. Can J Cardiol 2006;22:1121–6.

32. Ellis SG, Armstrong P, Betriu A et al. Facilitated percutaneous coronary intervention versus primary percutaneous coronary intervention: design and rationale of the Facilitated Intervention with Enhanced Reperfusion Speed to Stop Events (FINESSE) trial. Am Heart J 2004;47:E16.

33. Betriu A, Masotti M. Comparison of mortality rates in acute myocardial infarction treated by percutaneous coronary intervention versus fibrinolysis. Am J Cardiol 2005;95:100–1.

34. Boersma E. Does time matter? A pooled analysis of randomized clinical trials comparing primary percutaneous coronary intervention and in-hospital fibrinolysis in acute myocardial infarction patients. Eur Heart J 2006;27:779–88.

35. Pinto DS, Kirtane AJ, Nallamothu BK et al. Hospital delays in reperfusion for ST-elevation myocardial infarction: implications when selecting a reperfusion strategy. Circulation 2006;114:2019–25.

36. Herrmann HC. Update and rationale for ongoing acute myocardial infarction trials: combination therapy, facilitation, and myocardial preservation. Am Heart J 2006;151(Suppl 1):S30–9.

22

Antithrombotic treatment in vein graft interventions

Luis A Guzman and Theodore A Bass

Introduction

The first aortocoronary saphenous vein graft (SVG) implantation was performed in May 1967 by Garret and colleagues, with the subsequent pioneering work of Favaloro initiating the era of surgical revascularization of ischemic heart disease.[1,2] This major advance in surgical revascularization provided a significant improvement in angina relief and, in selected patients, improved long-term prognosis.[3,4] However, it has come to be recognized that SVG bypass surgery is of a palliative nature and does have some important limitations, including the fact that an accelerated atherosclerotic process develops within the graft over time, often resulting in untoward clinical sequelae. Several studies have reported up to 15% SVG occlusion during the first postsurgical year, with a further 1–2% closure rate between years 1 and 6. After 6 years, the attrition rate increases to 4–5% per year, as only 60% of the SVGs are patent by 10 years and less than 50% of these patent grafts remain free of significant obstruction.[3–8] Degenerative atherosclerotic SVG disease, as well as the progression of the native coronary vascular disease process, results in approximately 35% of patients requiring either reoperation or percutaneous revascularization 10–12 years after surgery.[9] The increased risk of a second bypass operation is well established, with a 3–5-fold increase in mortality and myocardial infarction.[7,10] With recognition of these limitations, SVG percutaneous intervention in patients with prior coronary bypass surgery (CABG) has been recommended. However, percutaneous treatment has similarly been associated with an increased periprocedural risk, as well as lower long-term patency as compared with interventions performed in native coronary arteries.[11] Coronary atheroembolism from the diseased vein graft appears to be the major cause of the increased risk associated with reoperations and vein graft percutaneous interventions.[7,10]

Pathogenesis of saphenous vein graft disease

Three pathophysiological processes are involved in the pathogenesis of SVG disease: thrombosis, intimal hyperplasia, and atherosclerosis. While these processes are interrelated, each appears to be temporally distinct, with thrombosis being the main mechanism of SVG occlusion during the first month after surgery, at an incidence of 3–12%.[6,7] This thrombotic occlusion is a consequence of several mechanisms, including vessel wall alterations during the vein harvesting process, changes in blood rheology and flow dynamics, and surgery-related technical factors. Intimal hyperplasia is the major contributor to disease progression between 1 month and 1 year. While this process rarely produces a significant degree of stenosis, it provides the basis for the later development of graft atheroma. Atherosclerosis is the dominant pathological process after the first year. Approximately 75–85% of acute coronary events in patients with prior CABG (unstable angina or acute non-ST-elevation or ST-elevation myocardial infarction (MI)) are caused by the atherosclerotic process developed in the SVG.[12] Although the fundamental process of atheroma development and the predisposition factors are similar in SVG and in native arteries, there are some differences that are considerations when contemplating percutaneous treatment strategies. Vein graft atherosclerosis tends to be diffuse, concentric, and friable. There is often a poorly developed or absent fibrous atheroma cap, with a little evidence of calcification.[13–17] There is a higher plaque lipid content, resulting from increased lipid uptake and slower lipolysis.[18,19] In addition, the compensatory enlargement (positive remodeling) described in coronary native arteries undergoing atherosclerotic disease progression does not appear to occur in the SVG atheromatous process.[20] Late thrombosis is a frequent event in old SVGs with advanced atherosclerosis.

Antithrombotic agents

Given the pivotal role of the thrombotic process contributing to SVG closure, several antithrombotic regimens have been evaluated in clinical practice in an attempt to decrease the incidence of SVG failure.

Antiplatelet agents

Aspirin

Aspirin is the most studied antiplatelet drug in the post-CABG patient population. Several randomized clinical trial have shown efficacy in preventing SVG occlusion. The Veterans Administration (VA) study has shown a significant reduction in SVG occlusion at 2 months and 1 year comparing aspirin therapy with placebo.[21,22] Importantly, the benefit appears to be more limited to those grafts placed to native vessels less than 2.0 mm in diameter noting no significant benefit in larger vessels. These finding have been confirmed in several other investigative trials.[23] The beneficial effect of aspirin appears to be time-dependent as well as dose-dependent. The benefits are appreciated when aspirin is given either before or during the first 24 hours of surgery, with no benefit being seen if the medication is started later than 3 days postoperatively. A high dose of aspirin does not appear to provide an incremental benefit. The meta-analysis by the Antiplatelets Trialists' Collaboration clearly demonstrated that doses between 75 and 325 mg are clinically as effective as higher doses.[23] While aspirin has been demonstrated to clearly provide long-term clinical benefits in patients with known coronary artery disease, it does not appear to favorably affect graft patency after 1 year of treatment. Goldman et al[24] reported in 455 patients that continued use of aspirin, 325 mg/day, for an additional 2 years after the initial year of therapy did not show any benefit in graft patency at the end of the third year (graft occlusion 17% for those with long-term aspirin, compared with 19.7% occlusion for the placebo group; $p=0.40$).

The occurrence of aspirin non-responsiveness and an increased risk of clinical events has recently been recognized in this group of patients. This phenomenon has also been identified in patients with a history of CABG surgery. In a small study, almost 42% of patients post CABG showed biochemical indicators suggesting a lack of effect of aspirin at a dose of 325 mg.[25] However, the clinical implications of aspirin non-responsiveness for graft failure are currently unknown. This topic is discussed in greater detail elsewhere in this book.

Dipyridamole

Dipyridamole has been used for many years in this setting to prevent graft occlusion. It has mainly been studied in combination with aspirin. A systematic review of the nine randomized trials published by the Antiplatelets Trialists' Collaboration showed no clear benefit on graft patency with the combination therapy compared with aspirin alone.[23]

Thienopyridines

Ticlopidine is the first drug from this pharmacological group to be used clinically. It has been evaluated in the context of CABG surgery in two randomized trials. The effect was evaluated at 3–12 months, showing a significant improvement in graft patency compared with placebo.[26,27] The patency rate at 8 months was 92.9% in the ticlopidine group versus 78.2% in the placebo group ($p<0.02$). It is important to note that these trials did not use aspirin in either arm and therefore did not answer the question of whether or not ticlopidine was better than aspirin or if dual therapy offered greater benefit than aspirin monotherapy. Although ticlopidine has been proposed as an alternative therapy for those patients with allergy to aspirin, its serious side-effects continue to limit its clinical use.

More recently, clopidogrel has been incorporated in clinical practice with a significantly better safety profile and better efficacy than ticlopidine.[28,29] However, its effect on graft patency has not been sufficiently evaluated. A recent report showed a tendency favoring greater vein graft patency in patients undergoing 'off-pump' surgery when aspirin and clopidogrel were used in combination (87%) compared with aspirin alone (66%).[30] There are also indications of clinical benefit using combination aspirin and clopidogrel therapy in post-CABG patients. A post hoc analysis of the CURE trial demonstrated that patients undergoing CABG surgery in the context of non-ST-elevation acute coronary syndrome, pretreated with aspirin and clopidogrel, had a better clinical outcome at 1 year compared with patients treated with aspirin alone: a 9.3% frequency of cardiovascular death, MI, or stroke for clopidogrel treatment versus 11.4% for placebo treatment (relative risk (RR) 0.80; 95% confidence interval (CI) 0.72–0.90).[31] However, there was an increase in bleeding complication, reoperations, and blood transfusion in the combination group, again raising significant safety concerns. Therefore, there is currently not enough evidence supporting the routine use of clopidogrel in combination with aspirin in the post-CABG patient population. However, we are learning more regarding the use of monotherapy clopidogrel in the post-CABG population. The CAPRIE trial reported an encouraging retrospective analysis of 1480 patients undergoing CABG randomized to clopidogrel or aspirin. The annual event rate of death, MI, stroke, and rehospitalization was 23% for the aspirin group and 15.9% for the clopidogrel group ($p=0.001$).[32] Therefore, in patients with an allergy or a contraindication to aspirin, the use of clopidogrel may well prove to be beneficial.

Oral anticoagulants

Several randomized studies have evaluated the effects on graft failure of the use of oral anticoagulants. No trial has demonstrated a benefit realized by greater graft patency resulting from using oral anticoagulants when compared with aspirin or a combination of aspirin and dipyridamole.[24,33,34] The largest published study, the Post Coronary Artery Bypass Graft Trial, provides the most definitive answer.[35] This trial randomized 1351 post-CABG patients to coumadin or placebo, using a 2×2 factorial design. Both groups received aspirin. The trial showed no reduction in graft failure on adding coumadin (disease progression 34% vs 32%; $p = 0.48$), and no indication of clinical improvement, with similar rates of MI (5.0% vs 5.0%) and the need for further revascularization (7.8% vs 7.9%).

Percutaneous interventions

Interventional cardiologists have long appreciated the many challenges involved in the percutaneous treatment of degenerated SVGs. Compared with treating native coronary arteries, balloon angioplasty of SVG lesions yielded significantly lower primary success rates and higher long-term restenosis rates.[36,37] The most challenging problem with SVG intervention remains the higher incidence of acute procedure complications – most notably related to the problem of distal plaque and thrombus embolization with ensuing MI.[38]

Stents in the prevention of restenosis

Enthusiasm triggered by the initial experience using bare metal stents to treat de novo coronary artery lesions translated into investigations examining the efficacy of these stents when deployed to treat SVG disease. These studies were especially important, given the disappointment among the interventional cardiovascular community regarding the results of balloon angioplasty techniques used to treat these complex, challenging lesions. The pivotal trial designed to answer this question was the SAVED study.[39] This investigation randomized a total of 220 patients to receive either conventional balloon angioplasty or a bare metal coronary stent. The study demonstrated significantly higher procedural success (92%) with the use of the stent as a primary approach, compared with a 69% primary success rate when balloon angioplasty was used as the initial interventional treatment strategy ($p < 0.001$). Long-term results were similarly somewhat encouraging. Angiographic restenosis was significantly decreased by the use of stents, with a net gain in luminal diameter at 6 months of 0.85±0.96 mm, compared with 0.54±0.91 mm for the balloon group ($p = 0.002$). Clinical outcomes, including freedom from death, MI,

repeated bypass surgery, or revascularization of the target lesion, were also significantly improved in the stent group (73% vs 58%; $p = 0.03$). Based on this study, stenting became the gold standard for the treatment of SVG, although the results did not measure up to the positive benchmarks realized with stenting native coronary arteries. Most notably, procedural complications and unacceptably high angiographic and clinical reoccurrence rates were noted to persist.

The advent of drug-eluting stents has significantly changed the restenosis problems. Multiple randomized studies have proven their efficacy in preventing restenosis.[40,41] In the context of SVG interventions, drug-eluting stents appear to also decrease the incidence of restenosis after stent implantation. The recently reported SSIR trial randomized 75 patients with 80 SVG lesions to a sirolimus-eluting stent (SES) or a bare metal stent (BMS).[42] In-stent late loss was significantly reduced with the SES compared with the BMS (0.38 ± 0.51 mm vs 0.79 ± 0.66 mm; ($p = 0.001$). Binary restenosis was reduced to 13.6% in the SES group, compared with 32.6% in the BMS group (RR 0.42; 95% CI 0.18–0.97; $p = 0.031$). Target lesion and vessel revascularization rates were significantly reduced: 5.3% versus 21.6% (RR 0.24; 95% CI 0.05–1.0; $p = 0.047$) and 5.3% versus 27% (RR 0.19; 95% CI 0.05–0.83; $p = 0.012$), respectively.

Embolic complications and prevention

Several studies have demonstrated an increased incidence of ischemic complications in the setting of SVG interventions. The incidences of Q and non-Q MI range from 5% to 20% as reported in various series.[38] These finding continue to compare unfavorably with the complication rates reported in trials involving native coronary intervention. Cardiac enzyme elevation and MI has been attributed to the increased incidence of distal embolization and the 'non-reflow' phenomenon often associated with SVG intervention (an incidence of 15–20%).[43] Experience has shown that these intraprocedural 'events' indeed have long-term adverse clinical implications for patients, including an associated higher 1-year mortality rate. Hong et al[38] found in 1056 patient with SVG interventions a 15% incidence of MI (creatine kinase MB isoenzyme (CK-MB) >5-fold baseline). During the 12 months' follow-up, this group of patients had an 11.7% mortality rate, compared with 4.8% in those SVG interventions with no procedurally related CK-MB elevation ($p < 0.05$).

There are several known predictors of these ischemic complications. Grafts older than 3 years have a higher incidence of ischemic complications. Angiographic evidence of severely disease graft, 'degenerated vein graft', and the presence of intraluminal thrombus are also important predictors.

Several approaches have been employed over the years with the intention of improving the result of the interventions in this setting, ranging from aggressive pharmacological interventions, including thrombolytic agents or glycoprotein IIb/IIIa (GPIIb/IIIa) inhibitors, to different device-based approaches.

Pharmacologic interventions

Antiplatelet agents and anticoagulants

The combination of dual antiplatelet treatment with aspirin and clopidogrel and intravenous heparin is considered the gold standard of antithrombotic treatment in the context of every percutaneous intervention, including lesions in SVGs. These agents are discussed in greater detail in other chapters of this book.

Thrombolytic agents

The significant success in opening thrombotic lesions in the context of acute MI with various thrombolytic agents led to the investigation of the use of similar pharmacological agents in the setting of vein graft interventions. Initial small, mostly single-center, anecdotal reports provided some encouraging preliminary results.[44] However, better-designed multicenter prospective trials failed to demonstrate clinical benefit from a strategy of local prolonged throbolytic drug infusion. In addition, significant safety concerns were noted, based on the observed increased incidence of severe bleeding complications and the high incidence of embolic complications and non-Q MI. Teirstein et al[45] randomized 107 patients with SVG occlusion to low versus high dose of intraarterial urokinase. Following completion of lytic infusion, 50% of patients in the high-dose group achieved TIMI grade ≥2, compared with only 24% in the low-dose group ($p=0.01$). However, after final angioplasty, the high-dose infusion group demonstrated only a small, non-significant, increase in procedural success: 72% versus 60%. There were no observed differences in hard clinical endpoints (death/MI) on comparing the two groups, with a 16% incidence of non-Q MI in both. Bleeding complications using either low- or high-dose strategies showed an unacceptably high rate, including a 12% incidence of major bleeds in both groups. The ROBUST trial[46] provided similar findings, including a procedural success rate of prolonged thrombolytic infusion of 69%, with an associated high mortality rate (6.5%) and a 22% incidence of MI. Major bleeding occurred in 20% of patients. Based on these results, local infusion of thrombolytics has been abandoned in the context of SVG coronary interventions.

Glycoprotein IIb/IIIa inhibitors

Several large, multicenter trials have provided a large amount of data demonstrating benefit resulting from the use of GPIIb/IIIa receptor blocking agents in the setting of percutaneous coronary interventions.[47–51] However, no such randomized studies have been performed to investigate the potential benefit of these class of agents treating patients undergoing SVG intervention. Subgroup analysis of larger studies has failed to demonstrate consistent, clear benefit with use of GPIIb/IIIa agents in the SVG population. Figure 22.1 summarizes these results.[47–51] In addition, Karha et al[52] recently reported similar findings from the Cleveland Clinic database with the use of more contemporary interventions, including stents and distal protection devices. The study included 1537 patients with SVG interventions; 941 patients were pretreated with GPIIb/IIIa inhibitors and 596 did not receive these. While the incidence of non-Q MI was quite elevated in both groups, there was no significant difference in the incidence on comparing the groups. After adjustment for baseline characteristics and the use of distal protection devices, there appeared to be no benefit in using GPIIb/IIIa inhibitors with respect to preventing MI or death (hazard ratio (HR) 0.92; 95% CI 0.69–1.23; $p=0.59$), suggesting again that these agents do not provide significant benefit in the setting of SVG interventions.

Investigators have looked into using a localized intragraft infusion of GPIIb/IIIa inhibitors prior to the planned interventional procedure to reduce thrombus burden and be able to perform a safer intervention.[53] These agents have similarly been used following an embolic or non-reflow

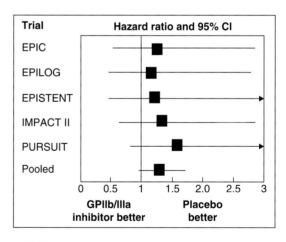

Figure 22.1
Meta-analysis of the effect of glycoprotein IIb/IIIa (GPIIb/IIIa) receptor blockers in the context of saphenous vein graft interventions. These pooled data includes a retrospective evaluation of 627 patients from randomized clinical trials using GPIIb/IIIa inhibitors in the context of SVG percutaneous treatment. EPIC, EPILOG, EPISTEN used abciximab as the active agent, IMPACT II used integrilin, and PURSUIT used tirofiban.[64]

complication as rescue treatment. However, these case reports or very small single-center experiences have provided little scientific evidence of clinical benefit.

Device approaches

Other techniques have also been tried in attempts to solve the many challenges presented by SVG intervention. These technologies have initially focused on strategies involving plaque removal. The use of directional atherectomy (DCA) in treating SVG disease was evaluated in the early 1990s, with suboptimal results. The CAVEAT II trial evaluated 300 SVG interventions against balloon angioplasty. This study showed similar angiographic success without any significant improvement in reducing the restenosis rate (50% for balloon vs 45% for DCA; $p=0.49$).[54] However, DCA use was found to show a very strong trend toward increase embolic events (5% for balloon vs 13% for DCA) and MI (10% vs 16%; $p=0.06$). The transluminal extraction catheter (TEC) was also evaluated with the intention of extract the friable and thrombotic material found in diseased SVGs in the hope of limiting untoward complications. Although no randomized study has adequately evaluated this device, data obtained from several registries have shown not very promising results, with an approximately 15% incidence of distal embolization and non-reflow.[55] Due to the high incidence of complications and the significant technical difficulties, this procedure has been abandoned.

Polytetrafluoroethylene (PTFE)-covered stents were deployed with the intention of avoiding distal embolization by covering the entire length of the disease graft. These attempts also failed to provide encouraging results. The RECOVERS study evaluated in 301 patients a PTFE-covered stent versus a bare metal stent. This study showed an increased incidence of acute events in the PTFE-stent group (10.9% for PTFE stents vs 4.1% for bare metal stents; $p=0.04$) and no improvement in 6-month restenosis rate (24% in both groups).[56]

Alternative methods of stent deployment have also been attempted. Direct stenting – the deployment of stents without balloon predilatation – has shown encouraging results, with a decrease in the incidence of acute complications, and it is a widely used deployment strategy in the interventional community.[57,58]

A number of techniques have been designed to capture emboli resulting from SVG interventional manipulation. Three different types of protection devices have been developed and studied in a clinical setting. Randomized clinical trials assessing these devices have shown consistent benefit in reducing the incidence of ischemic complications in the setting of SVG interventions. The filter distal protection device consists of a basket with pores of different sizes that allow blood but not atherosclerotic or thrombotic material to flow through the filter. The filter is placed distal to the stenosis prior to proceeding with the treatment of the lesion. After completion of the procedure, the filter is removed together with the trapped material. The second device employs distal balloon occlusion. In this case, the flow is completely interrupted while the procedure is performed. After completion, the material is aspirated, the balloon is removed, and flow is re-established. The third device is the proximal occlusion balloon. In this case, the balloon is placed proximally and the flow is interrupted before the lesion. After the procedure has been performed, the material is aspirated and the flow is then re-established.

Table 22.1 summarizes the results of the randomized studies evaluating these devices. The SAFER study evaluated the distal balloon protection system in 801 patients.[59] The study showed a significant decrease in the primary endpoint of death, MI, and urgent revascularization from 16.5% in patients without distal protection to 9.6% in those with distal protection ($p=0.004$). After this first pivotal trial, balloon occlusion was approved by the US Food and Drug Administration (FDA) for SVG intervention and became the standard of care in this setting. The subsequent trials used the distal balloon occlusion device as the gold standard

Table 22.1 *Major adverse clinical events (MACE) with the use of distal protection devices in the context of SVG percutaneous interventions*

Study	No. of patients	MACE rate (%)		
		Control	Protection Device	*p*-value
SAFER[59]	801	16.5	9.6	0.004
PRIDE[63]	631	10.1	11.2	0.62
FIRE[60]	651	11.6	9.9	0.53
PROXIMAL[61]	600	9.2	10	0.65

The primary endpoint in all trials was MACE (death, MI, urgent CABG, and/or repeat target vessel revascularization) at 30 days. SAFER was the only trial in which the control group comprised patients treated without distal protection. All of the other randomized trials used patients treated with Percusurge distal balloon occlusion as control group. The studies were performed to define efficacy and non-inferiority to the standard of care (the Percusurge device). SAFER used the Percusurge device (distal balloon occlusion). PRIDE used the TriActiv device (distal balloon occlusion); *p* for non-inferiority= 0.02. FIRE used the FilterWire EX device (filter distal protection); *p* for non-inferiority=0.0008. PROXIMAL used the Proxis device (proximal balloon occlusion).

for comparison. The FIRE trial compared the filter device with the distal balloon occlusion device in 651 patients in a randomized fashion, showing very similar results for both devices.[60] Recently, the results of the PROXIMAL trial also showed similar beneficial findings with the use of the proximal balloon occlusion device in this setting.[61] The type of device to be used appears to be more closely related to operator preference and experience and to lesion characteristics than to device performance. In a very carefully performed study, particulates retrieved with a vascular filtering device or an occlusion balloon were found to be similar in amount and characteristics.[62]

Summary

Aortocoronary SVG disease comprises different but inter-related processes, with thrombosis playing a major role in early as well as late graft failure. Prevention of graft failure includes several strategies. Improvements in vein harvesting and surgical technique are the main steps. Early antithrombotic treatment with aspirin appears to improve graft patency during the first year. Aspirin non-responsiveness and the role of combinations of antiplatelet agents are important areas for future research. Percutaneous treatment in this setting is still one of the major challenges in interventional cardiology. Multiple antithrombotic agents have been evaluated in this context with the intention of increasing procedural success and decreasing complications. However, no significant improvements in the initial results were observed on adding more aggressive drugs, with important safety concerns related to increased bleeding complications being noted when thrombolytic agents and/or GPIIb/IIIa inhibitors were used. Even though risk factors and clinical sequelae of SVG atherosclerosis are similar to those of native coronaries, significant pathological differences exist that predispose to the embolic complications in this setting. Recent incorporation of embolic protection devices appears to significantly improve procedural success, with an important decrease in ischemic complications. Stents, and more recently drug-eluting stents, appear to be very effective in preventing restenosis. However, progression of the atherosclerotic disease within the graft remains the main reason for long-term graft failure and a major challenge for future development.

References

1. Garrett H, Dennis E, DeBakey M. Aortocoronary bypass with saphenous vein graft. Seven-year follow-up. JAMA 1973;223:792–4.
2. Favaloro R. Saphenous vein graft in the surgical treatment of coronary artery disease. Operative technique. J Thorac Cardiovasc Surg 1969;58:178–85.
3. Yusuf S, Zucker D, Peduzzi P et al. Effect of coronary artery bypass graft surgery on survival: overview of 10 year results from randomized trials by the Coronary Artery Bypass Graft Surgery Trialists Collaboration. Lancet 1994;344:563–70.
4. Davis K, Chaitman B, Ryan T et al. Comparison of 15 year survival for men and women after initial medical or surgical treatment for coronary artery disease: a CASS registry study. J Am Coll Cardiol 1995;25:1000–9.
5. Campeau L, Enjalbert M, Lesperance J et al. The relation of risk factors to the development of atherosclerosis in saphenous vein bypass grafts and the progression of disease in the native circulation: a study 10 years after aortocoronary bypass surgery. N Engl J Med 1984;311:1329–32.
6. Bourassa M. Fate of venous grafts: the past, the present and the future. J Am Coll Cardiol 1991;5:1081–3.
7. Fitzgibbon G, Kafka H, Leach A et al. Coronary bypass graft fate and patient outcome: angiographic follow-up of 5,065 grafts related to survival and reoperation in 1,388 patients during 25 years. J Am Coll Cardiol 1996;28:616–26.
8. Alderman E, Corley S, Fisher L et al. Five-year angiographic follow-up of factors associated with progression of coronary artery disease in the Coronary Artery Surgery Study (CASS). J Am Coll Cardiol 1993;22:1141–54.
9. Weintraub W, Jones E, Craver J, Guyton R. Frequency of repeat coronary bypass or coronary angioplasty after coronary artery bypass surgery using saphenous venous grafts. Am J Cardiol 1994;73:103–12.
10. Loop F, Lytle B, Cosgrove D et al. Reoperation for coronary atherosclerosis: changing practice in 2509 consecutive patients. Ann Surg 1990;212:378–86.
11. Lefkovits J, Holmes DR, Califf RM et al. Predictors and sequelae of distal embolization during saphenous vein graft intervention from the CAVEAT-II trial. Coronary Angioplasty Versus Excisional Atherectomy Trial. Circulation 1995;92:734–40.
12. Chen L, Theroux P, Lesperance J et al. Angiographic features of vein grafts versus ungrafted coronary arteries in patients with unstable angina and previous bypass surgery. J Am Coll Cardiol 1996;28:1493–9.
13. Lie J, Lawrie G, Morris G. Aortocoronary bypass saphenous vein graft atherosclerosis: anatomic study of 99 vein grafts from normal and hyperlipoproteinemic patients up to 75 months postoperatively. Am J Cardiol 1977;40:906–14.
14. Kalan J, Roberts W. Morphologic findings in saphenous veins used as coronary arterial bypass conduits for longer than 1 year: necropsy analysis of 53 patients, 123 saphenous veins, and 1865 five-millimeter segments of veins. Am Heart J 1990;119:1164–84.
15. Neitzel G, Barboriak J, Pintar K, Qureshi I. Atherosclerosis in aortocoronary bypass grafts: morphologic study and risk factor analysis 6 to 12 years after surgery. Arteriosclerosis 1986;6:594–600.
16. Ratliff N, Myles J. Rapidly progressive atherosclerosis in aortocoronary saphenous vein grafts: possible immune-mediated disease. Arch Pathol Lab Med 1989;113:772–6.
17. Stary H, Bleakley Chandler A et al. A definition of advanced types of atherosclerotic lesions and a histological classification of atherosclerosis: a Report from the Committee on Vascular Lesions of the Council on Arteriosclerosis, American Heart Association. Circulation 1995;92:1355–74.
18. Shafi S, Palinski W, Born G. Comparison of uptake and degradation of low density lipoproteins by arteries and veins of rabbits. Atherosclerosis 1987;66:131–8.
19. Larson R, Hagen P, Fuchs J. Lipid biosynthesis in arteries, veins and venous grafts. Circulation 1974;50:III-139.
20. Nishioka T, Luo H, Berglund H et al. Absence of focal compensatory enlargement or constriction in diseased human coronary saphenous vein bypass grafts: an intravascular ultrasound study. Circulation 1996;93:683–90.

21. Goldman S, Copeland J, Moritz T et al. Improvement in early saphenous vein graft patency after coronary artery bypass surgery with antiplatelet therapy: results of a Veterans Administration Cooperative Study. Circulation 1988;6:1324–32.

22. Goldman S, Copeland J, Moritz T et al. Saphenous vein graft patency 1 year after coronary artery bypass surgery and effects of antiplatelet therapy: results of a Veterans Administration Cooperative Study. Circulation 1989;80:1190–7.

23. Antiplatelet Trialists' Collaboration. Collaborative overview of randomised trials of antiplatelet therapy – II: Maintenance of vascular graft or arterial patency by antiplatelet therapy. BMJ 1994;308:159–68.

24. Goldman S, Copeland J, Moritz T et al. Long-term graft patency (3 years) after coronary artery surgery: effects of aspirin: results of a VA cooperative study. Circulation 1994;89:1138–43.

25. Buchanan M, Brister S. Individual variation in the effects of aspirin on platelet function: implications for the use of ASA clinically. Can J Cardiol 1995;11:221–7.

26. Chevigne M, David J, Rigo P, Limet R. Effect of ticlopidine on saphenous vein bypass patency rates: a double-blind study. Ann Thorac Surg 1984;37:371–8.

27. Limet R, David J, Magotteaux P et al. Prevention of aorta–coronary bypass graft occlusion: beneficial effect of ticlopidine on early and late patency rates of venous coronary bypass grafts: a double-blind study. J Thorac Cardiovasc Surg 1987;94:773–83.

28. Bertrand ME, Rupprecht HJ, Urban P, Gershlick AH; CLASSICS Investigators. Double-blind study of the safety of clopidogrel with and without a loading dose in combination with aspirin compared with ticlopidine in combination with aspirin after coronary stenting : the clopidogrel aspirin stent international cooperative study (CLASSICS). Circulation 2000;102:624–9.

29. Bhatt DL, Bertrand BE, Berger PB et al. Meta-analysis of randomized and registry comparisons of ticlopidine with clopidogrel after stenting. J Am Coll Cardiol 2002;39:9–14.

30. Ibrahim K, Tjomsland O, Halvorsen D et al. Effect of clopidogrel on midterm graft patency following off-pump coronary revascularization surgery. Heart Surg Forum 2006;9:E581–6.

31. Clopidogrel in Unstable Angina to Prevent Recurrent Events Trial Investigators. Effects of clopidogrel in addition to aspirin in patients with acute coronary syndromes without ST-segment elevation. N Engl J Med 2001;345:494–502.

32. Bhatt DL, Chew DP, Hirsch AT et al. Superiority of clopidogrel versus aspirin in patients with prior cardiac surgery. Circulation 2001;103:363–8.

33. Gohlke H, Gohlke-Barwolf C, Sturzenhofecker P et al. Improved graft patency with anticoagulant therapy after aortocoronary bypass surgery: a prospective, randomized study. Circulation 1981;64:II-22–7.

34. Stein P, Dalen J, Goldman S et al. Antithrombotic therapy in patients with saphenous vein and internal mammary artery bypass grafts. Chest 1995;108:424S–30S.

35. The Post Coronary Artery Bypass Graft Trial Investigators. The effect of aggressive lowering of low-density lipoprotein cholesterol levels and low-dose anticoagulation on obstructive changes in saphenous-vein coronary-artery bypass grafts. N Engl J Med 1997;336:153–62.

36. de Feyter PJ, van Suylen RJ, de Jaegere PPT et al. Balloon angioplasty for the treatment of lesions in saphenous vein bypass grafts. J Am Coll Cardiol 1993;21:1539–49.

37. Platko WP, Holman J, Whitlow PL, Franco I. Percutaneous transluminal angioplasty of saphenous vein graft stenosis: long-term follow-up. J Am Coll Cardiol 1989;14:1645–50.

38. Hong M, Mehran R, Dangas G et al. Creatine kinase-MB enzyme elevation following successful saphenous vein graft intervention is associated with late mortality. Circulation 1999;100:2400–5.

39. Savage M, Douglas JJ, Fischman D et al. Stent placement compared with balloon angioplasty for obstructed coronary bypass grafts.

Saphenous Vein De Novo Trial Investigators. N Engl J Med 1997;337:740–7.

40. Morice MC, Serruys PW, Sousa JE et al; RAVEL Study Group. A randomized comparison of a sirolimus-eluting stent with a standard stent for coronary revascularization. N Engl J Med 2002;346:1773–80.

41. Moses JW, Leon MB, Popma JJ et al; SIRIUS Investigators. Sirolimus-eluting stents versus standard stents in patients with stenosis in a native coronary artery. N Engl J Med 2003;349:1315–23.

42. Vermeersch P, Agostoni P, Verheye S et al. Randomized double-blind comparison of sirolimus-eluting stent versus bare-metal stent implantation in diseased saphenous vein grafts: six-month angiographic, intravascular ultrasound, and clinical follow-up of the RRISC trial. J Am Coll Cardiol 2006;48:2423–31.

43. Piana RN, Paib GY, Moscucci M et al. Incidence and treatment of 'no-reflow' after percutaneous coronary intervention. Circulation 1994;89:2514–18.

44. Hartmann JR, McKeever LS, Stamato NJ et al. Recanalization of chronically occluded aortocoronary saphenous vein bypass grafts by extended infusion of urokinase: initial results and short-term clinical follow-up. J Am Coll Cardiol 1991;18:1517–23.

45. Teirstein P, Mann JT 3rd, Cundey PE Jr et al. Low- versus high-dose recombinant urokinase for the treatment of chronic saphenous vein graft occlusion. Am J Cardiol 1999;83:1623–8.

46. Hartmann J, McKeever LS, O'Neill W et al. Recanalization of chronically occluded aortocoronary saphenous vein bypass grafts with long-term, low dose direct infusion of urokinase (ROBUST): a serial trial. J Am Coll Cardiol 1996;27:60–6.

47. The EPIC Investigators. Use of a monoclonal antibody directed against the platelet glycoprotein IIb/IIIa receptor in high-risk coronary angioplasty. N Engl J Med 1994;330:956–61.

48. The EPILOG Investigators. Platelet glycoprotein IIb/IIIa receptor blockade and low-dose heparin during percutaneous coronary revascularization. N Engl J Med 1997;336:1689–96.

49. The EPISTENT Investigators. Randomised placebo-controlled and balloon-angioplasty-controlled trial to assess safety of coronary stenting with use of Platelet glycoprotein IIb/IIIa blockade. Evaluation of Platelet IIb/IIIa Inhibitor for Stenting. Lancet 1998;352:87–92.

50. The IMPACT-II Investigators. Randomised placebo-controlled trial of effect of eptifibatide on complications of percutaneous coronary intervention. Integrilin to Minimise Platelet Aggregation and Coronary Thrombosis – II. Lancet 1997;349:1422–8.

51. The PURSUIT Trial Investigators. Inhibition of platelet glycoprotein IIb/IIIa with eptifibatide in patients with acute coronary syndromes. Platelet Glycoprotein IIb/IIIa in Unstable Angina: Receptor Suppression Using Integrilin Therapy. N Engl J Med 1998;339: 436–43.

52. Karha J, Gurm H, Rajagopal V et al. Use of platelet glycoprotein IIb/IIIa inhibitors in saphenous vein graft percutaneous coronary intervention and clinical outcomes. Am J Cardiol 2006;98:906–10.

53. Barsness G, Buller C, Ohman E et al. Reduced thrombus burden with abciximab delivered locally before percutaneous intervention in saphenous vein grafts. Am Heart J 2000;139:824–9.

54. Holmes DJ, Topol E, Califf R et al. A multicenter, randomized trial of coronary angioplasty versus directional atherectomy for patients with saphenous vein bypass graft lesions. CAVEAT-II Investigators. Circulation 1995;91:1966–74.

55. Safian R, Grines C, May M et al. Clinical and angiographic results of transluminal extraction coronary atherectomy in saphenous vein bypass grafts. Circulation 1994;89:302–12.

56. Stankovic G, Colombo A, Presbitero P et al. Randomized evaluation of polytetrafluoroethylene-covered stent in saphenous vein grafts: the Randomized Evaluation of polytetrafluoroethylene COVERed stent in Saphenous vein grafts (RECOVERS) Trial. Circulation 2003;108:37–42.

57. Loubeyre C, Morice MC, Lefevre T et al. A randomized comparison of direct stenting with conventional stent implantation in selected patients with acute myocardial infarction. J Am Coll Cardiol 2002;39:15–21.

58. Lozano I, Lopez-Palop R, Pinar E et al. [Direct stenting in saphenous vein grafts. Immediate and long-term results.] Rev Esp Cardiol 2005;58:270–7. [in Spanish]

59. Baim D, Wahr D, George B et al. Saphenous vein graft Angioplasty Free of Emboli Randomized (SAFER) Trial Investigators. Randomized trial of a distal embolic protection device during percutaneous intervention of saphenous vein aorto-coronary bypass grafts. Circulation 2002;105:1285–90.

60. Stone G, Rogers C, Hermiller J et al. FilterWire Ex Randomized Evaluation Investigators. Randomized comparison of distal protection with a filter-based catheter and a balloon occlusion and aspiration system during percutaneous intervention of diseased saphenous vein aorto-coronary bypass grafts. Circulation 2003;108:548–53.

61. Rogers C. A prospective randomized comparison of proximal and distal protection in patients with diseased saphenous vein grafts. Presented at Transcatheter Cardiovascular Therapeutics, 2005.

62. Rogers C, Huynh R, Seifert P et al. Embolic protection with filtering or occlusion balloons during saphenous vein graft stenting retrieves identical volumes and sizes of particulate debris. Circulation 2004;109:1735–40.

63. Carrozza JP Jr, Mumma M, Breall J et al; PRIDE Study Investigators. Randomized evaluation of the TriActiv balloon-protection flush and extraction system for the treatment of saphenous vein graft disease. J Am Coll Cardiol 2005;46:1677–83.

64. Roffi M, Mukherjee D, Chew D et al. Lack of benefit from intravenous platelet glycoprotein IIb/IIIa receptor inhibition as adjunctive treatment for percutaneous interventions of aortocoronary bypass grafts: a pooled analysis of five randomized clinical trials. Circulation 2002;106:3063–7.

23

Antiplatelet therapy in diabetes mellitus

Dominick J Angiolillo, Piera Capranzano, and Carlos Macaya

Introduction

Cardiovascular disease is the leading cause of morbidity and mortality in patients with diabetes mellitus (DM).[1] DM is a pandemic currently affecting more than 150 million people worldwide and will double over the next 20 years.[2] This will be due almost exclusively to an increase in type 2 DM (T2DM). DM is associated with a two- to fourfold risk of developing coronary artery disease (CAD), peripheral arterial disease (PAD), and stroke.[3] Further, in over one-third of DM patients with atherosclerotic disease, two or more arterial districts are involved. Of note, patients with DM have a long-term cardiovascular risk similar to that observed among patients without DM but who have a prior history of myocardial infarction (MI).[4] Also, DM patients who already suffered an ischemic event have a higher rate of recurrence than patients without DM.[5,6]

Several mechanisms account for the increased atherothrombotic risk in DM patients.[1–6] T2DM patients frequently have other cardiovascular risk factors (hypertension, dyslipedemia, or obesity). However, this accounts for no more than 25% of their excess cardiovascular risk.[7] There are other factors specific for the diabetic population contributing to their increased atherthrombotic risk, which include hyperglycemia, insulin resistance, and proinflammatory and prothrombotic status.[8–10] In particular, the prothrombotic status is related to endothelial dysfunction, impaired fibrinolysis, increased coagulation factors, and increased platelet reactivity (Table 23.1). Since platelets play a key role in the development of atherothrombotic events, the dysfunctional status of platelets in DM patients may contribute to the enhanced athrothrombotic risk of these patients. This highlights the pivotal role of antiplatelet agents in both primary and secondary prevention of ischemic events in DM patients.

Aspirin

Aspirin as a primary prevention strategy in diabetes mellitus

The American Diabetes Association (ADA) recommends that a dosage of 75–162 mg of enteric-coated aspirin be used as a preventive strategy in high-risk diabetic individuals. Individuals are defined as being at high risk for cardiovascular events on the basis of the following risk factors:[11] a family history of CAD; cigarette smoking; hypertension; weight >120% of ideal body weight; microalbuminuria or macroalbuminuria; total cholesterol >200 mg/dl (low-density lipoprotein (LDL) cholesterol >100; high-density lipoprotein (HDL) cholesterol <55 mg/dl in women and <45 mg/dl in men; and triglycerides >200 mg/dl). The American Heart Association (AHA) has issued similar guidelines,[12] and recommends 75–160 mg/day of aspirin as a primary prevention strategy in high-risk individuals, defined as those with a 10-year risk of CAD greater than 10%.

These guidelines are supported by the results of several clinical trials. The Primary Prevention Project, in which low-dose aspirin (100 mg/day) was evaluated for the prevention of cardiovascular events in individuals ($n = 4495$) with one or more risk factors (hypertension, hypercholesterolemia, DM, obesity, family history of premature MI, or being elderly), showed that after a mean follow-up of 3.6 years, aspirin was found to significantly lower the frequency of cardiovascular death (from 1.4% to 0.8%; relative risk (RR) 0.56, 95% confidence interval (CI) 0.31–0.99) and total cardiovascular events (from 8.2% to 6.3%; RR 0.77, 95% CI 0.62–0.95).[13] USPHS (US Physicians' Health Study)[14] was a 5-year primary prevention trial in 22 701 healthy men that included 533 men with DM. Among DM

Table 23.1 *Mechanisms leading to the prothrombotic state in an individual with diabetes mellitus*

Impaired fibrinolysis	Impaired platelet function	Impaired coagulation	Endothelial dysfunction
↑ PAI	↑ Adhension	↑ Fibrinogen	↑ Adhesion molecules (VCAM, etc.)
↑ α_2-antiplasmin	↑ Aggregation	↑ vWF	↑ Leukocyte–endothelial interaction
↑ tPA	↑ Activation	↑ Thrombin	↑ Oxidative cell stress (induction of NFκB)
	↑ GPIIb/IIIa	↑ FVII, FVIII	↑ Impaired vasodilatation (↑ ET1, ↓ NO)
	↑ P-selectin	↑ ATIII	↑ Impaired endothelial regeneration
	↑ CD40L	↑ Sulfated heparins	

PAI, plasminogen activator inhibitor; tPa, tissue-type plasminogen activator; GPIIb/IIIa, glycoprotein IIb/IIIa; vWF, von Willebrand factor, FVII, FVIII, factors VII and VIII; ATIII, antithrombin III; VCAM, vascular cell adhesion molecule; NFκB, nuclear factors κB; ET1, endothelin 1; NO, nitric oxide.

subjects, 4.0% of those treated with 325 mg aspirin every other day had an MI, versus 10.1% of those who received placebo (RR 0.39). In ETDRS (Early Treatment Diabetic Retinopathy Study),[15] although aspirin did not prevent progression of retinopathy, it did produce a significant 28% reduction in risk for MI over 5 years ($p = 0.038$) without an excess of retinal or vitreous hemorrhage. The HOT (Hypertension Optimal Treatment) study[16] studied antihypertensive treatment in 18 790 hypertensive individuals, 1501 of whom had DM. Subjects were randomized to either low-dose aspirin (75 mg/day) or placebo therapy. Aspirin therapy resulted in an additional 15% reduction in the risk for cardiovascular events over that seen with antihypertensive therapy ($p = 0.03$). Fatal bleeding, including cerebral bleeding, was equally common in the aspirin and placebo groups, whereas nonfatal bleeding was more common with aspirin therapy.

Aspirin as a secondary prevention strategy in diabetes mellitus

The ADA recommends the use of aspirin (81–325 mg/day) as a secondary prevention measure in diabetic patients with atherosclerotic disease.[11] Two large meta-analyses of major secondary prevention trials by the Antithrombotic Trialists' Collaboration (ATC) have concluded that aspirin (or another oral antiplatelet drug) is protective in most patients who are at high risk for cardiovascular disease, including those with diabetes.[6,17] The ATC meta-analysis of 287 secondary prevention trials involved 212 000 high-risk patients who had acute or previous vascular disease or another condition that increased the risk of vascular occlusion.[6] Aspirin was the most frequently used agent, with

doses ranging from 75 to 325 mg/day. A low dose of aspirin (75–150 mg/day) was found to be at least as effective as higher daily doses. In the main high-risk groups (acute MI, past history of MI, past history of stroke or transient ischemic attack (TIA), acute stroke, and other relevant history of vascular disease), antiplatelet therapy significantly reduced the incidence of vascular events by 23%. Low doses of aspirin were as effective as high doses, but bleeding complications were reduced at the lower dosage levels. In the more than 4500 DM patients studied by the ATC, the incidence of vascular events was reduced from 23.5% with control treatment to 19.3% with antiplatelet therapy ($p < 0.01$),[17] while this fell from 17.2% to 13.7% ($p < 0.00001$) in the approximately 42 000 non-DM patients. Although the overall incidence of vascular events is much higher in patients with diabetes, the benefit of antiplatelet therapy in DM and non-DM patients was similar (42 vascular events were prevented for every 1000 DM patients and 35 events for every 1000 non-DM patients).

P2Y$_{12}$ receptor antagonists

Ticlopidine was evaluated for its effects on microvascular disease in DM patients in the TIMAD (Ticlopidine in Microangiopathy of Diabetes) study.[18] A total of 435 patients with non-proliferative diabetic retinopathy were randomized to receive ticlopidine, 250 mg twice daily, or placebo and were followed for up to 3 years. Ticlopidine significantly reduced annual microaneurysm progression by 67% based on fluorescein angiograms ($p = 0.03$), and among insulin-treated diabetic patients, it reduced annual microaneurysm progression by 85% ($p = 0.03$). Moreover, the insulin-treated diabetic patients had a trend for developing fewer new vessels. Overall progression of retinopathy was significantly less severe with ticlopidine ($p = 0.04$). This study supports the postulate that platelets are involved in the pathogenesis of microvascular disease in patients with DM. A similar study with aspirin in diabetic individuals, ETDRS, showed no effect on progression of retinopathy.[15]

The CAPRIE (Clopidogrel versus Aspirin in Patients at Risk of Ischemic Events) trial examined the effects of 75 mg clopidogrel once daily versus 325 mg aspirin once daily in a large secondary prevention population consisting of 19 185 patients with recent ischemic stroke, recent MI, or established PAD.[19] Patients were followed up for a mean of 1.9 years. Approximately 20% of these patients were known to have DM. The annual incidence of the primary endpoint (combined incidence of vascular death, MI, or ischemic stroke) was 5.32% with clopidogrel and 5.83% with aspirin, representing an 8.7% RR reduction with clopidogrel above aspirin ($p=0.043$). Bhatt et al.[20] retrospectively analyzed results in the diabetic subgroup in the CAPRIE study. Of 1 914 DM patients randomized to clopidogrel, 15.6% had the composite vascular primary endpoint, versus 17.7% of 1 952 DM patients randomized to aspirin therapy ($p=0.042$). This led to 21 vascular events prevented for every 1000 DM patients treated, which increased to 38 among patients with insulin-dependent DM. In non-DM patients, the composite vascular primary endpoint was non-statistically significant in patients randomized to treatment with clopidogrel (12.7%) versus aspirin (11.8%). Such superiority of clopidogrel compared with aspirin in DM patients has been attributed to the more potent antiplatelet effects of clopiodgrel over aspirin, thus allowing more efficient inhibition of the hyper-reactive diabetic platelet.[21] In addition, increased adenosine diphosphate (ADP) exposure of diabetic platelets may lead to persistence of enhanced platelet reactivity despite treatment with aspirin, which may be overcome with an ADP receptor antagonist such as clopidogrel. This aspect is linked with the 'aspirin resistance' concept. Aspirin resistance is used to explain the occurrence of a cardiovascular event in an individual receiving standard aspirin therapy. Resistance to antiplatelet therapy is an emerging clinical entity.[22] Numerous causes have been attributed to the aspirin resistance phenomenon, and several studies have shown it to be more frequently observed in patients with DM.[23]

The CURE (Clopidogrel in Unstable Angina to Prevent Recurrent Events) study examined outcomes with clopidogrel plus aspirin versus aspirin alone in patients ($n = 12 562$) with unstable angina or non-Q-wave MI.[24] Patients were randomized to receive either clopidogrel (300 mg loading dose and 75 mg thereafter) or placebo in addition to aspirin for up to 1 year. Patients on clopidogrel and aspirin experienced a significant 20% reduction in the first primary outcome (composite of vascular death, MI, or stroke) compared with patients receiving aspirin and placebo ($p < 0.001$).[20] Significantly more patients in the clopidogrel plus aspirin group had major bleeding (3.7% vs

2.7%), but there was no increase in life-threatening bleeds. There were 2840 patients with DM in the study. Patients on clopidogrel and aspirin experienced an approximately 17% reduction in the first primary outcome (95% CI 0.70–1.02). Thus, the effect in the diabetic subgroup was in the same direction as in the entire study, but had borderline statistical significance. Of note, the event rate was much higher in the diabetic cohort of patients: the primary composite cardiovascular endpoint occurred in 14.2% of patients on clopidogrel versus 16.7% of those on placebo. These high event rates may be in part attributed to the persistence of increased platelet reactivity in DM patients even when on dual antiplatelet therapy compared with non-DM patients. In fact, despite the clinical benefits achieved with the adjunctive use of clopidogrel in high-risk patients, laboratory and clinical experience with this drug has led to an understanding of some of its limitations. In particular, clopidogrel has been shown to be associated with a broad interindividual variability in its antiplatelet effects (see Chapter 8), and some patients, in particular diabetics, are more prone to have reduced antiplatelet effects.[25] Several functional studies have shown that both in the acute phase, following administration of a 300 mg loading dose of clopidogrel, and in the maintenance phase, while on 75 mg daily dose therapy, patients with T2DM have a lower degree of platelet inhibition compared with non-DM patients, which is even more marked in insulin-treated diabetics.[26,27] Therefore, inadequate platelet inhibition in DM patients treated with dual antiplatelet therapy may explain their higher risk of ischemic events, including stent thrombosis.[25,28] This phenomenon has been attributed to an upregulated status of the $P2Y_{12}$ pathway.[25] In the OPTIMUS (Optimizing antiPlatelet Therapy In diabetes MellitUS) study, which was performed in a selected cohort of T2DM patients with enhanced platelet reactivity, the use of a higher maintenance dose of clopidogrel (150 mg) improved platelet function profiles, although the majority of patients remained above the predefined therapeutic threshold.[29] This suggests that other more potent antithrombotic treatment regimens may be warranted in DM patients in order to enhance platelet inhibition. Future studies evaluating the clinical impact of novel strategies are warranted. Recent findings from TRITON–TIMI 38 (Trial to Assess Improvement in Therapeutic Outcomes by Optimizing Platelet Inhibition with Prasugrel–Thrombolysis in Myocardial Infarction), in which treatment with prasugrel, a third-generation thienopyridine that achieves potent $P2Y_{12}$ inhibition (see Chapter 9), led to better clinical outcomes, including reduced stent thrombosis rates, compared with clopidogrel;[30] the magnitude of this benefit was greatest in diabetic patients, a subgroup in which the clinical efficacy of prasugrel was not offset by increased bleeding.[30]

GPIIb/IIIa receptor antagonists

In a meta-analysis of six trials of intravenous glycoprotein (GP) IIb/IIIa inhibitors in ACS patients, in which 22% had DM ($n = 6458$), GPIIb/IIIa blockers significantly reduced mortality at 30 days from 6.2% to 4.6% ($p = 0.007$) in DM patients.[31] In all trials, patients were randomized to receive or not receive a GPIIb/IIIa inhibitor (tirofiban, lamifiban, eptifibatide, or abciximab) by bolus and then a constant infusion for 2–5 days after admission for ACS. Among the more than 22 000 patients in these trials who did not have DM, GPIIb/IIIa inhibitors did not improve survival. The effect of GPIIb/IIIa inhibitors in diabetic individuals was even greater in the 1279 patients who underwent percutaneous coronary intervention (PCI) during the index hospitalization; in these individuals, GPIIb/IIIa inhibitors reduced 30-day mortality from 4% to 1.2% ($p = 0.002$). Of note, these trials were performed in an era of limited use of clopidogrel, which has challenged the need for a GPIIb/IIIa receptor antagonist in DM patients. In fact, the ISAR–SWEET (Intracoronary Stenting and Antithrombotic Regimen: Is Abciximab a Superior Way to Eliminate Elevated Thrombotic Risk in Diabetics?) trial did not show any impact of bciximab on the 1-year risk of death and MI in DM patients ($n = 701$) undergoing PCI after pretreatment with a 600 mg loading dose of clopidogrel at least 2 hours before the procedure.[32] However, the ISAR–REACT 2 (Intracoronary Stenting and Antithrombotic: Regimen Rapid Early Action for Coronary Treatment 2) trial clearly showed that abciximab safely reduces the risk of adverse events (the primary endpoint was a composite of death, MI, or urgent target vessel revascularization occurring within 30 days) in patients with non-ST-elevation MI ACS undergoing PCI after pretreatment with 600 mg of clopidogrel, which was confined to patients with elevated troponin levels, but not to patients with ECG changes.[33] The benefit was observed across all subgroups, including DM. Overall, in accordance with current guidelines, these results continue to support the use of GPIIb/IIIa receptor antagonists in DM patients with ACS undergoing PCI.[34]

Conclusions

Patients with DM have an increased atherothrombotic risk. Antiplatelet therapy has a pivotal role in primary and secondary prevention of ischemic events in this high-risk patient population. However, despite the use of antiplatelet medication, DM patients have a risk of developing adverse clinical outcomes greater than that for non-diabetics. The dysfunctional status of diabetic platelets, as well as the different degrees of antiplatelet drug response in DM compared with non-DM patients, may contribute to their high risk of ischemic events, including stent thrombosis. While compliance with guidelines for antiplatelet drug management has clearly been shown to reduce morbidity and mortality in DM patients, there is accruing data showing that in these patients the degree of platelet inhibition achieved with standard treatment regimens may be inadequate. This supports the need for specific antiplatelet drug regimens, with either different dosages of current medication or development of novel antiplatelet drugs that are more specific to tackle the hyper-reactive diabetic platelet.[35,36]

References

1. American Diabetes Association. Role of cardiovascular risk factors in prevention and treatment of macrovascular disease in diabetes. Diabetes Care 1989;12:573–9.
2. King H, Aubert RE, Herman WH. Global burden of diabetes, 1995–2025: prevalence, numerical estimates, and projections. Diabetes Care 1998;21:1414–31.
3. Laakso MLS. Epidemiology of macrovascular disease in diabetes. Diabetes Rev 1997;5:294–315.
4. Haffner SM, Lehto S, Ronnema T et al. Mortality from coronary heart disease in subjects with type 2 diabetes and in nondiabetic subjects with and without prior myocardial infarction. N Engl J Med 1998;339:229–34.
5. Stein B, Weintraub WS, Gebhart SP et al. Influence of diabetes mellitus on early and late outcome after percutaneous coronary angioplasty. Circulation 1995;91:979–89.
6. Antithrombotic Trialists' Collaboration. Collaborative meta-analysis of randomised trials of antiplatelet therapy for prevention of death, myocardial infarction, and stroke in high risk patients. BMJ 2002;324:71–86.
7. Nesto RW. Correlation between cardiovascular disease and diabetes mellitus: current concepts. Am J Med 2004;116(Suppl 5A):11–22S.
8. Colwell JA, Nesto RW. The platelet in diabetes: focus on prevention of ischemic events. Diabetes Care 2003;26:2181–8.
9. Vinik AI, Erbas T, Park TS et al. Platelet dysfunction in type 2 diabetes. Diabetes Care 2001;24:1476–85.
10. Ferroni P, Basili S, Falco A, Davi G. Platelet activation in type 2 diabetes mellitus. J Thromb Haemost 2004;2:1282–91.
11. American Diabetes Association. Aspirin therapy in diabetes (Position Statement). Diabetes Care 2004;27(Suppl 1):S72–3.
12. Pearson TA, Blair SN, Daniels SR et al. AHA guidelines for primary prevention of cardiovascular disease and stroke: 2002 update. Consensus panel guide to comprehensive risk reduction for adult patients without coronary or other atherosclerotic vascular diseases (AHA Scientific Statement). Circulation 2002;106:388–91.
13. Collaborative Group of the Primary Prevention Project. Low-dose aspirin and vitamin E in people at cardiovascular risk: a randomized trial in general practice. Lancet 2001;357:89–95.
14. Steering Committee of the Physicians' Health Study Research Group. Final report on the aspirin component of the ongoing Physicians' Health Study. N Engl J Med 1989;321:129–35.
15. ETDRS Investigators. Aspirin effects on mortality and morbidity in patients with diabetes mellitus. Early Treatment Diabetic Retinopathy Study report 14. JAMA 1992;268:1292–300.
16. Hansson L, Zanchetti A, Carruthers SG et al, for the HOT Study Group. Effects of intensive blood-pressure lowering and low-dose aspirin in patients with hypertension: principal results of the Hypertension Optimal Treatment (HOT) randomised trial. Lancet 1998;351:1755–62.

17. Antiplatelet Trialists' Collaboration. Collaborative overview of randomised trials of antiplatelet therapy. I. Prevention of death, myocardial infarction, and stroke by prolonged antiplatelet therapy in various categories of patients. BMJ 1994;308:81–106.

18. TIMAD Study Group. Ticlopidine treatment reduces the progression of nonproliferative diabetic retinopathy. Arch Ophthalmol 1990;108:1577–83.

19. CAPRIE Steering Committee. A randomised, blinded, trial of clopidogrel versus aspirin in patients at risk of ischaemic events (CAPRIE). Lancet 1996;348:1329–39.

20. Bhatt D, Marso S, Hirsch A et al. Amplified benefit of clopidogrel versus aspirin in patients with diabetes mellitus. Am J Cardiol 2002;90:625–8.

21. Wang TH, Bhatt DL, Topol EJ. Aspirin and clopidogrel resistance: an emerging clinical entity. Eur Heart J 2006;27:647–54.

22. Savi P, Herbert JM. Clopidogrel and ticlopidine: P2Y12 adenosine diphosphate-receptor antagonists for the prevention of atherothrombosis. Semin Thromb Hemost 2005;31:174–83.

23. Watala C, Golanski J, Pluta J et al. Reduced sensitivity of platelets from type 2 diabetic patients to acetylsalicylic acid (aspirin) – its relation to metabolic control. Thromb Res 2004;113:101–13.

24. Yusuf S, Zhao F, Mehta SR et al. Clopidogrel in Unstable Angina to Prevent Recurrent Events Trial Investigators. Effects of clopidogrel in addition to aspirin in patients with acute coronary syndromes without ST-segment elevation. N Engl J Med 2001;345:494–502.

25. Angiolillo DJ, Fernandez Ortiz A, Bernardo E et al. Variability in individual responsiveness to clopidogrel: clinical implications, management, and future perspectives. J Am Coll Cardiol 2007; 49:1505–16.

26. Angiolillo DJ, Fernandez-Ortiz A, Bernardo E et al. Platelet function profiles in patients with type 2 diabetes and coronary artery disease on combined aspirin and clopidogrel treatment. Diabetes 2005;54:2430–5.

27. Angiolillo DJ, Bernardo E, Ramirez C et al. Insulin therapy is associated with platelet dysfunction in patients with type 2 diabetes mellitus on dual oral antiplatelet treatment. J Am Coll Cardiol 2006; 48:298–304.

28. Angiolillo DJ, Bernardo E, Sabate M et al. Impact of platelet reactivity on cardiovascular outcomes in patients with type 2 diabetes mellitus and coronary artery disease. J Am Coll Cardiol 2007; 50:1541–7.

29. Angiolillo DJ, Shoemaker SB, Desai B et al. Randomized comparison of a high clopidogrel maintenance dose in patients with diabetes mellitus and coronary artery disease: results of the Optimizing Antiplatelet Therapy in Diabetes Mellitus (OPTIMUS) study. Circulation 2007;115:708–16.

30. Wiviott SD, Braunwald E, McCabe CH et al. the TRITON–TIMI 38 Investigators. Prasugrel versus Clopidogrel in Patients with Acute Coronary Syndromes. N Engl J Med 2007;357:2001–15.

31. Roffi M, Chew DP, Mukherjee D et al. Platelet glycoprotein IIb/IIIa inhibitors reduce mortality in diabetic patients with non-ST-segment-elevation acute coronary syndromes. Circulation 2001;104: 2767–71.

32. Mehilli J, Kastrati A, Schuhlen H et al. Intracoronary Stenting and Antithrombotic Regimen: Is Abciximab a Superior Way to Eliminate Elevated Thrombotic Risk in Diabetics (ISAR–SWEET) Study Investigators. Randomized clinical trial of abciximab in diabetic patients undergoing elective percutaneous coronary interventions after treatment with a high loading dose of clopidogrel. Circulation 2004;110:3627–35.

33. Kastrati A, Mehilli J, Neumann FJ et al. Intracoronary Stenting and Antithrombotic: Regimen Rapid Early Action for Coronary Treatment 2 (ISAR–REACT 2) Trial Investigators. Abciximab in patients with acute coronary syndromes undergoing percutaneous coronary intervention after clopidogrel pretreatment: the ISAR-REACT 2 randomized trial. JAMA 2006;295:1531–8.

34. Smith SC Jr, Feldman TE, Hirshfeld JW Jr et al. ACC/AHA/SCAI 2005 guideline update for percutaneous coronary intervention: a report of the American College of Cardiology/American Heart Association Task Force on Practice Guidelines (ACC/AHA/SCAI Writing Committee to Update the 2001 Guidelines for Percutaneous Coronary Intervention). Circulation 2006;113:156–75.

35. Angiolillo DJ. Tackling the diabetic platelet: Is high clopidogrel dosing the answer? J Thromb Haemost 2006;4:2563–5.

36. Alfonso F, Angiolillo DJ. Platelet function assessment to predict outcomes after coronary interventions: hype or hope? J Am Coll Cardiol 2006;48:1751–4.

24

Stent thrombosis in the era of drug-eluting stents

Marco A Costa, Manel Sabaté, and Fernando Alfonso

Introduction

Drug-eluting stents (DES) represented a therapeutic milestone in the field of interventional cardiology. Clinical trials comparing DES with bare metal stents (BMS) have unequivocally demonstrated greater efficacy of these novel anti-proliferative devices to reduce restenosis and the need for repeat revascularization procedures.[1–10] However, the safety of DES has recently been questioned. In particular, DES have been associated with an enhanced risk of thrombotic events very late after treatment.[11] In this chapter, we will review the current understanding on pathophysiology and clinical aspects of stent thrombosis in the DES era.

Definition of stent thrombosis

Stent thrombosis is usually defined based on its temporal relationship with percutaneous coronary intervention (PCI). In the era of BMS, stent thrombosis was divided into acute (AST; <24 hours) or subacute (SAT; >24 hours but <30 days). The term late thrombosis (LST), defined as occurrence of target lesion thrombosis >30 days after PCI, was only introduced after the advent of intravascular brachytherapy.[12] As a result, there is a paucity of historical data on the occurrence of late thrombosis after balloon angioplasty or BMS. In the DES era, the term very late stent thrombosis (VLST) has been proposed to designate events occurring 1 year post PCI (Table 24.1).

Since 1999, rates of LST have been reported in major PCI trials; however, there are significant variations in the definition of stent thrombosis between studies. One should be careful when comparing data between trials and should always interpret the data in the context of each study's specific definitions. In general, SAT is usually defined as angiographic thrombus within the stented vessel at the time of the angiographic restudy. Any death not attributable to a non-cardiac cause in the first 30 days or any Q-wave myocardial infarction in the territory of the target vessel in the first 30 days should be considered a surrogate for stent thrombosis if vessel patency is not documented by angiography. The events have been usually defined as myocardial infarction occurring >30 days after the index procedure and attributable to the target vessel, with angiographic documentation (site-reported or by quantitative coronary angiography) of thrombus or total occlusion at the target site and freedom from an interim revascularization of the target vessel.

A new definition has recently been proposed by a group of investigators, industry and regulators known as the Academic Research Consortium (ARC). The major difference between the ARC and previous definitions (Table 24.2) is that the ARC also includes stent thrombosis occurring after repeat PCI during the follow-up period. Traditionally, patients with repeat revascularization were excluded from the thrombosis analysis because they have reached a clinical endpoint. The ARC definition provides a less biased and more clinically relevant comparison between potent anti-restenosis technologies, such as DES, and BMS. While the ARC definition represents an advance in clinical definition of stent thrombosis, it has limited value to discriminate the mechanisms of stent thrombosis and to define the thrombotic risk of each specific device, because it includes under the same category stent thrombosis occurring after repeat PCI and stent thrombosis occurring 'spontaneously', which may have entirely different pathophysiologies.

Incidence of stent thrombosis

It is likely that the true incidence of stent thrombosis exceeds current estimates, given that some patients are lost to follow-up or experience clinically silent events. Furthermore, study patients usually have lower risk than the real-world PCI population. Comparisons of the incidence of stent thrombosis between studies and devices have been hindered by short follow-up periods, differences in the use of antiplatelet drug regimens, requirements for angiographic re-evaluation, and patient population, among others.

Table 24.1 *Definition of stent thrombosis*

	Previous clinical trials	Academic Research Consortium (ARC) definition
Definition of timing		
Acute stent thrombosis	0–24 hours post stent implantation	0–24 hours post stent implantation
Subacute stent thrombosis	>24 hours–30 days post stent implantation	>24 hours–30 days post stent implantation
Late stent thrombosis	>30 days–1 year post stent implantation	>30 days–1 year post stent implantation
Very late stent thrombosis	N/A	>1 year post stent implantation
Evidence in defining stent thrombosis	Sudden onset of typical chest pain with electrocardiographic changes, indicating acute ischemia in the distribution of the target vessel. Complete or partial occlusion within the stented segment, with evidence of thrombus in angiography.	Three categories of evidence in defining stent thrombosis: 1. Confirmed/definite 2. Probable 3. Possible

Table 24.2 *Categories of evidence in the Academic Research Consortium (ARC) definition of stent thrombosis*

1. Confirmed/definite

Angiographic confirmed stent thrombosis is considered to have occurred if:
1. Thrombolysis in Myocardial Infarction (TIMI) flow is:
   (a) grade 0 with occlusion originating in the stent or in the segment 5 mm proximal or distal to the stent region in the presence of a thrombus
   (b) grade 1, 2, or 3 originating in the stent or in the segment 5 mm proximal or distal to the stent region in the presence of a thrombus

AND at least one of the following criteria, up to 48 hours, has been fulfilled:
2. New onset of ischemic symptoms at rest (typical chest pain with duration >20 minutes)
3. New ischemic ECG changes suggestive of acute ischemia
4. Typical rise and fall in cardiac biomarkers (>2× upper limit of normal value of creatine kinase)

2. Probable

Clinical definition of probable stent thrombosis is considered to have occurred in the following cases:
1. Any unexplained death within the first 30 days
2. Irrespective of the time after the index procedure, any myocardial infarction in the absence of any obvious cause that is related to documented acute ischemia in the territory of the implanted stent without angiographic confirmation of stent thrombosis

3. Possible

Clinical definition of possible stent thrombosis is considered to have occurred with any unexplained death beyond 30 days

Acute and subacute stent thrombosis

The incidence of AST and SAT in the era of second-generation BMS with high-pressure deployment under appropriate dual antiplatelet therapy is low overall varying from 0.4% in low-risk groups to 2.8% in higher-risk scenarios.[13–20] In a pooled analysis of six BMS clinical trials with a total of 6000 patients, the incidence of 30-day stent thrombosis was 0.9%. The incidence of 30-day stent thrombosis in the ARTS trial, which included only patients with multivessel BMS procedures, was 2.8%.[17] Overall, the incidences of AST and SAT with DES in large scale randomized clinical trials were comparable with that of BMS (Table 24.3).[21,22]

Late stent thrombosis

LST and VLST represent one of the major concerns associated with DES. There is a paucity of data regarding late thrombotic events after PCI procedures. Balloon angioplasty or BMS PCI have not been scrutinized for late thrombotic events until recently. Late and sudden thrombotic coronary occlusion after PCI became a known pathological entity only after the introduction of intracoronary brachytherapy.[12] Over the past few years, LST after BMS has been reported and shown to be related to severe in-stent restenosis.[23,24] The incidence of LST has also been shown to be similar between DES and BMS in various clinical trials

Table 24.3 *Incidence of stent thrombosis in clinical trials*

Trial	Type of study[a]	Follow-up duration (months)	Stent[b]	Duration of clopidogrel (months)	AST/SAT[c] (%)	Late stent thrombosis (%)	Very late stent thrombosis (%)
RAVEL[1]	RCT	12	SES ($n = 120$)	2	0	0	NA
			BMS ($n = 118$)		0	0	NA
SIRIUS[2]	RCT	12	SES ($n = 533$)	3	0.2 ($n = 1$)	0.2 ($n = 1$)	NA
			BMS ($n = 525$)		0.2 ($n = 1$)	0.6 ($n = 3$)	NA
E-SIRIUS[3]	RCT	9	SES ($n = 175$)	2	1.1 ($n = 2$)	0	NA
			BMS ($n = 177$)		0	0	NA
C-SIRIUS[4]	RCT	12	SES ($n = 50$)	2	2 ($n = 1$)	0	NA
			BMS ($n = 50$)		0	2 ($n = 1$)	NA
ASPECT[5]	RCT	6	PES ($n = 90$)	6	0	0	NA
			BMS ($n = 48$)		0	0	NA
ELUTES[6]	RCT	12	PES ($n = 153$)	6	0.7 ($n = 1$)	0	NA
			BMS ($n = 39$)		2.6 ($n = 1$)	0	NA
TAXUS-I[7]	RCT	12	PES ($n = 31$)	6	0	0	NA
			BMS ($n = 30$)		0	0	NA
TAXUS-II[8]	RCT	12	PES ($n = 266$)	6	0.4 ($n = 1$)	0.8 ($n = 2$)	NA
			BMS ($n = 270$)		0	0	NA
TAXUS-IV[9]	RCT	9	PES ($n = 662$)	6	0.3 ($n = 2$)	0.3 ($n = 2$)	NA
			BMS ($n = 652$)		0.6 ($n = 4$)	0.2 ($n = 1$)	NA
DELIVER[10]	RCT	9	PES ($n = 522$)	6	0.2 ($n = 1$)	0.2 ($n = 1$)	NA
			BMS ($n = 519$)		0.2 ($n = 1$)	0.2 ($n = 1$)	NA
DIABETES[36]	RCT	9	SES ($n = 80$)	12	0	0	NA
			BMS ($n = 80$)		1.3 ($n = 1$)	1.3 ($n = 1$)	NA
Ong et al.[21]	Retrospective study	6	SES ($n = 1017$)	3–6		0.3 ($n = 3$)	NA
			PES ($n = 989$)	6		0.5 ($n = 5$)	NA
Iakovou et al.[26]	RCT	9	SES ($n = 1062$)	3	0.4 ($n = 4$)	0.5 ($n = 5$)	NA
			PES ($n = 1167$)	6	0.8 ($n = 10$)	0.8 ($n = 10$)	NA
Bavry et al.[25]	Meta-analysis	9–24	SES	2–3	4.2 events/1000	3.5 events/1000	3.6 events/1000[d]
			BMS		3.5 event/1000	4.9 events/1000	0 events/1000
			PES	6	4.6 events/1000	6.3 events/1000[d]	5.9 events/1000[d]
			BMS		6.3 events/1000	1.1 events/1000	0 events/1000
			Overall DES		4.4 events/1000	5.0 events/1000	5.0 events/1000[d]
			Overall BMS		5.0 events/1000	2.8 events/1000	0 events/1000
Pfisterer et al.[11]	RCT	18	DES ($n = 545$)	6		1.4 ($n = 7$)	NA
			BMS ($n = 281$)			0.8 ($n = 2$)	NA
Stone et al.[27]	Meta-analysis	48	SES ($n = 870$)	2–3	NA	NA	0.6 ($n = 5$)[d]
			BMS ($n = 878$)		NA	NA	0
			PES ($n = 1749$)	6	NA	NA	0.5 ($n = 9$)[d]
			BMS ($n = 1757$)		NA	NA	0.1 ($n = 2$)

[a]RCT, randomized clinical trial.
[b]SES, sirolimus-eluting stent; BMS, bare metal stent; PES, paclitaxel-eluting stent.
[c]AST/SAT, acute stent thrombosis/subacute stent thrombosis.
[d]$p < 0.05$ vs BMS.

and recent meta-analyses. Angiographically documented LST rates may vary from 0.2% to 1.4% (Table 24.3). In a pooled analysis including 10 randomized studies, no differences in LST was found between sirolimus-eluting stents (SES), paclitaxel-eluting stents (PES), and BMS.[25] It should be realized that SES trials required 2–3 months' of dual antiplatelet therapy (aspirin plus thienopyridines), while PES mandates 6 months' treatment. In a large cohort of patients, likely representing real-world clinical experiences, LST was observed in 0.7% of patients who underwent successful implantation of SES or PES.[26]

Based on the ARC definition, the probable or definite 1-year incidence of stent thrombosis was in 0.6% for SES versus 1.3% for BMS in the pooled randomized trials. Similarly, overall, the 1-year incidence of stent thrombosis was 0.9% for PES versus 0.8% for BMS in the PES randomized trials. Taken together, the available data support the notion that currently available DES are not associated with increased risk of stent thrombosis during the first year after PCI.

Very late stent thrombosis

Recent meta-analyses have demonstrated a slight increase in the rate of VLST in patients receiving either PES or SES. One of these meta-analyses considered the RAVEL trial, the three SIRIUS trials, and the five TAXUS trials. In this regard, the incidences of stent thrombosis between the first and fourth years were 0.6% for SES, 0% for BMS ($p = 0.02$), 0.7% for PES, and 0.2% for BMS ($p = 0.02$).[27] Another meta-analysis of individual data on 4958 patients from 14 randomized trials comparing SES stent with BMS[28] demonstrated no differences in terms of death or the combined endpoint of death or myocardial infarction. However, over the 4-year period after the first year following the procedure, the overall risk of stent thrombosis was 0.6% (95% confidence interval (CI) 0.3–1.2) in the SES group and 0.05% (95% CI 0.01–0.4) in the BMS group ($p = 0.02$).

Pathophysiology
Predictors of stent thrombosis

The main factors associated with LST and VLST remain elusive. Prediction of when and if stent thrombosis will occur in a given patient is nearly impossible at present. However, some anatomical and clinical risk factors may indicate an increased risk of stent thrombosis (Figure 24.1), and special surveillance of such patient subsets seems appropriate. It is important to notice that the mechanisms and predictors of VLST, which is the thrombotic event being associated with DES, might be different from those associated with early or late stent thrombosis, and remain unknown.

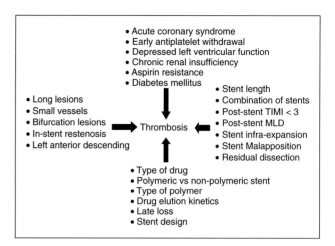

Figure 24.1
Clinical, angiographic, procedural, and stent-related predictors of thrombosis.

Previous reports[22,26] have implicated stent deployment techniques, premature discontinuation of antiplatelet therapy, bifurcation lesions, diabetes mellitus, and renal failure in the occurrence of early and late stent thrombosis. Delayed re-endothelialization, hypersensitivity reactions, and hypercoagulability have all been proposed as contributing biological factors. It is unlikely that any of these variables alone can cause stent thrombosis, as the incidence of each risk factor is much higher than the currently known rates of thrombosis after DES.

Re-endothelialization: fact or myth?

Necropsy examination of 23 patients who died more than 30 days after PCI suggested that DES were associated with less endothelialization than BMS.[29] Histological evidence of stent thrombosis was present in 14 of 23 patients treated with a DES, and features of delayed healing were observed in all patients. Additional predictors for LST were identified in 11 patients, including chronic inflammation, hypersensitivity, ostial and bifurcation stenting, malapposition, and penetration of the stent into a necrotic core.

The temporal appearance of the thrombotic events represents a challenge to our understanding of the re-endothelialization process. It should be realized that endothelial dysfunction represents the basis for atherosclerosis and coronary artery disease (CAD) development, and that endothelial cells are likely absent or dysfunctional at the time of PCI. Restoration of endothelial function to its level before CAD development should indeed be a main goal of PCI or other therapeutic strategies. Previous reports in the era of balloon angioplasty and BMS have already shown that endothelial function is not restored until late after PCI.[30] One should not expect DES using potent cell cycle inhibitors to accelerate this process, and expectations of full endothelial recovery before 3–6 months, although desirable, are unrealistic.

Figure 24.2 illustrates potential clinical scenarios associated with re-endothelialization after PCI. Whether functional re-endothelialization ever achieves 100% after PCI remains to be demonstrated (hypothesis 1, Figure 2). Nevertheless, current wisdom suggests that endothelial coverage should increase over time after PCI (hypothesis 2, Figure 2). The speed of endothelial recovery may be governed by local biological factors or drugs. There appears to be a period of lower incidence of stent thrombosis between 6 and 18 months after DES – the 'safest post-DES period'. This temporal aspect of stent thrombosis is puzzling if one attempts to link re-endothelialization and VLST, unless endothelium recovers for a period of time, and then become dysfunctional later after DES (hypothesis 3, Figure 2).

The concept that intimal hyperplasia, observed clinically as late lumen loss, represents a marker of re-endothelialization is largely speculative and incorrect. Endothelial cells represent an important biological barrier against intimal proliferation, and DES designed to expedite endothelial recovery have been proposed to prevent intimal hyperplasia. Indeed, enhanced neointimal hyperplasia observed after stenting has been associated with more pronounced and prolonged endothelial dysfunction.[31]

Stent deployment procedure

In the early 1990s, BMS were under intense scrutiny because of a high incidence of stent thrombosis.[32] Various antithrombotic treatment regimens were attempted at the time, but the results were mostly disappointing. A reduction in the incidence of SAT was only achieved after improvements in stent deployment techniques with the use of high-pressure balloon inflations.[33] Similarly, DES have been associated with the occurrence of delayed stent thrombosis, and multiple clinical risk factors and antithrombotic treatment regimens have been proposed.[26,34] An early hazard associated with suboptimal PCI is somewhat to be expected, but data from the STLLR trial ($n = 1574$), the only study ever to

evaluate the impact of stent deployment techniques in a prospective and blind fashion, suggested that geographical miss (lack of proper DES coverage of lesion or injured coronary segment) was associated not only with early thrombotic events, but a threefold increase in myocardial infarction (MI) >30 days after implantatuion of SES (Costa MA, personal communication, 2006).

AST and SAT have been associated with procedural factors such as dissection, incomplete lesion coverage, suboptimal stent deployment (underexpansion and malapposition), and excessive stent length (particularly in small vessels).[9,15,16,22,35,36] Whether intravascular ultrasound (IVUS) should be used to prevent stent thrombosis after DES implantation remains to be demonstrated in properly designed studies, but studies that utilize IVUS-guided DES deployment, such as the DIABETES series and RAVEL, have reported 0% of stent thrombosis at 1-year follow-up.[37–40] Similarly, the J-CYPHER study, which include a very large percentage of IVUS utilization, reported very low rates of SAT and LST (0.36% and 0.028%) (Kimura T, personal communication, 2006).

In comparison with BMS, late stent malapposition occurs more frequently after DES.[41] While acute stent malapposition has been implicated with SAT, the relationship between late malapposition and LST has not been fully established to date. The low incidence of both phenomena and the difficulty of evaluating stent apposition in patients presenting with stent thrombosis are challenges in proving such a relationship.

Judicious stent deployment technique is imperative, because poor PCI strategies directly and independently impact clinical outcomes. Operators should pay special attention to match the length and size of the DES to the lesion and vessel. Proper positioning of the stent, rather than the absolute stent length, is important.

Anatomical and clinical factors

A relationship between stent thrombosis and DES length has been reported.[22] Bifurcation PCI remains a technical challenge, even in the DES era. In particular, treatment of bifurcations with two DES appears to be associated with a higher risk of stent thrombosis.[42,43] The presence of a bifurcation lesion has also been shown to be an independent predictor of stent thrombosis.[21,26,29]

Stent thrombosis is also more prevalent in certain patient subsets.[21] Renal failure, low ejection fraction, and diabetes are independent predictors of stent thrombosis. In the e-CYPHER registry, insulin-dependent diabetes, acute coronary syndrome at presentation, and advanced age were clinical predictors, whereas low TIMI flow grade after PCI, multivessel PCI, and severely calcified or totally occluded lesions were angiographic or procedural predictors of stent thrombosis at 12 months.[44]

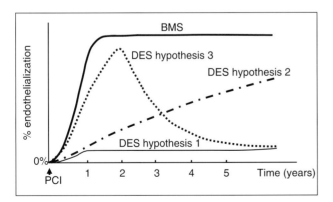

Figure 24.2
Potential clinical scenarios associated with re-endothelialization after percutaneous coronary intervention (PCI).

Antiplatelet therapy

Increased platelet reactivity, related to discontinuation of antiplatelet therapy and/or to antiplatelet drug resistance, has been associated with AST and SAT.[45] The occurrence of stent thrombosis was shown in four cases between 335 and 375 days after DES implantation, and all of these patients were reported to have discontinued antiplatelet therapy in the days prior to the event.[46] Others have found that premature discontinuation of antiplatelet therapy represents an independent factor for stent thrombosis occurring within 9 months after DES PCI,[26] although a temporal relationship between stent thrombosis and discontinuation of therapy was not established in this report.

Discontinuation of clopidogrel within the first month in patients with acute MI treated with DES occurred in 13.6%.[47] Patients no longer taking thienopyridines at 1 month were older, less likely to have completed high school, and less likely to be married, had low socioeconomic status, more pre-existing cardiovascular disease and were not counseled about medication use at hospital discharge. These patients were at increased risk of death in the subsequent 11 months. Overall, these observations should be utilized in clinical decision-making processes by the interventionalist when defining the stent (BMS or DES) to be used. Somewhat alarming is the realization that stent thrombosis may also occur in stable patients taking antiplatelet monotherapy months after appropriate discontinuation of clopidogrel[48] and in those taking dual antiplatelet therapy.

Extended-duration clopidogrel therapy appears to play a more important role after DES than after BMS implantation.[34,49] Previous studies have established the clinical long-term benefit of prolonged dual antiplatelet therapy in acute coronary syndrome/PCI patients.[34,50] However, the clinical benefits associated with long-term dual antiplatelet therapy are attributed to the global 'systemic' effects of enhanced platelet inhibition, as they reduce the cumulative risk of death, MI, and stroke. Indeed, enhanced platelet inhibition with dual antiplatelet therapy has a 'local' impact at the site of stent implantation, but whether the observed clinical effects of prolonged use of clopidogrel in DES-treated patients is directly related to a decrease in stent thrombosis remains to be determined.[34]

In the BMS era, dual antiplatelet therapy was used for a very short period (<15 days) or even omitted, without undesirable thrombotic consequences.[33,51] As discussed above, one should not expect full endothelial function recovery 15 days after PCI. The lack of a peak in the incidence of stent thrombosis events between 15 days and 30 days after BMS PCI is somewhat puzzling, if one considers endothelialization as the main biological factor associated with thrombosis after PCI.

It is important to realize that these previous DES reports did not investigate VLST, but rather SAT and LST. Whether prolonged dual antiplatelet therapy is relevant to preventing VLST remains to be defined. It is possible that dual antiplatelet therapy plays a more important role in preventing early thrombotic events versus VLST. Furthermore, none of these reports were designed to establish the direct temporal relationship between stent thrombosis and antiplatelet therapy. The most appropriate period to discontinue thienopyridines after DES, and whether dual antiplatelet therapy should be maintained beyond 12 months post procedure, remain to be proven.

Antiplatelet drug resistance

Several studies have shown the clinical implications of individual response variability to antiplatelet therapy.[45] In addition to post-stent ischemic events (e.g., MI), these clinical outcomes have also included stent thrombosis.[45,52–54] However, to date, these studies have been limited to assessment of thrombotic events associated with BMS and occurring in the early phases after stent implantation (<30 days). The phenomenon of individual response variability to antiplatelet therapy may explain the persistence in some patients of enhanced platelet reactivity despite the use of dual antiplatelet therapy, thus contributing to the occurrence of stent thrombosis. However, these studies have been primarily focused on individual responsiveness to clopidogrel and have not fully explored aspirin-induced antiplatelet effects. This is of note because VSLT, which is currently the main concern with DES, typically occurs in patients while on sole aspirin therapy. Functional studies, however, have shown that response to aspirin may vary as well and that such responsiveness may also vary over time. Thus, changes in the degree of platelet inhibition in patients treated with aspirin may have an impact on VLST. In a recent study by Wenaweser et al,[55] aspirin, but not clopidogrel, resistance was found to be associated with stent thrombosis.

Currently, there is increasing concern regarding how to manage patients with antiplatelet drug resistance. However, to date, there is still a lack of consensus on both how to measure and which cut-off value should be considered to properly define this phenomenon, limiting any well-founded therapeutic recommendation. Current guidelines state (class IIb indication with level of evidence C) that only in patients in whom stent thrombosis may be catastrophic or lethal (unprotected left main, bifurcating left main, and last patent coronary vessel) may the dose of clopidogrel be increased to 150 mg/day if <50% inhibition of platelet aggregation is demonstrated.[56] However, although the functional ex vivo effects of high clopidogrel maintenance dosing have been evaluated,[57] this has yet to be assessed in a clinical scenario. To date, there are no recommendations of any class regarding modification of aspirin dose in patients with inadequate aspirin-induced antiplatelet effects.

Hypersensitivity to polymer/drug

Hypersensitivity reactions to DES polymer or drug are rare events and difficult to establish clinically. Localized hypersensitivity to DES has been suggested recently from necropsy studies showing eosinophilic infiltrate.[58] There were 262 reports of hypersensitivity symptoms in the FDA database of 5783 reports. Of these reports, 10 were certainly ($n = 1$) or probably ($n = 9$) caused by DES. Intrastent eosinophilic inflammation, thrombosis, and lack of intimal healing were confirmed in four necropsies.[59] Whether these adverse reactions occur early or late after DES deployment also remain to be established. Hypersensitivity reaction, given its rare frequency and potential delayed appearance, represents a good explanation for the unknown mechanisms associated with VLST, although such a link remains largely speculative.

Clinical considerations

Stent thrombosis after DES may have catastrophic consequences. Approximately 70% of patients with DES thrombosis experience MI, and the fatality rate ranges from 15% to 45%.[21,22,26] Among 126 patients who experienced stent thrombosis in the e-CYPHER registry, 53 (42.1%) died, and 55 (43.7%) suffered an MI.[44] Although concerns have been raised regarding the safety of DES, the overall incidence of this catastrophic event is low and, in the first year following stent implantation, is similar to that observed in patients treated with BMS. Similarly to stent thrombosis occurring with BMS, stent deployment technique and compliance with antiplatelet therapy have an important role in early DES thrombosis. Thus, optimizing stent deployment and complying with current guidelines on the duration of dual antiplatelet therapy (12 months for any DES) will allow physicians to pursue the benefits of using DES without any increase in risk compared with BMS.[22,56] However, DES thrombosis may occur in patients taking dual antiplatelet therapy, and, most alarmingly, available data show a potential for more thrombotic events starting beyond the first year after DES implantation (VLST). Importantly, current data have allowed us to evaluate the risk of VLST up to 4 years, but when and if this risk will cease is still unknown.

The occurrence of VLST has been shown to be in most cases unrelated to cessation of dual antiplatelet therapy, as it often occurs many months after clopidogrel withdrawal. Overall, this raises to question whether continuation of dual antiplatelet therapy out to 1 year would have any benefit in terms of prevention of stent thrombosis that occurs more than 2 years after DES implantation. In addition, one should not underestimate the bleeding risks and overall costs associated with prolonged dual antiplatelet therapy. In fact, major bleeding rates are 3.7% in the first year alone.[60,61] Given, the temporal pattern of VLST with DES and the non-negligible economic and safety considerations associated with prolonged dual antiplatelet therapy, lifetime antiplatelet therapy should not be universally recommended to all patients treated with DES. Better understanding of the pathophysiology of VLST, which, as underscored in this chapter, may differ from earlier thrombotic events, may allow better identification of patients in whom prolonged dual antiplatelet therapy may be justified, or even recommencement of dual antiplatelet therapy after a certain time lapse (e.g., 18 months) from DES implantation.

Conclusions

Despite the net clinical benefit associated with the use of DES, the risk of VLST remains a concern. The safety profiles of DES do not seem to differ from those of BMS in the acute and subacute phases following coronary intervention. The main factors associated with LST and VLST remain elusive, and no single factor can claim sole responsibility for the occurrence of stent thrombosis, which is likely the result of a multifactorial process. A better understanding of the pathophysiology of this phenomenon, which has potentially catastrophic consequences, will help in the development of strategies and technologies for its prevention.

References

1. Morice MC, Serruys PW, Sousa JE et al. A randomized comparison of a sirolimus-eluting stent with a standard stent for coronary revascularization. N Engl J Med 2002;346:1773–80.
2. Moses JW, Leon MB, Popma JJ et al. Sirolimus-eluting stents versus standard stents in patients with stenosis in a native coronary artery. N Engl J Med 2003;349:1315–23.
3. Schofer J, Schluter M, Gershlick AH et al. Sirolimus-eluting stents for treatment of patients with long atherosclerotic lesions in small coronary arteries: double-blind, randomised controlled trial (E-SIRIUS). Lancet 2003;362:1093–9.
4. Schampaert E, Cohen EA, Schluter M et al. The Canadian study of the sirolimus-eluting stent in the treatment of patients with long de novo lesions in small native coronary arteries (C-SIRIUS). J Am Coll Cardiol 2004;43:1110–15.
5. Hong MK, Mintz GS, Lee CW et al. Paclitaxel coating reduces in-stent intimal hyperplasia in human coronary arteries: a serial volumetric intravascular ultrasound analysis from the Asian Paclitaxel-Eluting Stent Clinical Trial (ASPECT). Circulation 2003;107:517–20.
6. Gershlick A, De Scheerder I, Chevalier B et al. Inhibition of restenosis with a paclitaxel-eluting, polymer-free coronary stent: the European evaLUation of pacliTaxel Eluting Stent (ELUTES) trial. Circulation 2004;109:487–93.
7. Grube E, Silber S, Hauptmann KE et al. TAXUS I: six- and twelve-month results from a randomized, double-blind trial on a slow-release paclitaxel-eluting stent for de novo coronary lesions. Circulation 2003;107:38–42.
8. Colombo A, Drzewiecki J, Banning A et al. Randomized study to assess the effectiveness of slow- and moderate-release polymer-based paclitaxel-eluting stents for coronary artery lesions. Circulation 2003;108:788–94.

9. Stone GW, Ellis SG, Cox DA et al. A polymer-based, paclitaxel-eluting stent in patients with coronary artery disease. N Engl J Med 2004;350:221–31.

10. Lansky AJ, Costa RA, Mintz GS et al. Non-polymer-based paclitaxel-coated coronary stents for the treatment of patients with de novo coronary lesions: angiographic follow-up of the DELIVER clinical trial. Circulation 2004;109:1948–54.

11. Pfisterer M, Brunner-La Rocca HP, Buser PT et al. Late clinical events after clopidogrel discontinuation may limit the benefit of drug-eluting stents: an observational study of drug-eluting versus bare-metal stents. J Am Coll Cardiol 2006;48:2584–91.

12. Costa MA, Sabate M, van der Giessen WJ et al. Late coronary occlusion after intracoronary brachytherapy. Circulation 1999;100:789–92.

13. Karrillon GJ, Morice MC, Benveniste E et al. Intracoronary stent implantation without ultrasound guidance and with replacement of conventional anticoagulation by antiplatelet therapy. 30-day clinical outcome of the French Multicenter Registry. Circulation 1996;94:1519–27.

14. Moussa I, Di Mario C, Reimers B et al. Subacute stent thrombosis in the era of intravascular ultrasound-guided coronary stenting without anticoagulation: frequency, predictors and clinical outcome. J Am Coll Cardiol 1997;29:6–12.

15. Cutlip DE, Baim DS, Ho KK et al. Stent thrombosis in the modern era: a pooled analysis of multicenter coronary stent clinical trials. Circulation 2001;103:1967–71.

16. Cheneau E, Leborgne L, Mintz GS et al. Predictors of subacute stent thrombosis: results of a systematic intravascular ultrasound study. Circulation 2003;108:43–7.

17. Serruys PW, Unger F, Sousa JE et al. Comparison of coronary-artery bypass surgery and stenting for the treatment of multivessel disease. N Engl J Med 2001;344:1117–24.

18. Werner GS, Gastmann O, Ferrari M et al. Risk factors for acute and subacute stent thrombosis after high-pressure stent implantation: a study by intracoronary ultrasound. Am Heart J 1998;135:300–9.

19. De Servi S, Repetto S, Klugmann S et al. Stent thrombosis: incidence and related factors in the R.I.S.E. Registry (Registro Impianto Stent Endocoronarico). Catheter Cardiovasc Interv 1999;46:13–18.

20. Schuhlen H, Kastrati A, Dirschinger J et al. Intracoronary stenting and risk for major adverse cardiac events during the first month. Circulation 1998;98:104–11.

21. Ong AT, Hoye A, Aoki J et al. Thirty-day incidence and six-month clinical outcome of thrombotic stent occlusion after bare-metal, sirolimus, or paclitaxel stent implantation. J Am Coll Cardiol 2005;45:947–53.

22. Moreno R, Fernandez C, Hernandez R et al. Drug-eluting stent thrombosis: results from a pooled analysis including 10 randomized studies. J Am Coll Cardiol 2005;45:954–9.

23. Farb A, Burke AP, Kolodgie FD, Virmani R. Pathological mechanisms of fatal late coronary stent thrombosis in humans. Circulation 2003;108:1701–6.

24. Hayashi T, Kimura A, Ishikawa K. Acute myocardial infarction caused by thrombotic occlusion at a stent site two years after conventional stent implantation. Heart 2004;90:e26.

25. Bavry AA, Kumbhani DJ, Helton TJ et al. Late thrombosis of drug-eluting stents: a meta-analysis of randomized clinical trials. Am J Med 2006;119:1056–61.

26. Iakovou I, Schmidt T, Bonizzoni E et al. Incidence, predictors, and outcome of thrombosis after successful implantation of drug-eluting stents. JAMA 2005;293:2126–30.

27. Stone GW, Moses JW, Ellis SG et al. Safety and efficacy of sirolimus- and paclitaxel-eluting coronary stents. N Engl J Med 2007;356:998–1008.

28. Kastrati A, Mehilli J, Pache J et al. Analysis of 14 trials comparing sirolimus-eluting stents with bare-metal stents. N Engl J Med 2007;356:1030–9.

29. Joner M, Finn AV, Farb A et al. Pathology of drug-eluting stents in humans: delayed healing and late thrombotic risk. J Am Coll Cardiol 2006;48:193–202.

30. Grewe PH, Deneke T, Machraoui A et al. Acute and chronic tissue response to coronary stent implantation: pathologic findings in human specimen. J Am Coll Cardiol 2000;35:157–63.

31. van Beusekom HM, Whelan DM, Hofma SH et al. Long-term endothelial dysfunction is more pronounced after stenting than after balloon angioplasty in porcine coronary arteries. J Am Coll Cardiol 1998;32:1109–17.

32. Serruys PW, Strauss BH, Beatt KJ et al. Angiographic follow-up after placement of a self-expanding coronary-artery stent. N Engl J Med 1991;324:13–17.

33. Colombo A, Hall P, Nakamura S et al. Intracoronary stenting without anticoagulation accomplished with intravascular ultrasound guidance. Circulation 1995;91:1676–88.

34. Eisenstein EL, Anstrom KJ, Kong DF et al. Clopidogrel use and long-term clinical outcomes after drug-eluting stent implantation. JAMA 2007;297:159–68.

35. Orford JL, Lennon R, Melby S et al. Frequency and correlates of coronary stent thrombosis in the modern era: analysis of a single center registry. J Am Coll Cardiol 2002;40:1567–72.

36. Togni M, Windecker S, Cocchia R et al. Sirolimus-eluting stents associated with paradoxic coronary vasoconstriction. J Am Coll Cardiol 2005;46:231–6.

37. Sabate M, Jimenez-Quevedo P, Angiolillo DJ et al. Randomized comparison of sirolimus-eluting stent versus standard stent for percutaneous coronary revascularization in diabetic patients: the diabetes and sirolimus-eluting stent (DIABETES) trial. Circulation 2005;112:2175–83.

38. Regar E, Serruys PW, Bode C et al. Angiographic findings of the multicenter Randomized Study With the Sirolimus-Eluting Bx Velocity Balloon-Expandable Stent (RAVEL): sirolimus-eluting stents inhibit restenosis irrespective of the vessel size. Circulation 2002;106:1949–56.

39. van Hout BA, Serruys PW, Lemos PA et al. One year cost effectiveness of sirolimus eluting stents compared with bare metal stents in the treatment of single native de novo coronary lesions: an analysis from the RAVEL trial. Heart 2005;91:507–12.

40. Sousa JE, Costa MA, Abizaid AC et al. Sustained suppression of neointimal proliferation by sirolimus-eluting stents: one-year angiographic and intravascular ultrasound follow-up. Circulation 2001;104:2007–11.

41. Serruys PW, Degertekin M, Tanabe K et al. Intravascular ultrasound findings in the multicenter, randomized, double-blind RAVEL (RAndomized study with the sirolimus-eluting VElocity balloon-expandable stent in the treatment of patients with de novo native coronary artery Lesions) trial. Circulation 2002;106:798–803.

42. Ge L, Airoldi F, Iakovou I et al. Clinical and angiographic outcome after implantation of drug-eluting stents in bifurcation lesions with the crush stent technique: importance of final kissing balloon post-dilation. J Am Coll Cardiol 2005;46:613–20.

43. Colombo A, Moses JW, Morice MC et al. Randomized study to evaluate sirolimus-eluting stents implanted at coronary bifurcation lesions. Circulation 2004;109:1244–9.

44. Urban P, Gershlick AH, Guagliumi G et al. Safety of coronary sirolimus-eluting stents in daily clinical practice: one-year follow-up of the e-Cypher registry. Circulation 2006;113:1434–41.

45. Angiolillo DJ, Fernandez-Ortiz A, Bernardo E et al. Variability in individual responsiveness to clopidogrel: clinical implications, management and future perspectives. J Am Coll Cardiol 2007;49:1505–16.

46. McFadden EP, Stabile E, Regar E et al. Late thrombosis in drug-eluting coronary stents after discontinuation of antiplatelet therapy. Lancet 2004;364:1519–21.

47. Spertus JA, Kettelkamp R, Vance C et al. Prevalence, predictors, and outcomes of premature discontinuation of thienopyridine therapy

after drug-eluting stent placement: results from the PREMIER registry. Circulation 2006;113:2803–9.

48. Ong AT, McFadden EP, Regar E et al. Late angiographic stent thrombosis (LAST) events with drug-eluting stents. J Am Coll Cardiol 2005;45:2088–92.

49. Eisenstein EL, Anstrom KJ, Kong DF et al. Clopidogrel use and long-term clinical outcomes after drug-eluting stent implantation. JAMA 2007;297:159–68.

50. Yusuf S, Zhao F, Mehta SR et al. Effects of clopidogrel in addition to aspirin in patients with acute coronary syndromes without ST-segment elevation. N Engl J Med 2001;345:494–502.

51. Berger PB, Bell MR, Hasdai D et al. Safety and efficacy of ticlopidine for only 2 weeks after successful intracoronary stent placement. Circulation 1999;99:248–53.

52. Barragan P, Bouvier JL, Roquebert PO et al. Resistance to thienopyridines: clinical detection of coronary stent thrombosis by monitoring of vasodilator-stimulated phosphoprotein phosphorylation. Catheter Cardiovasc Interv 2003;59:295–302.

53. Ajzenberg N, Aubry P, Huisse MG et al. Enhanced shear-induced platelet aggregation in patients who experience subacute stent thrombosis: a case-control study. J Am Coll Cardiol 2005;45:1753–6.

54. Gurbel PA, Bliden KP, Samara W et al. Clopidogrel effect on platelet reactivity in patients with stent thrombosis: results of the CREST study. J Am Coll Cardiol 2005;46:1827–32.

55. Wenaweser P, Dorffler-Melly J, Imboden K et al. Stent thrombosis is associated with an impaired response to antiplatelet therapy. J Am Coll Cardiol 2005;45:1748–52.

56. Grines CL, Bonow RO, Casey DE Jr et al. Prevention of premature discontinuation of dual antiplatelet therapy in patients with coronary artery stents: a science advisory from the American Heart Association, American College of Cardiology, Society for Cardiovascular Angiography and Interventions, American College of Surgeons, and American Dental Association, with representation from the American College of Physicians. Circulation 2007;115:813–18.

57. Angiolillo DJ, Shoemaker SB, Desai B et al. Randomized comparison of a high clopidogrel maintenance dose in patients with diabetes mellitus and coronary artery disease: results of the Optimizing Antiplatelet Therapy in Diabetes Mellitus (OPTIMUS) study. Circulation 2007;115:708–16.

58. Virmani R, Guagliumi G, Farb A et al. Localized hypersensitivity and late coronary thrombosis secondary to a sirolimus-eluting stent: Should we be cautious? Circulation 2004;109:701–5.

59. Nebeker JR, Virmani R, Bennett CL et al. Hypersensitivity cases associated with drug-eluting coronary stents: a review of available cases from the Research on Adverse Drug Events and Reports (RADAR) project. J Am Coll Cardiol 2006;47:175–81.

60. Collet JP, Montalescot G, Blanchet B et al. Impact of prior use or recent withdrawal of oral antiplatelet agents on acute coronary syndromes. Circulation 2004;110:2361–7.

61. Diener HC, Bogousslavsky J, Brass LM et al. Aspirin and clopidogrel compared with clopidogrel alone after recent ischaemic stroke or transient ischaemic attack in high-risk patients (MATCH): randomised, double-blind, placebo-controlled trial. Lancet 2004;364:331–7.

25

Bleeding complications: anticoagulant and antiplatelet therapy control

Ken Kozuma and Takaaki Isshiki

Introduction

Treatment of coronary artery disease is usually initiated with antithrombotic agents, since fatal coronary events are always associated with atherothrombosis. In addition, with the rapid progress in interventional cardiology, the importance of antiplatelet and anticoagulant agents is increasing. Percutaneous coronary intervention (PCI) necessarily damages the arterial wall and dislodges atherosclerotic plaques. Therefore, the use of antithrombotic drugs is essential to prevent thrombus formation. Heparin has been used as a basic agent. It has been demonstrated that underdosing of heparin lead to thrombotic complications during PCI.[1] Other anticoagulant therapy is mainly required when severe flow disturbance or turbulence exists in the heart, and is not necessary for atherosclerotic plaque. Specifically, valvular heart disease (including prosthetic valves), aortic graft disease, and atrial fibrillation are the common indications for anticoagulant therapy besides heparin, whereas antiplatelet therapy is more effective in reducing the complications of coronary artery disease.

The standard antiplatelet therapy for ischemic heart disease is aspirin. Clopidogrel has also become standard medication for acute coronary syndrome ACS and PCI with stenting. Glycoprotein (GP) IIb/IIIa receptor inhibitors are agents that decrease acute ischemic complications in patients with ACS and in those undergoing PCI. Although the use of antithrombotic agents is associated with reduced ischemic complications, it also increases the risk for bleeding and blood transfusion.[2,3]

Increased risk of bleeding is a major adverse effect of anticoagulant and antiplatelet therapy in the management of coronary artery disease. It has been reported that the rate of minor bleeding was 13% among patients undergoing PCI in the USA, with more than 5% requiring blood transfusion.[3,4] One of the major complications related to PCI is bleeding, since an arterial sheath is placed in the patient's groin (except for the transradial approach).

Bleeding complications are increasingly recognized as independent predictors of short- and longer-term mortality and therapies associated with reduced bleeding risk may improve survival. Therefore, balancing the competing risks of recurrent ischemia and bleeding has emerged as a key clinical issue. This chapter describes bleeding complications related to anticoagulant and antiplatelet therapy, mainly with PCI.

Types and classification of bleeding complications

Types of bleeding complications are listed in Table 25.1. Arterial access is inherently related to the risk of arterial bleeding at the puncture site. The incidence of hematoma in ACS patients is thought to be 4–5% in PCI. In the case of an asymptomatic simple groin hematoma, no treatment is usually necessary. In contrast, hematoma with hypotension or hemorrhagic shock can be a life-threatening event. Immediate aggressive compression of the puncture site with immediate volume expansion and transfusion may be required. A pseudoaneurysm is a new cavity between the artery and skin. It is formed by continuous bleeding and is recognized by physical examination as a sharp egg-shaped, pulsating beat with a systolic murmur. When it is smaller than 10 cm, it can usually be treated by prolonged repeated compression. The rare large pseudonaneurysm require surgical treatment. Retroperitoneal bleeding is a rare complication, but carries a high mortality. It is caused either by direct damage to the arteries induced by devices or by an inappropriately high puncture site. This complication may lead to the development of hemorrhagic shock, since bleeding can continue silently. An urgent computed tomography scan is useful for the diagnosis of retroperitoneal bleeding. Surgical treatment is usually needed. Cardiac tamponade is a relatively rare complication. This complication usually caused

Table 25.1 *Bleeding complications*

- Bleeding complications at the arterial puncture site during and after PCI:
  - Simple groin hematoma
  - Groin hematoma withhypotension or hemorrhagic shock
  - Pseudoaneurysm of the femoral artery
- Retroperitoneal bleeding
- Cardiac tamponade
- Intracranial bleeding
- Gastrointestinal bleeding
- Bleeding complications after cardiac surgery

by perforation by guidewires or dilatation catheters. Immediate pericardial drainage, stent graft, and/or cardiac surgery are needed for the stabilization. The risk of intracranial hemorrhage can occur in any setting of antithrombotic treatment for coronary artery disease. An elderly low-weight woman is a predictor for a high incidence of intracranial bleeding. Physicians have to be careful in using antithrombotic agents. Gastrointestinal bleeding is also not related to PCI procedures but rather to the antithrombotic therapy. When gastrointestinal bleeding occurs in patients with a recently implanted stent, physicians are faced with a difficult decision. There is always a dilemma whether to continue or discontinue antiplatelet therapy. This must be managed by an individual balance between the cardiac and gastrointestinal risks to the patient.

A wide variety of classifications have been used in clinical studies. In most studies, bleeding is categorized as major and minor. Various definitions such as hospitalization, requiring surgery or intervention, intracranial, or retroperitoneal were included or not included in the category of major bleeding, depending on the trial. Therefore, it sometimes seems difficult to compare the results of clinical trials with regard to the safety of the antithrombotic treatments. Among them, two classifications are commonly utilized[5] to assess bleeding severity; Thrombolysis in Myocardial Infarction (TIMI)[6] and Global Utilization of Streptokinase or Tissue Plasminogen Activator Outcomes (GUSTO)[7] (Table 25.2). Data from four multicenter randomized clinical trials of patients who had ACS ($n = 26\,452$) have been used to determine an association between bleeding severity as measured by the GUSTO scale and 30-day and 6-month mortality rates using Cox proportional hazards modelling that incorporated bleeding as a time-dependent covariate. There were stepwise increases in the adjusted hazards of 30-day mortality (mild bleeding, hazard ratio (HR) 1.6, 95% confidence interval (CI) 1.3–1.9; moderate bleeding, HR 2.7, 95% CI 2.3–3.4; severe bleeding, HR 10.6, 95% CI 8.3–13.6) and 6-month mortality (mild bleeding, HR 1.4, 95% CI 1.2–1.6; moderate bleeding, HR 2.1, 95% CI 1.8–2.4; severe bleeding, HR 7.5, 95% CI 6.1–9.3) as bleeding severity increased. A comparison has recently been made between the TIMI and GUSTO classifications.[5]

The TIMI classification is more popular, because the definition is clear using numerical changes in hemoglobin and hematocrit. However, the GUSTO classification takes blood transfusion as an important predictor for an adverse outcome. Combination of both scales may be appropriate for the assessment of bleeding complications.

Clinical impact of bleeding complications

The majority of bleeding events are not life-threatening. However, major hemorrhage is associated with the severity of worse clinical outcomes. In patients with ACS from the Global Registry of Acute Coronary Events (GRACE), mortality is significantly higher than in patients without major bleeding (18.6% vs 5.1%; $p < 0.001$) (Figure 25.1).[2] Therefore, it is absolutely imperative to reduce bleeding complication during PCI for patients' outcome. Transradial intervention is one of the solutions to this problem.[8] Arterial closure devices have been developed to relief patients' pain and the effort of manual compression at the vascular access site. However, meta-analyses have suggested an increased risk of access site complications when these devices are used.

What are the subgroups of patients who have an increased risk of bleeding complications? It has been reported that emergency patients are at increased risk,[9] particularly after thrombolysis. In addition, predictors for major bleeding have been demonstrated as being female, elderly, or of low body weight, use of heparin after the procedure, and renal insufficiency (Table 25.3).[2,10] A large observational study investigating over 10 000 patients who underwent PCI in the USA revealed the frequency and predictors of bleeding complications (Table 25.4). In this study, major bleeding according to the TIMI criteria occurred in 5.4% of the patients and minor bleeding in 12.7%.[3] A blood transfusion was required in 5.4%. Significant predictive factors for bleeding were intra-aortic balloon pumps, procedural hypotension, and renal insufficiency. Major bleeding was associated with higher in-hospital and 1-year mortality than no or minor bleeding. In patients who needed blood transfusion, 1-year mortality was higher than among patients without transfusion as well.[3,11]

Bleeding complications also affect length of hospital stay and financial costs. In the EPIC and IMPACT-II trials, minor bleeding prolonged the median length of stay by 1–2 days, whereas major bleeding prolonged it by 4 days.[12,13] Bleeding complications also result in additional costs, which may cancel the effects of reducing clinical events by the antithrombotic drugs.[14] For example, the REPLACE-2 study demonstrated that lower rates of bleeding seen with bivalirudin than with heparin plus a GPIIb/IIIa inhibitor reduced in-hospital costs by $405 per patient.[15] Economic assessment may vary among countries because of various financial systems for medical care and hospital stay.

Table 25.2	Classification of bleeding severity	
Classification	Severity	Criteria
TIMI[6]	Major	Intracranial bleeding
		Overt bleeding, with a decrease in hemoglobin ≥5 g/dl or decrease in hematocrit ≥15%
	Minor	Spontaneous gross hematoma
		Spontaneous hematemesis
		Observed bleeding, with decrease in hemoglobin ≥3 g/dl but <5 g/dl, or decrease in hematocrit ≥10%
		No observed bleeding, with decrease in hemoglobin ≥4 g/dl but <5 g/dl, or decrease in hematocrit ≥12%
	Minimal	Any blood loss insufficient to meet criteria listed above
GUSTO[7]	Severe	Intracranial bleeding or substantial hemodynamic compromise requiring treatment
	Moderate	Need for transfusion
	Mild	Bleeding that does not meet criteria for either severe or moderate bleeding

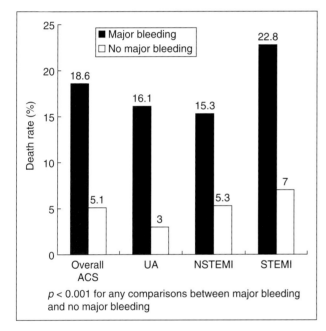

Figure 25.1
In-hospital death rates in patients who developed or did not develop major bleeding: results from the GRACE registry.[2] ACS, acute coronary syndrome; UA, unstable angina; STEMI, ST-segment-elevation myocardial infarction; NSTEMI, non-ST-segment elevation myocardial infarction.

Influence of anticoagulant and antiplatelet therapies on bleeding complications

Current antithrombotic therapy is mainly divided into two categories: thrombin inhibitors and antiplatelet drugs. Thrombin inhibitors also have two basic types: indirect thrombin inhibitors such as heparin and low-molecular-weight heparins (LMWH), which are unable to inhibit clot-bound thrombin, and direct thrombin inhibitors such as bivalirudin, lepirudin and argatroban. LMWHs were developed as fragments of unfractionated heparin (UFH) produced by chemical or enzymatic processes. More recently, direct thrombin inhibitors such as bivalirudin have been introduced into the clinical field. The effects of heparin, LMWH, and direct thrombin inhibitors have been demonstrated in many clinical fields. Antiplatelet agents are mainly categorized into aspirin, GPIIb/IIIa inhibitors, adenosine diphosphate (ADP) inhibitors, and others such as phosphodiesterase inhibitors.

The standard anticoagulant therapy in coronary artery disease is UFH. Heparin is the most common drug used during PCI, and in certain subgroups of patients the use of GPIIb/IIa has become standard. Aspirin is essentially given to all patients with coronary artery disease. Thienopyridines have usually been used for patients undergoing PCI. These medications are well supported by guidelines in order to avoid bleeding complications.

Heparin

Heparin is an essential agent for PCI, and its dose is adjusted by a monitoring of the activated clotting time (ACT). Bleeding complications with heparin are thought to be associated with excess dose.[16] However, the optimum ACT to prevent bleeding complications has not been established so far, since the anticoagulant effects vary from patient to patient. In general, 250–300 s or 300–350 s may be appropriate, depending on the device, according to ACC/AHA guidelines, although 200–250 s and 350–375 s are recommended in other studies. Important considerations for bleeding complications are patient-related factors such as renal failure, chronic alcohol abuse, and old age. In addition, timing of sheath removal is very important to prevent bleeding complication. An ACT of 150–180 s is advised for sheath removal.[10]

Table 25.3 *Factors significantly associated with major bleeding in all acute coronary syndrome patients (n=24 045): results from the GRACE registry*[2]

Variable	Adjusted odds ratio	95% confidence interval	*p*-value
Age (per 10-year increase)	1.28	1.21–1.37	<0.0001
Female sex	1.43	1.23–1.66	<0.0001
History of renal insufficiency	1.48	1.19–1.84	0.0004
History of bleeding	2.83	1.94–4.13	<0.0001
Mean arterial pressure (per 20 mmHg ↓)	1.11	1.04–1.19	0.0016
Diuretics	1.69	1.44–1.99	<0.0001
Low-molecular-weight heparin only	0.70	0.57–0.85	0.0003
Thrombolytics only	1.43	1.14–1.78	0.0017
GPIIb/IIIa inhibitors only	1.93	1.59–2.35	<0.0001
Thrombolytics and GPIIb/IIIa inhibitors	2.38	1.69–3.35	<0.0001
Intravenous inotropic agents	2.05	1.68–2.50	<0.0001
Other vasodilators	1.35	1.09–1.68	0.0068
Right heart catheterization	2.48	1.98–3.11	<0.0001
Percutaneous coronary intervention	1.63	1.36–1.94	<0.0001

LMWH has been shown to have lower rates of in-hospital mortality and major bleeding than UFH. The REDUCE trial has demonstrated a reduction is composite major adverse cardiovascular events (MACE: death, MI, and re-PCI) at 24 hours by using LMWH compared with UFH.[17] In the FRISC study, patients with ACS were randomized to LMWH or placebo. The LMWH group demonstrated a 63% reduction in death or MI.[18] Both trials were successful in showing short-term efficacy, but failed in the mid-term outcomes. Difficulty in anticoagulation monitoring is one of the major disadvantages of LMWH, since optimum dosing has not been established. Although anticoagulation monitoring is not possible during PCI, it has been demonstrated that LMWH has the potential to be at least as safe as intravenous UFH in terms of risk of bleeding complications.[19]

Oral anticoagulant treatment

Oral anticoagulant treatment (OAT) is intended to reduce the risk of thromboembolism in various clinical settings. In brief, routine OAT is not indicated for ischemic heart disease. Anticoagulation therapy is required in patients with atrial fibrillation, mechanical heart valves, previous thromboembolism, or other conditions. Addition of both aspirin and thienopiridines for patients with anticoagulation therapy (triple therapy) increases the risk of bleeding.[20,21] Especially related to the combination of antiplatelet therapy, a high mortality rate (approximately 30%) due to intracranial hemorrhage has been reported with OAT.[22] The optimum anticoagulation level for patients with aspirin and thienopyridines has not been established.

Direct thrombin inhibitors

Bivalirudin, lepirudin, desirudin, and argatroban are induced in this category. Bivalirudin has become one of the major antithrombotic agents used in patients undergoing PCI. It is associated with reduced bleeding risks, ischemic events, and costs.[23–26] In the REPLACE-2 trial, patients were randomized into two groups: bivalirudin with provisional GPIIb/IIIa inhibitors and heparin plus planned GPIIb/IIIa inhibitors.[27] MACE rates were not different between the two groups, but major bleeding rates within 30 days were lower in the bivalirudin group (2.4% vs 4.1%; *p* < 0.001). Major bleeding was a significant predictor of 1-year mortality in this trial. The PROTECT trial also demonstrated a reduction in the rates of minor bleeding and transfusion in the bivalirudin plus eptifibatide group compared with the heparin or enoxaparin group, although major bleeding was not different.[28] Furthermore, in the recent ACUITY trial, bivalirudin alone showed similar rates of ischemic events to heparin plus a GPIIb/IIIa inhibitor and significantly lower rates of bleeding (Figure 25.2).[29] Bivalirudin may improve the outcomes of patients undergoing PCI by reducing bleeding complications.[30]

Antiplatelet agents
Aspirin

Antiplatelet agents produce a hemostatic defect, which can increase the risk of mucocutaneous bleeding. The risk of major bleeding associated with antiplatelet agents is difficult to estimate, since the incidence is very low in

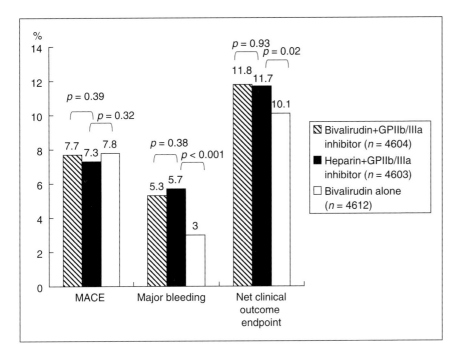

Figure 25.2
Clinical outcomes at 30 days: results from the ACUITY trial.[29] Bivalirudin plus a GPIIb/IIIa inhibitor and heparin plus a GPIIb/IIIa inhibitor were equivalent in terms of major adverse cardiovascular events (MACE: death, myocardial infarction, or unplanned revascularization for ischemia), major bleeding, and net clinical outcome (combination of composite ischemia or major bleeding). Bivalirudin alone demonstrated a lower incidence of major bleeding and net clinical outcome endpoint.

individual trials. The Antithrombotic Trialist's Collaboration performed a meta-analysis of 287 studies with 135 000 patients comparing antiplatelet therapy versus control. The overall rate of major bleeding was 1.13% in the antiplatelet therapy group, with an increase in risk of 1.6. The antithrombotic effect of aspirin due to inhibition of thromboxane A_2 is dose-independent in the range from 30 to 1300 mg. In contrast, gastroenteric toxicity due to the inhibition of cyclooxygenase (COX) and to direct chemical toxicity is dose-dependent. The risk of hospitalization for bleeding and/or gastroenteric perforations due to aspirin is similar to that of other antiplatelet agents and significantly higher than in the general population.[31] The benefit–risk ratio of antiplatelet agents therapy depends on the absolute risk of thrombotic and hemorrhagic events in individual patients. For example, antiplatelet therapy is beneficial for patients with a high risk of thrombotic events such as ACS, but is more harmful for patients with active gastrointestinal bleeding.

Thienopyridines

The thienopyridines, such as ticlopidine, plasgrel, and clopidogrel, are oral inhibitors of ADP-induced platelet aggregation. Intravenous ADP inhibitors are now under development. These medications are the standard regimen for patients with ACS, with or without PCI, and have potent effects in inhibiting platelet aggregation. Although clopidogrel alone is not closely associated with a high incidence of major bleeding,[32] the risk of major bleeding such as intracranial hemorrhage is relatively high in combination therapy with aspirin and anticoagulants.

GPIIb/IIIa inhibitors

GPIIb/IIIa inhibitors, such as abciximab, tirofiban, and eptifibatide, decrease ischemic events but may increase the risk of bleeding complications.[33,34] In a meta-analysis of randomized trials of abciximab as adjunctive therapy in PCI, the risk of major bleeding was higher than in the control group (odds ratio 1.89). An adjusted heparin dosage (70 U/kg) without maintenance infusion reduced the bleeding risk equivalent to the risk of heparin infusion alone.[35,36] Another meta-analysis of abciximab in ST-elevation MI has shown a reduction of mortality in the short and long term without increasing the risk of major bleeding in patients undergoing PCI.[37] The current recommended target ACT for GPIIb/IIIa inhibitors is <300 s.[38] Modifications, including reduced dosing, weight-adjusted heparin, and avoidance of postprocedural heparin, have improved the rates of bleeding complications (Table 25.5).

Implications and treatment of bleeding complications

Once bleeding complications occur, active efforts should be made to identify the cause of bleeding and to achieve hemostasis. Then treatment of the bleeding source as soon as possible is essential. Access site bleeding, intracranial hemorrhage, gross hematuria and gastrointestinal bleeding are major manifestations of bleeding complications. If ACT is prolonged, heparin or LMWH should be stopped and may be reversed by protamine. However, antithrombotic

Table 25.4 *Multivariate analysis for bleeding and transfusion predictors*[a]

Predictive variable	Odds ratio	95% confidence interval	p-value
Major bleeding predictors			
Intra-aortic balloon pump (any)	3.0	2.2–4.1	0.0001
Procedural hypotension	2.9	2.0–4.3	0.0001
Age:[a]			
>80 years	1.9	1.4–2.7	0.0001
70–80 years	1.6	1.2–2.0	0.0002
Abciximab	1.8	1.2–2.6	0.003
Chronic renal insufficiency	1.5	1.1–1.9	0.002
Systemic hypertension history	1.3	1.0–1.6	0.032
Transfusion predictors			
Retroperitoneal bleeding	9.6	3.4–26.7	0.0001
Gastrointestinal bleeding	8.2	4.9–13.5	0.0001
Hematoma	3.6	2.8–4.6	0.0001
Age ≥80 years	1.8	1.3–2.4	0.0001
Recurrent typical chest pain	1.4	1.0–1.8	0.045
Hematocrit nadir	0.6	0.5–0.7	0.0001

[a]Odds ratio was calculated comparing with patients <50 years old.

Table 25.5 *Major bleeding complications in large trials of GPIIb/IIIa inhibitors*

Study	Year	GPIIb/IIIa inhibitor	Major bleeding
EPIC	1994	Abciximab ($n = 708$)	14%
IMPACT-II	1997	Eptifibatide ($n = 2682$)	5.1%
RESTORE	1997	Tirofiban ($n = 1071$)	5.3%
CAPTURE	1997	Abciximab ($n = 630$)	3.8%
EPILOG	1997	Abciximab standard-dose ($n = 935$)	3.5%
		Abciximab low-dose ($n = 918$)	2.0%
EPISTENT	1998	Abciximab ($n = 1590$)	1.5%
ISAR-2	2000	Abciximab ($n = 201$)	3.5%
ESPRIT	2000	Eptifibatide ($n = 1040$)	1.3%
ADMIRAL	2001	Abciximab ($n = 151$)	0.7%
CADILLAC	2002	Abciximab ($n = 528$)	0.6%
TARGET	2002	Abciximab ($n = 2411$)	0.8%
		Tirofiban ($n = 2398$)	0.9%
PROTECT–TIMI-30	2006	Eptifibatide ($n = 527$)	3.2%

agents such as bivalirudin and GP IIb/IIIa inhibitors do not have any specific antidotes.

The occurrence of bleeding complications may lead to a series of events that put the patient at an increased risk of death. Among these, cessation of antithrombotic therapy, in particular antiplatelet agents, potentially leading to an increased risk of thrombosis, plays a key role.

Other consequences of bleeding include hypotension, anemia, and reduction in oxygen delivery. Despite the potential risks, antithrombotic therapy should be discontinued if bleeding leads to hypotension or if bleeding is vigorous. This should be followed by hemodynamic support with fluid repletion and vasopressor therapy as necessary. All of these actions, however, set the patient at risk for recurrent ischemia and myocardial infarction. Once anemia occurs as a result of bleeding, the patient continues to be at risk.

Anemia has several effects on the myocardium. Mild-to-moderate anemia (hemoglobin 7.0–10.0 g/dL) leads to increased cardiac output, primarily through reduced blood viscosity leading to reduced afterload. Under these conditions, myocardial oxygen demand does not change. The myocardium has a high oxygen-extraction ratio, however, and can augment oxygen delivery only by increasing coronary blood flow. Such an increase may not be possible in patients with fixed coronary artery stenoses. In the normal healthy heart, oxygen consumption and oxygen extraction are relatively constant at hematocrit levels between 20–60%. There are considerable experimental data suggesting that a hemoglobin level of 7 g/dL is tolerated without myocardial ischemia if there is no obstructive coronary artery disease. With coronary artery obstruction, however, ischemia can occur with even mild anemia in experimental studies. One target for therapy, therefore, is to raise hemoglobin levels in order to augment oxygen delivery. This can be achieved by erythropoietin and red blood cell (RBC) transfusion. There is no data, however, on the use of erythropoietin for acute anemia that occurs in the setting of PCI patients. RBC transfusion is the most readily available method to increase hematocrit in anemic patients.

Because reduced blood volume and reduced oxygen delivery can lead to myocardial ischemia in patients with obstructive coronary artery disease, it is commonly believed that these patients require higher hemoglobin levels in order to prevent adverse events. While clinical studies suggest that raising hemoglobin levels via transfusion increases oxygen delivery, studies also show that measures of tissue oxygenation either decrease or do not change. The reason for this paradox (greater oxygen delivery but no improvement in tissue use) is unclear, but alterations in erythrocyte nitric oxide biology in stored blood may provide a partial explanation. Nitric oxide (NO), a gas essential to oxygen exchange, is depleted in stored RBCs, which may cause them to function as NO 'sinks,' leading to vasoconstriction and platelet aggregation. Of note, transfusion has been associated with increased mortality and myocardial infarction. According to the American College of Physicians guidelines, routine transfusion should be avoided until the hematocrit falls below 21%. If the platelet count is lower than 100 000/mm3, platelet transfusion should be considered.

Given the prognostic implications of bleeding and the adverse effects associated with potential treatment strategies (e.g. transfusions), the best therapeutic strategy is "prevention" of bleeding complications. Prevention of bleeding complications is also most cost efficient. Particular attention should be given to those patients at high risk of bleeding, such as the elderly and patients with renal insufficiency. Tailoring antithrombotic medications according to an individual's thrombotic/bleeding risk should be implemented. Development of new drugs that provide reliable antithrombotic effects (reducing ischemic risk) while simultaneously reducing bleeding may provide important advances in management of PCI/ACS patients.

Conclusions

Bleeding complications associated with antithrombotic therapy have a major impact on patient outcome, especially in the setting of ACS. The TIMI and GUSTO criteria are current standard definitions in several studies. However, a broader standard definition including any significant bleeding may be needed for comparisons of the safety of antithrombotic agents. Contemporary antithrombotic medications such as GPIIb/IIIa inhibitors tend to increase the risk of bleeding complications. Direct thrombin inhibitors such as bivalirudin may be an alternative medication to the combication of heparin and GPIIb/IIIa inhibitors.

It is nevertheless important for physicians to perceive bleeding complications as having a serious impact on patient outcomes and to make the best possible effort for their prevention. The most important criteria is that the benefit of an antithrombotic therapy should exceed the risk of bleeding complications due to that therapy.

References

1. Chew DP, Bhatt DL, Lincoff AM et al. Defining the optimal activated clotting time during percutaneous coronary intervention: aggregate results from 6 randomized, controlled trials. Circulation 2001;103:961–6.
2. Moscucci M, Fox KA, Cannon CP et al. Predictors of major bleeding in acute coronary syndromes: the Global Registry of Acute Coronary Events (GRACE). Eur Heart J 2003;24:1815–23.
3. Kinnaird TD, Stabile E, Mintz GS et al. Incidence, predictors, and prognostic implications of bleeding and blood transfusion following percutaneous coronary interventions. Am J Cardiol 2003;92:930–5.
4. Lauer MA, Karweit JA, Cascade EF et al. Practice patterns and outcomes of percutaneous coronary interventions in the United States: 1995 to 1997. Am J Cardiol 2002;89:924–9.
5. Rao SV, O'Grady K, Pieper KS et al. A comparison of the clinical impact of bleeding measured by two different classifications among patients with acute coronary syndromes. J Am Coll Cardiol 2006;47:809–16.
6. Rao AK, Pratt C, Berke A et al. Thrombolysis in Myocardial Infarction (TIMI) trial – phase I: hemorrhagic manifestations and changes in plasma fibrinogen and the fibrinolytic system in patients treated with recombinant tissue plasminogen activator and streptokinase. J Am Coll Cardiol 1988;11:1–11.
7. Berkowitz SD, Granger CB, Pieper KS et al. Incidence and predictors of bleeding after contemporary thrombolytic therapy for myocardial infarction. The Global Utilization of Streptokinase and Tissue Plasminogen activator for Occluded coronary arteries (GUSTO) I Investigators. Circulation 1997;95:2508–16.
8. Louvard Y, Benamer H, Garot P et al. Comparison of transradial and transfemoral approaches for coronary angiography and angioplasty in octogenarians (the OCTOPLUS study). Am J Cardiol 2004;94:1177–80.
9. Al-Mallah M, Bazari RN, Jankowski M et al. Predictors and outcomes associated with gastrointestinal bleeding in patients with acute coronary syndromes. J Thromb Thrombolysis 2007;23:51–5.
10. Smith SC Jr, Dove JT, Jacobs AK et al. ACC/AHA guidelines for percutaneous coronary intervention (revision of the 1993 PTCA guidelines) – executive summary: a report of the American College of Cardiology/ American Heart Association Task Force on Practice Guidelines (Committee to Revise the 1993 Guidelines for Percutaneous Transluminal Coronary Angioplasty) endorsed by the Society for Cardiac Angiography and Interventions. Circulation 2001;103:3019–41.
11. Rao SV, Jollis JG, Harrington RA et al. Relationship of blood transfusion and clinical outcomes in patients with acute coronary syndromes. JAMA 2004;292:1555–62.
12. Blankenship JC, Hellkamp AS, Aguirre FV et al. Vascular access site complications after percutaneous coronary intervention with abciximab in the Evaluation of c7E3 for the Prevention of Ischemic Complications (EPIC) trial. Am J Cardiol 1998;81:36–40.
13. Mandak JS, Blankenship JC, Gardner LH et al. Modifiable risk factors for vascular access site complications in the IMPACT II trial of angioplasty with versus without eptifibatide. Integrilin to Minimize Platelet Aggregation and Coronary Thrombosis. J Am Coll Cardiol 1998;31:1518–24.

14. Mark DB, Talley JD, Topol EJ et al. Economic assessment of platelet glycoprotein IIb/IIIa inhibition for prevention of ischemic complications of high-risk coronary angioplasty. EPIC Investigators. Circulation 1996;94:629–35.

15. Cohen DJ, Lincoff AM, Lavelle TA et al. Economic evaluation of bivalirudin with provisional glycoprotein IIB/IIIA inhibition versus heparin with routine glycoprotein IIB/IIIA inhibition for percutaneous coronary intervention: results from the REPLACE-2 trial. J Am Coll Cardiol 2004;44:1792–800.

16. Brener SJ, Moliterno DJ, Lincoff AM et al. Relationship between activated clotting time and ischemic or hemorrhagic complications: analysis of 4 recent randomized clinical trials of percutaneous coronary intervention. Circulation 2004;110:994–8.

17. Karsch KR, Preisack MB, Baildon R et al. Low molecular weight heparin (reviparin) in percutaneous transluminal coronary angioplasty. Results of a randomized, double-blind, unfractionated heparin and placebo-controlled, multicenter trial (REDUCE trial). Reduction of Restenosis After PTCA, Early Administration of Reviparin in a Double-Blind Unfractionated Heparin and Placebo-Controlled Evaluation. J Am Coll Cardiol 1996;28:1437–43.

18. Fragmin during Instability in Coronary Artery Disease (FRISC) Study Group. Low-molecular-weight heparin during instability in coronary artery disease. Lancet 1996;347:561–8.

19. Borentain M, Montalescot G, Bouzamondo A et al. Low-molecular-weight heparin vs. unfractionated heparin in percutaneous coronary intervention: a combined analysis. Catheter Cardiovasc Interv 2005;65:212–21.

20. Karjalainen PP, Porela P, Ylitalo A et al. Safety and efficacy of combined antiplatelet-warfarin therapy after coronary stenting. Eur Heart J 2007;28:726–32.

21. Hart RG, Tonarelli SB, Pearce LA. Avoiding central nervous system bleeding during antithrombotic therapy: recent data and ideas. Stroke 2005;36:1588–93.

22. Cantalapiedra A, Gutierrez O, Tortosa JI et al. Oral anticoagulant treatment: risk factors involved in 500 intracranial hemorrhages. J Thromb Thrombolysis 2006;22:113–20.

23. Bittl JA, Strony J, Brinker JA et al. Treatment with bivalirudin (Hirulog) as compared with heparin during coronary angioplasty for unstable or postinfarction angina. Hirulog Angioplasty Study Investigators. N Engl J Med 1995;333:764–9.

24. Bittl JA, Chaitman BR, Feit F et al. Bivalirudin versus heparin during coronary angioplasty for unstable or postinfarction angina: final report reanalysis of the Bivalirudin Angioplasty Study. Am Heart J 2001;142:952–9.

25. Direct Thrombin Inhibitor Trialists' Collaborative Group. Direct thrombin inhibitors in acute coronary syndromes: principal results of a meta-analysis based on individual patients' data. Lancet 2002;359:294–302.

26. Milkovich G, Gibson G. Economic impact of bleeding complications and the role of antithrombotic therapies in percutaneous coronary intervention. Am J Health Syst Pharm 2003;60(14 Suppl 3): S15–21.

27. Lincoff AM, Bittl JA, Harrington RA et al. Bivalirudin and provisional glycoprotein IIb/IIIa blockade compared with heparin and planned glycoprotein IIb/IIIa blockade during percutaneous coronary intervention: REPLACE-2 randomized trial. JAMA 2003; 289:853–63.

28. Gibson CM, Morrow DA, Murphy SA et al. A randomized trial to evaluate the relative protection against post-percutaneous coronary intervention microvascular dysfunction, ischemia, and inflammation among antiplatelet and antithrombotic agents: the PROTECT–TIMI-30 trial. J Am Coll Cardiol 2006;47:2364–73.

29. Stone GW, McLaurin BT, Cox DA et al. Bivalirudin for patients with acute coronary syndromes. N Engl J Med 2006;355:2203–16.

30. Manoukian SV, Feit F, Mehran R et al. Impact of major bleeding on 30-day mortality and clinical outcomes in patients with acute coronary syndromes: an analysis from the ACUITY Trial. J Am Coll Cardiol 2007;49:1362–8.

31. Garcia Rodriguez LA, Cattaruzzi C, Troncon MG et al. Risk of hospitalization for upper gastrointestinal tract bleeding associated with ketorolac, other nonsteroidal anti-inflammatory drugs, calcium antagonists, and other antihypertensive drugs. Arch Intern Med 1998;158:33–9.

32. Cay S, Yilmaz MB, Korkmaz S. Intracranial bleeding associated with clopidogrel. Cardiovasc Drugs Ther 2005;19:157–8.

33. Blankenship JC. Bleeding complications of glycoprotein IIb–IIIa receptor inhibitors. Am Heart J 1999;138:287–96.

34. Cho L, Topol EJ, Balog C et al. Clinical benefit of glycoprotein IIb/IIIa blockade with abciximab is independent of gender: pooled analysis from EPIC, EPILOG and EPISTENT trials. Evaluation of 7E3 for the Prevention of Ischemic Complications. Evaluation in Percutaneous Transluminal Coronary Angioplasty to Improve Long-Term Outcome with Abciximab GP IIb/IIIa blockade. Evaluation of Platelet IIb/IIIa Inhibitor for Stent. J Am Coll Cardiol 2000;36:381–6.

35. The EPILOG Investigators. Platelet glycoprotein IIb/IIIa receptor blockade and low-dose heparin during percutaneous coronary revascularization. N Engl J Med 1997;336:1689–96.

36. de Queiroz Fernandes Araujo JO, Veloso HH, Braga De Paiva JM et al. Efficacy and safety of abciximab on acute myocardial infarction treated with percutaneous coronary interventions: a meta-analysis of randomized, controlled trials. Am Heart J 2004;148:937–43.

37. De Luca G, Suryapranata H, Stone GW et al. Abciximab as adjunctive therapy to reperfusion in acute ST-segment elevation myocardial infarction: a meta-analysis of randomized trials. JAMA 2005;293: 1759–65.

38. Lincoff AM, Tcheng JE, Califf RM et al. Standard versus low-dose weight-adjusted heparin in patients treated with the platelet glycoprotein IIb/IIIa receptor antibody fragment abciximab (c7E3 Fab) during percutaneous coronary revascularization. PROLOG Investigators. Am J Cardiol 1997;79:286–91.

26

Heparin-induced thrombocytopenia: etiopathogenesis, clinical presentation, and management

Theodore E Warkentin

Overview

Heparin-induced thrombocytopenia (HIT) is a common adverse event in certain patient populations, especially postoperative patients receiving thromboprophylaxis with unfractionated heparin (UFH) for 1–2 weeks.[1,2] Although HIT is an immune disorder, it has certain atypical features, such as the transient formation of antibodies that recognize a 'self' protein – platelet factor 4 (PF4) – bound to heparin.[3] Indeed, this lack of immunologic 'memory' permits safe re-exposure to heparin even in a patient with a history of HIT, for indications such as cardiac surgery.[4] The clinical importance of HIT results from its strong association with thrombosis, both venous and arterial.[5] Although HIT is not a rare condition, an emerging issue is *over*diagnosis of HIT, particularly since certain widely used tests will detect both pathogenic and non-pathogenic antibodies.[6] HIT is also a potentially preventable disease: the risk of HIT is lower with low-molecular-weight heparin (LMWH) compared with UFH.[1,2]

Definition

HIT can be defined as any event, most often thrombocytopenia with or without thrombosis, in which the presence of platelet-activating, anti-PF4/heparin antibodies of immunoglobulin G (IgG) class can be implicated. HIT is a *clinicopathologic syndrome*, since both clinical and laboratory features are important (Figure 26.1).

HIT and the cardiologist

Both UFH and LMWH are commonly prescribed by cardiologists (see Chapter 15). Typical uses include thrombosis prevention (or extension) in medical patients (acute coronary syndrome (ACS), ST-elevation myocardial infarction

(STEMI), congestive heart failure (CHF), and acute atrial fibrillation) or surgical patients (post-cardiac surgery and post-ventricular assist device insertion) or during invasive procedures (cardiac catheterization or percutaneous coronary intervention (PCI)). UFH is also the mainstay of intraoperative anticoagulation during cardiac surgery, both 'on-pump' and 'off-pump'. However, to what extent any particular cardiologist will encounter HIT depends upon the type of practice. For example, a cardiologist involved in the postoperative management of cardiac surgery patients will encounter HIT, especially if UFH thromboprophylaxis is employed. But a cardiologist who only gives heparin briefly for invasive procedures, or who predominantly uses LMWH for medical thromboprophylaxis, will rarely encounter HIT.

Etiopathogenesis

HIT results when antibodies of IgG class are formed that recognize multimolecular complexes of PF4 and heparin on platelet surfaces, and that are able to activate platelets. In vivo platelet activation leads to a marked increase in thrombin generation. The concurrence of increased thrombin generation and increased risk of venous and arterial thrombosis classifies HIT as an *acquired hypercoagulability disorder*. Figure 26.2 summarizes HIT pathogenesis.[7]

Platelet factor 4/heparin complexes

Amiral et al[8] discovered that HIT antibodies recognize PF4 bound to heparin. PF4 is a 70-amino-acid (7780 Da) member of the C-X-C subfamily of chemokines, and is found in platelet α-granules and on endothelial cells. Four PF4 molecules self-associate to form compact tetramers of globular structure (about 31 000 Da). PF4 is rich in the basic amino acids

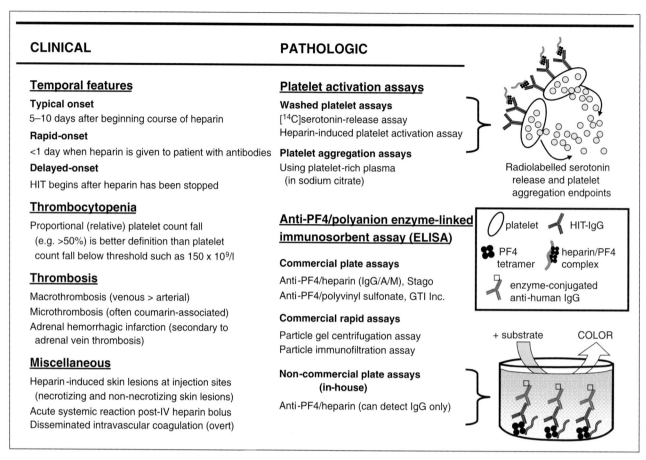

CLINICAL

Temporal features

Typical onset
5–10 days after beginning course of heparin

Rapid-onset
<1 day when heparin is given to patient with antibodies

Delayed-onset
HIT begins after heparin has been stopped

Thrombocytopenia
Proportional (relative) platelet count fall
(e.g. >50%) is better definition than platelet
count fall below threshold such as 150 x 10⁹/l

Thrombosis
Macrothrombosis (venous > arterial)
Microthrombosis (often coumarin-associated)
Adrenal hemorrhagic infarction (secondary to
adrenal vein thrombosis)

Miscellaneous
Heparin-induced skin lesions at injection sites
(necrotizing and non-necrotizing skin lesions)
Acute systemic reaction post-IV heparin bolus
Disseminated intravascular coagulation (overt)

PATHOLOGIC

Platelet activation assays

Washed platelet assays
[^{14}C]serotonin-release assay
Heparin-induced platelet activation assay

Platelet aggregation assays
Using platelet-rich plasma
(in sodium citrate)

Radiolabelled serotonin
release and platelet
aggregation endpoints

Anti-PF4/polyanion enzyme-linked immunosorbent assay (ELISA)

Commercial plate assays
Anti-PF4/heparin (IgG/A/M), Stago
Anti-PF4/polyvinyl sulfonate, GTI Inc.

Commercial rapid assays
Particle gel centrifugation assay
Particle immunofiltration assay

**Non-commercial plate assays
(in-house)**
Anti-PF4/heparin (can detect IgG only)

platelet   HIT-IgG
PF4   heparin/PF4
tetramer   complex
enzyme-conjugated
anti-human IgG

+ substrate   COLOR

Figure 26.1
HIT is a clinicopathologic syndrome. The left column lists the main clinical features of HIT. The right column lists various assays used to detect HIT antibodies. At least one clinical feature, together with detection of HIT antibodies, characterizes a patient with HIT.

lysine and arginine, which form a 'ring of positive charge' to which heparin binds, forming ultralarge PF4/heparin complexes, particularly with UFH.[9] HIT antigens are formed maximally when the molar ratio of PF4 to heparin is about 1:1 to 2:1.

The immune response against PF4/heparin complexes is polyspecific, as several neoepitopes are formed. Only some of these antibodies are *pathogenic*, i.e., they are of IgG class and are present in sufficient titer and with sufficient affinity for certain epitopes on PF4/heparin so as to effect platelet activation. Since HIT neoepitopes are on PF4 (not heparin), HIT can be considered an 'autoimmune' disorder. PF4 can also bind to platelets via platelet surface glycosaminoglycans such as chondroitin sulfate,[10] possibly explaining why HIT sometimes occurs a few days after heparin has been stopped ('delayed-onset HIT').[11]

IgG-induced platelet activation

PF4/heparin complexes bind to platelets by the negative charge of the polysulfated heparin. When IgG antibodies

bind to these complexes, the resulting PF4/heparin/IgG immune complexes bind to platelet FcγIIa receptors, leading to FcγIIa receptor clustering and resulting strong platelet activation, including the formation of procoagulant, platelet-derived microparticles.[12]

Only antibodies of IgG class can activate platelets. Nevertheless, anti-PF4/heparin antibodies of IgA and IgM class are frequently generated in patients who receive heparin. The detection of these non-pathogenic antibodies by commercial anti-PF4/heparin immunoassays is one reason why these assays lack high diagnostic specificity.[6]

Atypical immune response

There are several unusual aspects to HIT immunopathogenesis. As mentioned, HIT antibodies are transient, and become undetectable within a few weeks or months.[3] Further, HIT antibodies are usually not restimulated when a patient with previous HIT is re-exposed to heparin and, if antibodies are regenerated, they are not formed more quickly than 5 days following reexposure.[3] Also puzzling is

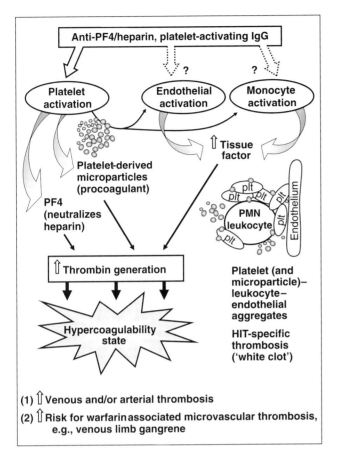

Figure 26.2
Pathogenesis of HIT: a central role for thrombin generation. The figure illustrates two explanations for thrombosis in HIT. (1) Activation of platelets (plt) by anti-platelet factor 4 (PF4)/heparin IgG antibodies (HIT antibodies), leading to formation of procoagulant, platelet-derived microparticles, and neutralization of heparin by PF4 released from activated platelets, leads to marked increase in thrombin ('hypercoagulability state') characterized by an increased risk of venous and arterial thrombosis, as well as an increased risk for coumarin-induced venous limb gangrene. (2) However, it is also possible that unique pathogenic mechanisms operative in HIT explain unusual thromboses, such as arterial 'white clots'. For example, HIT antibodies have been shown to activate endothelium and monocytes (leading to cell surface tissue factor expression), although this stimulation may be largely 'indirect' through poorly defined mechanisms involving platelet activation and, possibly, formation of platelet-derived microparticles. Further, aggregates of platelets and polymorphonuclear (PMN) leukocytes have been described in HIT. To what extent these cooperative interactions between platelets, platelet-derived microparticles, PMN leukocytes, monocytes, and endothelium lead to arterial (or venous) thrombotic events in HIT, either in large or small vessels, remains unclear. (From Warkentin TE.[7] with permission.)

the very fast onset of HIT, which can begin as early as five days after starting heparin, even for the first time.[3]

Hypercoagulability disorder

Thrombin–antithrombin complexes (a marker of in vivo thrombin generation) are greatly elevated in many patients with HIT.[13,14] In vivo activation of platelets, endothelium, and perhaps even monocytes, helps to explain these pro-thrombotic effects of HIT antibodies.[7]

Laboratory testing for HIT antibodies

There are two classes of assays to detect HIT antibodies: (a) platelet activation assays, and (b) PF4-dependent antigen assays (immunoassays).[15]

Platelet activation assays

Beginning in the 1970s, HIT antibodies were first detected based upon their ability to cause heparin-dependent activation and aggregation of normal donor platelets, using conventional platelet aggregometry. However, this method has limited sensitivity, and can yield false-positive results, especially when testing plasma from critically ill patients. Moreover, it allows only a few tests to be performed at any one time, limiting the number of control conditions that can be studied, thereby compromising test specificity. These assays are now infrequently performed.

In 1986, the platelet [14C]serotonin-release assay (SRA) was developed (Figure 26.1). This test uses 'washed' platelets from normal donors resuspended in divalent cation-containing buffer, and detects HIT antibodies by measuring release of radiolabelled serotonin (which is taken up into platelet-dense granules) induced by patient serum under various conditions. Selection of suitable platelet donors, and using a variety of control conditions, maximizes test sensitivity and specificity. Further enhancement of test specificity is achieved by studying several control maneuvers simultaneously in the microtiter plates. This SRA is considered the 'gold standard' for detecting clinically relevant platelet-activating, anti-PF4/heparin antibodies, and has superior operating characteristics (sensitivity-specificity tradeoff) compared with enzyme-linked immunosorbent assays (ELISAs).[6,16] Similar washed platelet assays that utilize non-radioactive platelet activation endpoints, such as platelet aggregation, are available in Europe. Washed platelet activation assays are technically demanding, and are performed by relatively few laboratories.

PF4/heparin ELISA

Two commercially available ELISAs are available that detect antibodies reactive against PF4/polyanion complexes.[15]

These detect the three major immunoglobulin classes (IgG, IgM, and IgA) against PF4 bound either to heparin (Asserachrom, Stago, France) or to polyvinyl sulfonate (GTI, Brookfield, WI). In-house anti-PF4/heparin ELISAs that only detect antibodies of IgG class have been described[6] (Figure 26.1).

Rapid immunoassays

Two rapid assays for HIT have been developed.[15] One – the particle gel immunoassay – utilizes PF4/heparin complexes bound to red, high-density polystyrene beads; after addition of patient serum or plasma, the anti-PF4/heparin antibodies bind to the antigen-coated beads. A secondary anti-human immunoglobulin antibody is added into the sephacryl gel to facilitate particle agglutination. The principle of this (and other gel centrifugation assays) is that upon centrifugation, the agglutinated beads (indicating the presence of anti-PF4/heparin antibodies) do not migrate through the sephacryl gel, whereas non-agglutinated beads (indicating absence of antibodies) pass through the gel, thus forming a red band at the bottom. This method is available to blood banks that utilize a gel centrifugation technology system. Currently, the particle gel immunoassay is available in Europe and Canada, and is under active investigation in the USA.

Another rapid immunoassay, the HealthTEST Heparin/Platelet factor 4 Antibody Assay (Akers Laboratories, Inc., Thorofare, NJ) received approval by the US Food and Drug Administration (FDA) for use in detecting anti-PF4/heparin antibodies. This assay utilizes a system known as Particle ImmunoFiltration Assay (PIFA), wherein patient serum is added to a reaction well containing dyed particles coated with PF4. Subsequently, non-agglutinated – but not agglutinated – particles – will migrate through the membrane filter. Thus, a negative test is shown by a blue color in the result well, whereas no color indicates a positive test. FDA approval was granted based upon the assay being judged by the FDA as substantially equivalent to the commercial ELISA from GTI Inc. The operating characteristics of the PIFA are poor.[16a]

Iceberg model

The 'iceberg model'[1,17] provides a conceptual framework for understanding the relationship between seroconversion and clinical events (Figure 26.3). For example, only a subset of anti-PF4/heparin IgG antibodies have platelet-activating properties, and only those antibodies with platelet-activating properties have the potential to cause HIT. Further, a high risk of thrombosis is seen among antibody-positive patients who develop thrombocytopenia, rather than among antibody-positive patients without a significant fall in platelet count.

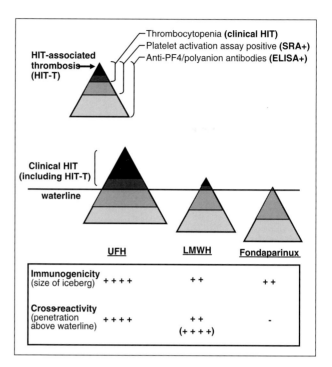

Figure 26.3
Iceberg model of HIT. The top schematic 'iceberg' shows the relationship between HIT antibodies detected by antigen assay (PF4/polyanion enzyme-linked immunosorbent assay: ELISA), washed platelet activation assay (serotonin-release assay: SRA), thrombocytopenia, and HIT-associated thrombosis. Although the antigen assay is more sensitive for detecting HIT antibodies, it is less specific for clinical HIT than the washed platelet activation assay. The bottom schematic icebergs illustrate relative risks of antibody formation and clinical HIT for three anticoagulant polysaccharides: unfractionated heparin (UFH), low-molecular-weight heparin (LMWH), and fondaparinux. Note that the reduction in risk of HIT with fondaparinux is theoretical, and has not been established through clinical trials. The data also suggest a *dissociation* in immunogenicity and cross-reactivity between these sulfated polysaccharides. UFH is most immunogenic (largest iceberg), whereas LMWH and fondaparinux exhibit similar immunogenicity. However, in contrast to UFH and LMWH, which can form well the antigens recognized by HIT antibodies, fondaparinux only poorly forms antigens with PF4 in vitro that are recognized by HIT antibodies. Note that LMWH is indicated by ++ and ++++ to indicate that its cross-reactivity appears to differ in vivo (++) and in vitro (++++). From Warkentin TE.[17] with permission.

Diagnostic interpretation

Tests vary in their sensitivity and specificity for detecting clinically significant HIT antibodies. In general, platelet activation assays using washed platelets have high sensitivity and specificity for clinical HIT. PF4/polyanion antigen assays also have high sensitivity, but lower specificity compared with platelet activation assays. For both classes of test, diagnostic specificity is higher when there is a 'strong' positive test result, for example serotonin release >80% (platelet activation assay) or >1.5 absorbance units (ELISA). In our view, the combination of two negative complementary assays (washed platelet activation assay and antigen assay) essentially rules out HIT.

Clinical presentations

The clinical picture of HIT is dominated by two features: thrombocytopenia and thrombosis.

Thrombocytopenia

Definition and severity of thrombocytopenia

Thrombocytopenia, defined as a 50% or greater fall in the platelet count, is the most common clinical manifestation of HIT, and occurs in at least 90% of patients. For surgical patients, the peak postoperative platelet count – not the preoperative platelet count – is the appropriate platelet count 'baseline'.[2]

For 90% of patients with HIT, the platelet count nadir falls between 15 and $150 \times 10^9/l$. The median platelet count nadir is about $60 \times 10^9/l$.[5,18] Especially in postoperative patients who develop thrombocytopenia, HIT can result in a large proportional fall in platelet count that may not decline to less than $150 \times 10^9/l$.[3]

Timing of thrombocytopenia

In 70% of patients, HIT is recognized based upon a fall in platelet count that occurs 5–10 days after starting heparin (first day of heparin = day 0).[3] This is called *typical-onset HIT*. In about 25–30% of patients, HIT is recognized because the platelet count falls occurs abruptly within 24 hours of starting heparin, or after increasing the dose of heparin. Such *rapid-onset* HIT[3] results when heparin is given to a patient who already has circulating HIT antibodies because of a very recent immunizing exposure to heparin, usually within the past few weeks. Rarely (<5%), HIT is characterized by a fall in the platelet count that begins several days *after* heparin has been stopped (*delayed-onset HIT*).[11]

Some exposures to heparin are more immunogenic than others. Consider a patient who receives small doses of UFH during heart catheterization, and who then undergoes cardiac surgery 4 days later. It is far more likely for HIT to occur 5–10 days after the surgery, and not 5–10 days after the preceding heart catheterization. This is because UFH administered during cardiac surgery is a highly immunogenic scenario. Figure 26.4(a) illustrates the typical temporal profile of HIT following cardiac surgery.[19]

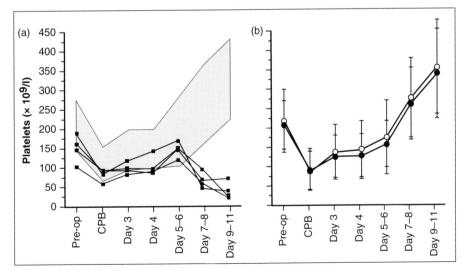

Figure 26.4
HIT and anti-PF4/heparin antibodies in a post-cardiac surgery population. (a) The shaded area indicates the median (± 2 SD) platelet count range in patients who tested negative for HIT antibodies. HIT is indicated by a platelet count fall that begins on or after day 5 of cardiac surgery. (b) Open circles and closed circles indicate the mean platelet counts of patients testing negative and positive, respectively, for anti-PF4/heparin antibodies. Pre-op, preoperative; CPB, cardiopulmonary bypass. (From Pouplard C, et al.[19] with permission.)

HIT-Associated thrombosis

Many – if not most – patients recognized with HIT develop thrombotic complications associated with their episode of HIT, often as their presenting feature.[18] Among the remaining patients recognized with 'isolated HIT' (i.e., thrombocytopenia without thrombosis), about half develop thrombosis during follow-up. HIT is strongly associated with thrombosis (odds ratio (OR) about 20–40).

Venous thrombosis (including adrenal hemorrhagic infarction)

The most common thrombotic event is venous thromboembolism: deep vein thrombosis (DVT: 50% of patients), pulmonary embolism (PE: 25%), upper-limb DVT (10% if a central venous catheter is used,[20]) and sometimes (<1%) unusual events such as cerebral venous (dural sinus) thrombosis.[5]

Adrenal hemorrhagic necrosis occurs in 3–5% of patients with HIT, and results from adrenal vein thrombosis, with resulting adrenal gland infarction.[5] If adrenal necrosis is bilateral, shock can result, which is preventable with corticosteroid therapy. Unilateral adrenal necrosis typically presents with flank or abdominal pain.

Arterial thrombosis

Arterial thrombosis most often manifests as an ischemic lower limb, acute stroke, or acute myocardial infarction. Interestingly, this rank order (aorto-ileofemoral > cerebrovascular > coronary arteries) is the opposite of that seen with typical atherothrombosis. Surgical removal of occluding platelet-rich 'white clots' can salvage the limb in some circumstances.

Limb ischemic syndromes, including venous limb gangrene

Thrombosis of limb arteries or veins leads to limb amputation in about 5–15% of patients with HIT. Occlusion of large arteries by platelet-rich 'white clots' with absent arterial pulses is the classic explanation for limb loss. In recent years, however, the syndrome of venous limb gangrene has increasingly been appreciated. Here, there is limb ischemia with palpable pulses, usually in the setting of DVT.[5,13] Most often, venous gangrene results from coumarin (e.g., warfarin) anticoagulation, whereby microvascular thrombosis results from warfarin-induced depletion of protein C (a vitamin K-dependent natural anticoagulant factor) during the intense hypercoagulability state of HIT. Affected patients have a *supra*therapeutic International Normalized Ratio (INR >3.5), which represents a surrogate marker for severe protein C depletion. Rarely, microvascular thrombosis leading to limb ischemia occurs in the absence of warfarin treatment.[5]

Disseminated intravascular coagulation

Although disseminated intravascular coagulation (DIC), as defined by increased levels of thrombin–antithrombin complexes and crosslinked fibrin degradation products (fibrin D-dimers), occurs in virtually all patients with HIT, *overt DIC*, as defined by low fibrinogen or elevated INR levels, is seen in only 10–15% of patients.[5] Overt DIC often indicates more severe HIT (e.g., severe thrombocytopenia) and may reflect a greater risk for microvascular thrombosis.

Other sequelae of HIT
Heparin-induced skin lesions

About 10–20% of patients who develop HIT while receiving subcutaneous injections of heparin manifest skin lesions at the heparin injection sites.[5,21] These range from painful, erythematous plaques to frank skin necrosis. Not all patients evince thrombocytopenia, but among those who do, the risk of arterial thrombosis appears unusually high.

Acute system reactions

Acute onset of inflammatory (fever, chills, or flushing), pulmonary (tachypnea, dyspnea, or respiratory arrest), cardiac (tachycardia, chest pain or tightness, or cardiac arrest), neurologic (headache or transient global amnesia) or gastrointestinal (large-volume diarrhea) symptoms or signs beginning 5–30 minutes after an intravenous heparin bolus is strongly suggestive of acute HIT.[5,22] Measuring the postbolus platelet count will reveal an abrupt decrease. About 5–10% of patients with HIT have such 'acute systemic reactions' as their presenting feature.

Cardiac sequelae of HIT

Table 26.1 lists the reported cardiac sequelae of HIT.[5] One study suggested that in post-coronary bypass surgery patients who develop HIT, occlusion of saphenous vein (but not artery) grafts is especially common.[23]

Differential diagnosis

Both heparin use and thrombocytopenia are common in hospitalized patients. Thus, the concurrence of these two events does not necessarily indicate HIT. Indeed, thrombocytopenia due to platelet consumption and hemodilution is

Table 26.1   *Cardiac complications of HIT*

- Myocardial infarction (and related sequelae, e.g., cardiogenic shock)

- Occlusion of saphenous vein graft post coronary artery bypass surgery

- Intra-atrial thrombus (can affect right or left heart chambers)

- Intraventricular thrombus (can affect right or left heart chambers)

- Prosthetic valve thrombosis

- Right heart failure secondary to massive pulmonary embolism

- Tachycardia, hypertension, chest pain, or cardiac (cardiorespiratory) arrest post intravenous heparin bolus

Adapted from Warkentin TE. Clinical picture of heparin-induced thrombocytopenia. In: Warkentin TE, Greinacher A, eds. Heparin-Induced Thrombocytopenia, 4th edn. New York: Informa Healthcare USA Inc., 2007: 21–66.

a common reason for a hematologist to be consulted for a post-cardiac surgery patient. Other common reasons for thrombocytopenia in hospitalized patients receiving heparin include septicemia, multiorgan system failure, and DIC (of multiple etiologies). Although several dozen drugs can cause immune-mediated thrombocytopenia (e.g., quinine, quinidine, rifampin, vancomycin, and sulfa antibiotics), these typically result in a platelet count fall to less than 20×10^9/l, together with petechiae and purpura, thus giving a different clinical presentation compared with HIT. Abciximab, tirofiban, or eptifibatide (glycoprotein (GP) IIb/IIIa antagonists) are far more likely than heparin to explain an abrupt drop in platelet count to less than 20×10^9/l following heart catheterization – even if the patient has previously received heparin but not the GPIIb/IIIa antagonist! This is because pre-existing GPIIb/IIIa antagonist-dependent antibodies are a relatively common explanation for abrupt onset of severe thrombocytopenia in this patient population.[24]

Frequency

Table 26.2 lists the factors that influence the frequency of HIT.[1,2,5,6,25,26] The type of heparin, type of patient population, and duration of heparin treatment are the most important factors. Thus, UFH thromboprophylaxis extending for a week or more after cardiac surgery is a common scenario for HIT (estimated frequency 1–2%), whereas a medical patient receiving a few days of LMWH for ACS has a very low frequency of HIT (probably <0.1%).[1,27] Female gender confers a somewhat greater risk of HIT (OR 1.5–2.0).[25]

Anti-PF4/heparin antibodies are commonly formed after cardiac surgery, with reported frequencies ranging from

Table 26.2   *Risk factors for HIT*[1,2,5,6,25,26]

Risk factor	Influence of risk of HIT (higher risk > lower risk)
Type of heparin	Bovine lung UFH > porcine intestinal UFH > porcine LMWH > fondaparinux[a]
Type of patient population	Postoperative > medical > obstetric, neonates
Duration of heparin use	11–14 days[b] > 5–10 days > less than 5 days
Dose of heparin	Prophylactic dose[c] ≥ therapeutic dose > heparin 'flushes'
Patient gender	Females > males

[a]In theory, fondaparinux should have a lower (perhaps negligible) frequency of HIT compared with LMWH, although this remains unproven.[26]
[b]Risk of HIT appears to decline beyond day 14,[1,5] unless heparin therapy is interrupted for surgery or an invasive procedure.
[c]The highest frequencies of HIT have been reported in association with prophylactic-dose heparin,[1,2] but whether this reflects a greater risk with this particular dose of heparin or rather other clinical factors (e.g., postoperative state) is uncertain. In contrast, HIT associated with heparin 'flushes' is rare.

30% to 65%. Only a minority of these are platelet-activating and thus have the potential to cause HIT.[1,16,19,28] The clinical irrelevance of most anti-PF4/heparin antibodies is illustrated in Figure 26.4(b), which shows that the platelet count profiles for patients positive and negative for anti-PF4/heparin antibodies (by commercial ELISA) are essentially identical.[19] This underscores the importance of interpreting a positive test for anti-PF4/heparin antibodies in the appropriate clinical context (see the subsection above on *Diagnostic interpretation*).

One non-randomized comparison of UFH with LMWH antithrombotic prophylaxis after cardiac surgery suggests that the risk of HIT may be less with LMWH,[19] perhaps because in vivo cross-reactivity of HIT antibodies with LMWH is less than with UFH. However, post-cardiac surgery thromboprophylaxis with LMWH is not an approved indication, and data regarding its effectiveness in this clinical setting are limited.

Treatment

Treatment principles

Table 26.3 lists six treatment principles, which can be classified as two *Do's* (stop heparin, initiate alternative non-heparin anticoagulation), two *Don'ts* (avoid/postpone warfarin, avoid platelet transfusions), and two *diagnostics*

Table 26.3   *Six treatment principles for strongly suspected or confirmed HIT*

Two *Do's*	1. *Do* stop heparin
	2. *Do* give alternative, non-heparin anticoagulant
Two *Don'ts*	3. *Don't* give warfarin during acute HIT (postpone warfarin until HIT is substantially resolved (platelet count $>150 \times 10^9/l$; give vitamin K if warfarin has already been given when HIT is recognized)
	4. *Don't* give prophylactic platelet transfusions
Two *Diagnostics*	5. *Test* for HIT antibodies
	6. *Test* for lower-limb DVT

(test for HIT antibodies; investigate for lower-limb DVT). In some patients, special adjunctive measures are needed, such as surgical thrombectomy for large artery occlusion. In HIT patients with coronary, cerebral, or peripheral arterial occlusive disease, adjunctive antiplatelet therapy may be helpful, although HIT can occur even in a patient receiving aspirin and clopidogrel.[29]

HIT is a profound hypercoagulability state, and simply stopping heparin does not prevent a high risk of symptomatic thrombosis over the next few days or weeks.[18] Accordingly, if there is sufficiently strong clinical suspicion for HIT, heparin cessation should be accompanied by administration of an alternative non-heparin anticoagulant.[4] If the clinical suspicion of HIT is not sufficiently great, other approaches can be acceptable, such as simply continuing the heparin or using an alternative non-heparin anticoagulant in prophylactic doses. For example, in Canada, low-dose danaparoid (750 U twice or thrice daily by subcutaneous (SC) injection) is appropriate in such patients (danaparoid is not available in the USA). In a patient who has good renal function, low-dose lepirudin (15 mg SC twice daily) or fondaparinux (2.5 mg SC once daily) might be appropriate as 'off-label' approaches when the risk of HIT is not considered sufficiently great to justify therapeutic-dose anticoagulation, but at the same time is not judged to be so low so as to allow continued treatment with heparin.[4]

Despite its lower risk of HIT, LMWH is contraindicated for treatment of HIT. Coumarins (e.g., warfarin) are also contraindicated during the acute thrombocytopenic phase of HIT (see below).

In general, patients with clinically suspected HIT should undergo laboratory testing for HIT antibodies. If the clinical suspicion for HIT is moderate or high, we recommend that patients undergo investigation for lower-limb DVT.[4] In most cases, initial treatment decisions are made prior to receiving the results of HIT antibody tests. The high negative predictive value of the washed platelet activation assays and the ELISAs means that heparin can be restarted if a patient tests negative in one or both of these tests.

Direct thrombin inhibitors

Direct thrombin inhibitors (DTIs) inhibit thrombin without requiring a cofactor (in contrast, UFH and LMWH inhibit thrombin *indirectly* by catalyzing neutralization of thrombin by antithrombin). Three DTIs – lepirudin, argatroban, and bivalirudin, are available in the USA. Lepirudin and argatroban are approved for the treatment of HIT (including HIT-associated thrombosis), whereas argatroban and bivalirudin are approved for anticoagulation during PCI in a patient in whom heparin is contraindicated because of HIT.

Lepirudin

Lepirudin (Refludan) is a 65-amino-acid protein closely resembling the structure of hirudin (leech anticoagulant), but manufactured using recombinant technology. It is a *bivalent* DTI, as it binds both to thrombin's fibrinogen-binding site, and to the apolar binding site, thereby blocking access to thrombin's active (catalytic) site. The affinity ($K_i = 60$ pmol/l) and specificity of lepirudin for thrombin are extremely high, with essentially irreversible binding. Lepirudin only minimally prolongs the INR,[30] and is monitored in most situations by the activated partial thromboplastin time (aPTT).

Clearance of hirudin occurs primarily by the kidneys. The usual half-life (80 minutes) can be greatly prolonged in a patient with renal failure. Most lepirudin distributes into the extravascular space (volume of distribution 0.30 liter/kg). Thus, during extended high dosing (e.g., cardiac surgery), lepirudin accumulates in the extravascular space, providing a pool from which ongoing redistribution back into the intravascular compartment occurs, resulting in high drug levels for some time.

Recent studies suggest that the standard recommended dosing regimen (0.40 mg/kg bolus, followed by an initial infusion of 0.15 mg/kg/h, adjusted by aPTT[14]) is too high.[31,32] This is because drug accumulation will occur even with minor degrees of renal insufficiency, which is common in the elderly population that often develops HIT. Thus, current dosing recommendations are to avoid the initial bolus in most situations, and to begin with a lower infusion rate (0.05–0.10 mg/kg/h), and to perform aPTT levels at 4-hour intervals until it is clear that the patient is in a steady state. Even lower doses of lepirudin are appropriate when there is substantially impaired renal function. For example, a constant infusion of only 0.005–0.10 mg/kg/h (about 3–7% of the approved dose), or intermittent low-dose boluses (e.g., 0.005–0.01 mg/kg) with frequent aPTT monitoring are appropriate when renal function is severely impaired, such as during chronic renal replacement therapy.

Laboratory monitoring is usually performed using the aPTT (usual target range 1.5–2.5 times the 'baseline' aPTT, which is usually the mean of the laboratory normal range). Depending upon the thromboplastin reagent used, however, this target range may not be optimal. For example, the aPTT–lepirudin concentration relationship may not be linear at high therapeutic aPTT levels. It might be useful, therefore, for laboratories to determine an aPTT–lepirudin standard curve by 'spiking' normal pooled plasma with various concentrations of lepirudin.[33] Appropriate lepirudin plasma levels range from 0.2 to 0.4 μg/ml (antithrombotic prophylaxis in non-HIT situations), to 0.5–0.8 μg/ml (isolated HIT), to 0.6–1.4 μg/ml (HIT plus thrombosis). A more accurate laboratory monitoring method that is usually used in situations in which high lepirudin concentrations are required (e.g., during cardiac surgery) is the ecarin clotting time.

Bleeding is the most important adverse effect of hirudin. Major bleeding occurred in 18.8–20.4% of patients receiving lepirudin during therapy of HIT, with five hemorrhagic deaths (2.4%) in the most recent prospective study (HAT-3) of 205 patients,[31] and seven hemorrhagic deaths (3.9%) in a recent retrospective study of 181 patients treated with lepirudin.[32] There is no antidote to reverse the effects of lepirudin.

Lepirudin is immunogenic, and antihirudin antibodies form commonly 1–4 weeks after beginning treatment. Fatal anaphylaxis has been reported, typically post lepirudin bolus in a patient who has recently received this drug.[33]

New or progressive thrombosis occurred in 4–12% (mean 7.9%) of patients treated with the standard dosing regimen of lepirudin in the three prospective cohort studies of HIT-associated thrombosis; this was lower than the event rate (30.8%) seen in the historical controls.[31] Lepirudin also appeared effective for treating isolated HIT.[34]

Argatroban

Argatroban (marketed as Argatroban in the USA and Novastan elsewhere) is a small-molecule arginine derivative. Pharmacological features includes its reversible thrombin inhibition, short half-life (40–50 minutes), hepatobiliary metabolism, lack of immunogenicity, and prolongation of the INR.[30,35–37]

Argatroban is a univalent DTI, since it binds reversibly only to the active (catalytic) site of thrombin (cf. lepirudin). The affinity of argatroban to thrombin ($K_i = 40$ nmol/l) is less than that of lepirudin, and its lower specificity for thrombin suggests that argatroban should be termed thrombin-*selective*, rather than thrombin-*specific*. The relatively high molar concentrations of argatroban required for an anticoagulant effect explains its disproportionate prolongation of the INR.[30]

Argatroban and its metabolites undergo hepatobiliary excretion. In normal individuals, the elimination half-life is about 40–50 minutes. The volume of distribution is 0.17 liter/kg. Thus, like lepirudin, it distributes mostly in the extravascular space. It is about 50% serum protein-bound.

Argatroban is given by intravenous infusion, with the approved initial dosing at 2 μg/kg/min, with a 75% reduction (to 0.5 μg/kg/min) for patients with hepatic insufficiency.[35,38] As with lepirudin, growing clinical experience suggests that the recommended dosing may be too high, and many physicians begin with lower doses (e.g., 0.5–1.0 μg/kg/min), especially in critically ill patients or those with renal insufficiency.[38] Monitoring of the anticoagulant action of argatroban is with the aPTT, with the usual target range being 1.5–3.0 times the baseline aPTT value (maximum 100 s). For patients undergoing hemodialysis, an argatroban 250 μg/kg bolus dose can be given at the start of dialysis, followed by a continuous 2 μg/kg/min infusion (or, if the patient is already at steady state on argatroban, simply maintaining the infusion with no need for additional bolus dosing).[39–41]

Bleeding is the most important adverse effect of argatroban. Major bleeding occurred in about 5% of patients enrolled in the clinical trials evaluating argatroban for HIT. Minor bleeding was reported in about 40% of patients. As with lepirudin, no antidote exists. Unlike hirudin, argatroban is not immunogenic.

New or progressive thrombosis occurs in 13.1–19.4% of patients treated with argatroban for HIT-associated thrombosis, which is lower than the rate (34.8%) seen in historical controls.[35,36] New thrombosis occurred in 5.8–8.1% of patients who received argatroban for isolated HIT (23.0% in controls).[35,36]

Use of argatroban for PCI is discussed below.

Bivalirudin

Bivalirudin (Angiomax) is a 'hirulog' (an analogue of hirudin) combining a 12-amino-acid sequence that binds to the fibrinogen-binding site on thrombin with a tetrapeptide sequence that recognizes the active site of thrombin, linked by a tetraglycine 'spacer'.[42] It exhibits much lower affinity for thrombin ($K_i = 2$ nmol/l) than lepirudin. Further, its inhibition of thrombin reverses over time, as thrombin cleaves bivalirudin at its Arg^3–Pro^4 bond. On account of such enzymic (non-organ) metabolism, only about 20% of bivalirudin clearance is renal. These differences from lepirudin probably explain the generally lower rates of bleeding observed with bivalirudin, compared with lepirudin, in studies of patients with ACS.

To date, minimal 'off-label' experience with bivalirudin for HIT has been reported. One evaluation of bivalirudin in 40 patients with clinically suspected HIT indicated favorable results (no details were given).[42] Only two patients were given intravenous boluses. Initial infusion rates generally ranged from 0.15 to 0.20 mg/kg/h (mean infusion rate

0.165 mg/kg/h). The target aPTT was a 1.5- to 2.5-fold prolongation of the baseline value. Thus, a reasonable regimen might be to initiate therapy at 0.15 mg/kg/h (no initial bolus), with subsequent adjustments according to aPTT.

Use of bivalirudin for PCI is discussed below.

DTI–coumarin overlap

Use of warfarin and other coumarins can lead to microvascular thrombosis in patients with acute HIT, and has been implicated in the pathogenesis of skin necrosis and venous limb gangrene.[5,13] Caution is therefore required in managing DTI–warfarin overlap, including postponing initiation of warfarin until the platelet count has substantially recovered (preferably to >150 × 10^9/l), beginning with low warfarin doses (first dose ≤ 5 mg), ensuring at least a 5-day overlap period with the DTI, and maintaining DTI therapy until the platelet count has reached a stable plateau within the normal platelet count range.[4] It is important to note that argatroban itself prolongs the INR to a considerable extent,[30] and so the target INR range during argatroban-warfarin cotherapy is somewhat greater than the usual therapeutic range (2.0 to 3.0) during warfarin monotherapy.

Indirect factor Xa inhibitors

There are two indirect factor Xa inhibitors: danaparoid and fondaparinux. Only the latter is currently marketed in the USA.

Danaparoid (Orgaran) is a mixture of anticoagulant glycosaminoglycans, predominantly (low-sulfated) heparan sulfate and dermatan sulfate. The anti factor Xa to antithrombin ratio is about 22. It is the only anticoagulant evaluated by randomized clinical trial for treatment of HIT, proving more effective than Dextran-70.[43] When used in therapeutic doses (usually 200 U/h intravenously, following a loading dose that depends upon patient weight), it was as effective as lepirudin in a non-randomized comparison, with less bleeding.[44] Danaparoid is less effective in HIT when used in prophylactic doses (e.g., 750 U twice or thrice daily),[44] which ironically is its approved dose for HIT in some jurisdictions. In our view, the low-dose protocol is useful in non-HIT clinical situations in which an alternative to heparin for antithrombotic prophylaxis is desired. However, when HIT is strongly suspected, we recommend that it be given in therapeutic dosing.[4,45] Although 15–40% of HIT sera exhibit weak cross-reactivity with danaparoid in vitro, this is rarely clinically significant, thus justifying its use without prior cross-reactivity testing.[4]

Fondaparinux (Arixtra) is a synthetic antithrombin-binding pentasaccharide anticoagulant with anti-factor Xa (and anti-factor IXa) activity, but no antithrombin activity. HIT antibodies do not cross-react with fondaparinux,[26] and thus in theory it should be effective in patients with HIT. However, minimal experience and uncertainty regarding optimal dosing in patients with HIT are relevant issues. Interestingly, fondaparinux appears to interact with PF4 in such a way as to promote formation of anti-PF4/heparin antibodies that, however, do not appear to react against PF4/fondaparinux.[26]

Since both danaparoid and fondaparinux have long anti-factor Xa half-lives (25 and 17 hours, respectively), and since neither prolongs the INR, this facilitates a smooth transition to warfarin therapy. No antidote exists for either drug.

Adjunctive therapies

There are situations where various adjunctive therapies might be appropriate for HIT. Surgical thrombectomy can be limb-saving in situations of acute large artery occlusion by platelet-rich 'white clots'. Pharmacologic thrombolysis (combined with anticoagulation) may be helpful in patients with severe pulmonary embolism. Plasmapheresis (replacing with fresh frozen plasma) or high-dose intravenous gammaglobulin are unproven but potentially useful treatment adjuncts to anticoagulation in patients with very severe HIT. Although inferior vena cava filters are sometimes used to manage patients with severe HIT, in our view these do not obviate the need for anticoagulation in HIT, and may contribute to lower limb thrombosis and possibly even limb ischemia and gangrene. We do not advocate their use in HIT. In our experience, severe venous limb ischemia complicating HIT is sometimes diagnosed clinically to represent 'compartment syndrome', leading to treatment with fasciotomy. However, reversal of warfarin anticoagulation (if warfarin has been given) and aggressive anticoagulation may be more important than fasciotomy when the underlying pathologic process is progressive macro- and microvascular thrombosis in veins and venules.

PCI and HIT

Two of the DTIs – argatroban and bivalirudin – are approved for anticoagulation during PCI in patients in whom heparin is contraindicated because of acute, subacute, or previous HIT. Table 26.4 lists the recommended dosing regimens for PCI.[46–48] For both agents, high procedural success rates have been reported in the setting of HIT.[46,47]

Cardiac surgery and HIT

For patients with previous HIT (HIT antibodies no longer detectable) who require cardiac surgery, it is recommended that UFH be given in the usual doses for cardiac surgery.[4,27] This is based on the following rationale: (a) repeat formation of HIT antibodies does not appear to occur more often

Table 26.4 *Dosing regimens for direct thrombin inhibitors for percutaneous coronary intervention (PCI)*

Direct thrombin inhibitor	Dosing regimen
Argatroban	350 µg/kg initial intravenous bolus; intravenous infusion, 25 µg/kg/min to maintain the activated clotting time (ACT) between 300 and 450 s[a,b]
Bivalirudin	0.75 mg/kg initial intravenous bolus; 1.75 mg/kg/h for the duration of the procedure[c]

[a]Patients with clinically relevant hepatic disease were not studied in the registration trials (Arg-216, -310, and -311) of argatroban in patients with or at risk of HIT undergoing PCI.

[b]Results from a multicenter, prospective pilot study in patients without HIT suggest that a reduced dose of argatroban (e.g., 250 or 300 µg/kg bolus followed by a 15 µg/kg/min infusion) may be appropriate if used in combination with GPIIb/IIIa inhibition during PCI.[48]

[c]If the creatinine clearance is <30 ml/min, reduction of the infusion rate to 1.0 mg/kg/h should be considered. If the patient is on hemodialysis, the infusion should be reduced to 0.25 mg/kg/h. No reduction in the bolus dose is needed.

in patients with a previous history of HIT; (b) if antibodies are regenerated, these take at least 5 days following surgery to reach significant levels (at a time when alternative, non-heparin anticoagulation can be given); (c) relative little experience with non-heparin anticoagulants exists. UFH is also a reasonable option for a patient with a weak-positive PF4/polyanion ELISA (<0.75 OD units) and a negative washed platelet activation assay.

For patients with acute HIT, or whose platelets have recovered but who still have detectable HIT antibodies (subacute HIT), several treatment options exist:[3,4,27] (i) await disappearance of HIT antibodies, and use heparin; (ii) give a non-heparin anticoagulant (e.g., bivalirudin, lepirudin, or danaparoid); or (iii) combine heparin with an antiplatelet agent (e.g., a prostacyclin analogue or a GPIIb/IIIa inhibitor) for intraoperative anticoagulation. For bivalirudin, well-studied protocols have been reported for both off-pump and on-pump cardiac surgery (non-HIT patients),[49,50] as has some experience in patients with HIT.

Acknowledgments

Studies described in this chapter[1–7,9,11–13,15–18,20,21,25–30,45] were supported by operating grants from the Heart and Stroke Foundation of Ontario from 1993 to 2005 (A2449, T2967, B3763, T4502, T5207, and T6157). We thank Jo-Ann I Sheppard for preparing the figures.

References

1. Lee DH, Warkentin TE. Frequency of heparin-induced thrombocytopenia. In: Warkentin TE, Greinacher A, eds. Heparin-induced Thrombocytopenia, 4th edn. New York: Informa Healthcare USA Inc, 2007:67–116.

2. Warkentin TE, Roberts RS, Hirsh J, Kelton JG. An improved definition of immune heparin-induced thrombocytopenia in postoperative orthopedic patients. Arch Intern Med 2003;163:2518–24.

3. Warkentin TE, Kelton JG. Temporal aspects of heparin-induced thrombocytopenia. N Engl J Med 2001;344:1286–92.

4. Warkentin TE, Greinacher A, Koster A et al. Treatment and prevention of heparin-induced thrombocytopenia: ACCP evidence-based clinical practice guidelines (8th edition). Chest 2008; in press.

5. Warkentin TE. Clinical picture of heparin-induced thrombocytopenia. In: Warkentin TE, Greinacher A, eds. Heparin-Induced Thrombocytopenia, 4th edn. New York: Informa Healthcare USA Inc, 2007:21–66.

6. Warkentin TE, Sheppard JI, Moore JC et al. Laboratory testing for the antibodies that cause heparin-induced thrombocytopenia: How much class do we need? J Lab Clin Med 2005;146:341–6.

7. Warkentin TE. An overview of the heparin-induced thrombocytopenia syndrome. Semin Thromb Hemost 2004;30:273–83.

8. Amiral J, Bridey F, Dreyfus M et al. Platelet factor 4 complexed to heparin is the target for antibodies generated in heparin-induced thrombocytopenia. Thromb Haemost 1992;68:95–6.

9. Greinacher A, Gopinadhan M, Günther JU et al. Close approximation of two platelet factor 4 tetramers by charge neutralization forms the antigens recognized by HIT antibodies. Arterioscler Thromb Vasc Biol 2006;26:2386–93.

10. Rauova L, Zhai L, Kowalska MA et al. Role of platelet surface PF4 antigenic complexes in heparin-induced thrombocytopenia pathogenesis: diagnostic and therapeutic implications. Blood 2006;107:2346–53.

11. Warkentin TE, Kelton JG. Delayed-onset heparin-induced thrombocytopenia and thrombosis. Ann Intern Med 2001;135:502–6.

12. Warkentin TE, Hayward CPM, Boshkov LK et al. Sera from patients with heparin-induced thrombocytopenia generate platelet-derived microparticles with procoagulant activity: an explanation for the thrombotic complications of heparin-induced thrombocytopenia. Blood 1994;84:3691–9.

13. Warkentin TE, Elavathil LJ, Hayward CPM et al. The pathogenesis of venous limb gangrene associated with heparin-induced thrombocytopenia. Ann Intern Med 1997;127:804–12.

14. Greinacher A, Eichler P, Lubenow N, Kwasny H, Luz M. Heparin-induced thrombocytopenia with thromboembolic complications: meta-analysis of two prospective trials to assess the value of parenteral treatment with lepirudin and its therapeutic aPTT range. Blood 2000;96:846–51.

15. Warkentin TE, Sheppard JI. Testing for heparin-induced thrombocytopenia antibodies. Transfus Med Rev 2006;20:259–72.

16. Warkentin TE, Sheppard JI, Horsewood P et al. Impact of the patient population on the risk for heparin-induced thrombocytopenia. Blood 2000;96:1703–8.

16a. Warkentin TE, Sheppard JI, Raschke R, Greinacher A. Performance characteristics of a rapid assay for anti-PF4/heparin antibodies, the Particle ImmunoFiltration Assay. J Thromb Haemost 2007;5:2308–10 (Epub 2007 Aug 3).

17. Warkentin TE. HIT: lessons learned. Pathophysiol Haemost Thromb 2006;35:50–7.

18. Warkentin TE, Kelton JG. A 14-year study of heparin-induced thrombocytopenia. Am J Med 1996;101:502–7.

19. Pouplard C, May MA, Regina S et al. Changes in platelet count after cardiac surgery can effectively predict the development of pathogenic heparin-dependent antibodies. Br J Haematol 2005;128:837–41.

20. Hong AP, Cook DJ, Sigouin CS, Warkentin TE. Central venous catheters and upper-extremity deep-vein thrombosis complicating immune heparin-induced thrombocytopenia. Blood 2003;101:3049–51.

21. Warkentin TE, Roberts RS, Hirsh J, Kelton JG. Heparin-induced skin lesions and other unusual sequelae of the heparin-induced thrombocytopenia syndrome: a nested cohort study. Chest 2005;127:1857–61.

22. Mims MP, Manian P, Rice L. Acute cardiorespiratory collapse from heparin: a consequence of heparin-induced thrombocytopenia. Eur J Haematol 2004;72:366–9.

23. Liu JC, Lewis BE, Steen LH et al. Patency of coronary artery bypass grafts in patients with heparin-induced thrombocytopenia. Am J Cardiol 2002;89:979–81.

24. Aster RH, Curtis BR, Bougie DW et al. Thrombocytopenia associated with the use of GPIIb/IIIa inhibitors: positive paper of the ISTH working group on thrombocytopenia and GPIIb/IIIa inhibitors. J Thromb Haemost 2006;4:678–9.

25. Warkentin TE, Sheppard JI, Sigouin CS et al. Gender imbalance and risk factor interactions in heparin-induced thrombocytopenia. Blood 2006;108:2937–41.

26. Warkentin TE, Cook RJ, Marder VJ et al. Anti-platelet factor 4/heparin antibodies in orthopedic surgery patients receiving antithrombotic prophylaxis with fondaparinux or enoxaparin. Blood 2005;106:3791–6.

27. Warkentin TE, Greinacher A. Heparin-induced thrombocytopenia and cardiac surgery. Ann Thorac Surg 2003;76:2121–31.

28. Warkentin TE, Sheppard JI. No significant improvement in diagnostic specificity of an anti-PF4/polyanion immunoassay with use of high heparin confirmatory procedure. J Thromb Haemost 2006;4:281–2.

29. Selleng K, Selleng S, Raschke R et al. Immune heparin-induced thrombocytopenia can occur in patients receiving clopidogrel and aspirin. Am J Hematol 2005;78:188–92.

30. Warkentin TE, Greinacher A, Craven S et al. Differences in the clinically effective molar concentrations of four direct thrombin inhibitors explain their variable prothrombin time prolongation. Thromb Haemost 2005;94:958–64.

31. Lubenow N, Eichler P, Lietz T, Greinacher A; HIT Investigators Group. Lepirudin in patients with heparin-induced thrombocytopenia – results of the third prospective study (HAT-3) and a combined analysis of HAT-1, HAT-2, and HAT-3. J Thromb Haemost 2005;3:2428–36.

32. Tardy B, Lecompte T, Boelhen F et al. Predictive factors for thrombosis and major bleeding in an observational study in 181 patients with heparin-induced thrombocytopenia treated with lepirudin. Blood 2006;108:1492–6.

33. Greinacher A. Lepirudin for the treatment of heparin-induced thrombocytopenia. In: Warkentin TE, Greinacher A, eds. Heparin-Induced Thrombocytopenia, 4th edn. New York: Informa Healthcare USA Inc, 2007:345–78.

34. Lubenow N, Eichler P, Lietz T et al. Lepirudin for prophylaxis of thrombosis in patients with isolated heparin-induced thrombocytopenia: an analysis of 3 prospective studies. Blood 2004;104:3072–7.

35. Lewis BE, Wallis DE, Berkowitz SD et al. ARG-911 Study Investigators. Argatroban anticoagulant therapy in patients with heparin-induced thrombocytopenia. Circulation 2001;103:1838–43.

36. Lewis BE, Wallis DE, Leya F et al. Argatroban anticoagulation in patients with heparin-induced thrombocytopenia. Arch Intern Med 2003;163:1849–56.

37. Lewis BE, Wallis DE, Hursting MJ et al. Effects of argatroban therapy, demographic variables, and platelet count on thrombotic risks in heparin-induced thrombocytopenia. Chest 2006;129:1407–16.

38. Levine RL, Hursting MJ, McCollum D. Argatroban therapy in heparin-induced thrombocytopenia with hepatic dysfunction. Chest 2006;129:1167–75.

39. Murray PT, Reddy BV, Grossman EJ et al. A prospective comparison of three argatroban treatment regimens during hemodialysis in end-stage renal disease. Kidney Int 2004;66:2446–53.

40. Tang IY, Cox DS, Patel K et al. Argatroban and renal replacement therapy in patients with heparin-induced thrombocytopenia. Ann Pharmacother 2005;39:231–6.

41. Reddy BV, Grossman EJ, Trevino SA et al. Argatroban anticoagulation in patients with heparin-induced thrombocytopenia requiring renal replacement therapy. Ann Pharmacother 2005;39:1601–5.

42. Bartholomew JR. Bivalirudin for the treatment of heparin-induced thrombocytopenia. In: Warkentin TE, Greinacher A, eds. Heparin-Induced Thrombocytopenia, 4th edn. New York: Informa Healthcare USA Inc, 2007:409–39.

43. Chong BH, Gallus AS, Cade JF et al. Prospective randomised open-label comparison of danaparoid with dextran 70 in the treatment of heparin-induced thrombocytopaenia with thrombosis: a clinical outcome study. Thromb Haemost 2001;86:1170–5.

44. Farner B, Eichler P, Kroll H, Greinacher A. A comparison of danaparoid and lepirudin in heparin-induced thrombocytopenia. Thromb Haemost 2001;85:950–7.

45. Lubenow N, Warkentin TE, Greinacher A et al. Results of a systematic evaluation of treatment outcomes for heparin-induced thrombocytopenia in patients receiving danaparoid, ancrod, and/or coumarin explain the rapid shift in clinical practice in the 1990s. Thromb Res 2006;117:507–15.

46. Lewis B, Matthai WH, Cohen M et al. ARG-216/310/311 investigators. Argatroban anticoagulation during percutaneous coronary intervention in patients with heparin-induced thrombocytopenia. Cathet Cardiovasc Intervent 2002;57:177–84.

47. Mahaffey KW, Lewis BE, Wildermann NM et al. ATBAT Investigators. The Anticoagulant Therapy with Bivalirudin to Assist in the Performance of Percutaneous Coronary Intervention in Patients with Heparin-Induced Thrombocytopenia (ATBAT) study: main results. J Invasive Cardiol 2003;15:611–16.

48. Jang IK, Lewis BE, Matthai WH, Kleiman NS. Argatroban anticoagulation in conjunction with glycoprotein IIb/IIIa inhibition in patients undergoing percutaneous coronary intervention: an open-label, nonrandomized pilot study. J Thromb Thrombolysis 2004;18:31–7.

49. Dyke CM, Smedira NG, Koster A et al. A comparison of bivalirudin to heparin with protamine reversal in patients undergoing cardiac surgery with cardiopulmonary bypass: the EVOLUTION-ON study. J Thorac Cardiovasc Surg 2006;131:533–9.

50. Merry AF, Raudkivi PJ, Middleton NG et al. Bivalirudin versus heparin and protamine in off-pump coronary artery bypass surgery. Ann Thorac Surg 2004;77:925–31.

27

Antithrombotic therapies for patients with cerebrovascular, peripheral arterial, and coronary artery disease

Sahil A Parikh and Joshua A Beckman

Introduction

Patients with extracoronary atherosclerotic vascular disease have the highest risk of death from coronary heart disease.[1,2] In patients with peripheral arterial disease (PAD), the risk of death is 15–30% at 5 years of follow-up, with 75% of these fatal events resulting from cardiovascular disease.[3] Similarly, patients with cerebrovascular disease (CVD) demonstrate elevated cardiovascular risk. In the Asymptomatic Carotid Surgery Trial (ACST), a 60-year-old patient with an asymptomatic, unilateral carotid artery stenosis had a 25% 10-year mortality rate.[4] In fact, patients with symptomatic PAD or CVD may have greater rates of cardiovascular death than patients initially presenting to medical attention for coronary heart disease. In one study, the annual mortality rate was higher among patients with PAD (8.2%) and stroke (11.3%) than after a myocardial infarction (6.3%) (Figure 27.1).[5]

Adverse atherosclerotic sequelae result from the process of atherothrombosis.[6] Rupture of an unstable plaque incites a cascade of events initiated by the aggregation of platelets with attendant thrombosis and vascular occlusion.[6] In addition, patients with PAD have long been recognized as having elevated markers of thrombogenicity.[7] Thus, with increasing awareness of atherosclerosis as a systemic disease, more aggressive strategies for the prevention of atherothrombotic events have evolved to include antithrombotic therapy.[3] In this chapter, we will relate evidence for the rational application of antithrombotic therapy for primary or secondary prevention of atherothrombotic events in the 'high-risk patient', the patient with extracoronary atherosclerotic vascular disease. Our discussion will consider antiplatelet, antithrombin, and anticoagulant therapy. In addition, we will review the role of primary prevention of stroke.

Antiplatelet therapy

Antiplatelet agents have repeatedly been studied and applied clinically for the prevention and treatment of atherothrombotic events in the coronary circulation. This rationale is well delineated elsewhere in this book. The role of antiplatelet therapy in the high-risk patient has likewise been extensively studied for the prevention of adverse cardiovascular events, including myocardial infarction (MI), stroke, and critical limb ischemia. Aspirin, the most common antiplatelet agent, is joined by the thienopyridines ticlopidine and clopidogrel and thromboxane synthase antagonists such as picotamide. In this section, we will review the impact of antiplatelet therapy and each specific class of agents for the prevention of atherothrombotic events in these high-risk patients. In addition, we will particularly review the role of antiplatelet therapy in the primary prevention of stroke in those patients without known atherosclerosis.

While many clinical studies have been performed in high-risk patient populations, the most informative assessment of the role of antiplatelet therapy comes from a meta-analysis performed by the Antithrombotic Trialists' Collaboration (ATC).[8,9] The most recent ATC meta-analysis considered 287 studies including 135 000 patients in comparisons of antiplatelet therapy with control and 77 000 patients in comparisons between different antiplatelet regimens.[9] Patients were considered to be at 'high annual risk' of >3% per year of vascular events due to pre-existing vascular disease.[9] The principal outcome measure was a 'serious vascular event', with a composite endpoint of non-fatal MI, non-fatal stroke, or vascular death. In sum, the relative risk reduction in these high-risk patients of serious vascular events due to the addition of antiplatelet therapy was approximately 25%. The absolute risk reduction

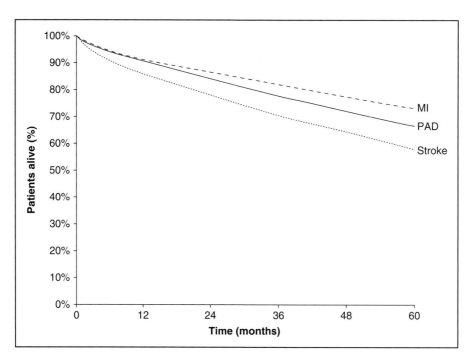

Figure 27.1
Survival among patients with peripheral arterial disease (PAD) compared with patients suffering a stroke or myocardial infactarction (MI). (Reproduced from Caro J et al.[5])

of vascular events was 2.5% for patients taking antiplatelet therapy (absolute risk 10.7%) versus control (absolute risk 13.2%). Therefore, the number of high-risk patients needed to treat (NNT) with antiplatelet therapy to prevent a single 'serious vascular event' was 40. Antiplatelet therapy in its myriad forms was effective in reducing events in patients with both prior and acute MI, with prior and acute stroke, and with known peripheral arterial disease. These data are shown in Figure 27.2.

When considering individual components of the composite endpoint in this meta-analysis, there are significant reductions of events in each vascular bed. For example, antiplatelet therapy reduced the relative risk of non-fatal MI by 34% and that of non-fatal MI or coronary heart disease-related death by 26%. The relative risk of stroke was reduced by 25%, in which a smaller rise in hemorrhagic stroke was offset by a larger reduction of ischemic stroke. Finally, in patients with PAD, there was a relative risk reduction of 23% for subsequent serious vascular events. Thus, in both primary and secondary prevention of MI and stroke, as well as in vascular events associated with PAD, antiplatelet therapy proved dramatically effective.

Aspirin

Aspirin is by far the most widely studied antiplatelet medication for the prevention of atherothrombotic events.[10] Aspirin permanently inactivates the cyclooxygenase (COX)

activity of prostaglandin H synthase 1 and 2 (COX-1 and COX-2, respectively), which catalyze the first step in the synthesis of such platelet aggregation-stimulating compounds as thromboxane A_2 and prostacyclin.[10] At a cost of a few pennies per dose, it has also proven to be a potent agent in reducing morbidity and mortality in these high-risk patients. In the most recent ATC meta-analysis, all doses of aspirin were shown to decrease adverse cardiovascular events, including MI, stroke or vascular death, by approximately 25% in patients with a wide variety of atherosclerotic disease.[9] A summary of the effects of aspirin therapy on the risk of vascular events is provided in Figure 27.3. Specifically, doses of <75 mg, 75–150 mg, 160–325 mg, and 500–1500 mg gave relative reductions of adverse cardiovascular events of 13%, 32%, 26%, and 19%, respectively. Thus, doses of aspirin 75–150 mg daily were as effective as doses > 150 mg daily.[9] Further analysis also noted that all doses < 325 mg led to similar rates of extracranial bleeding, approximately doubling the baseline risk.[9] These data suggest that the daily administration of 75–100 mg of aspirin to high-risk patients significantly reduces major cardiovascular events at the expense of a mild increase in the risk of bleeding.

Thienopyridines

The thienopyridines have also been studied as alternative antiplatelet agents compared with aspirin monotherapy.

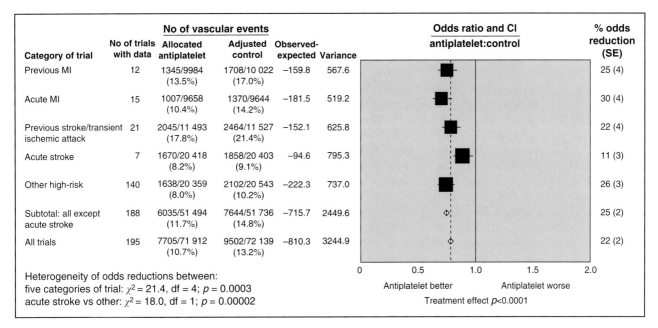

Category of trial	No of trials with data	No of vascular events				Odds ratio and CI antiplatelet:control	% odds reduction (SE)
		Allocated antiplatelet	Adjusted control	Observed-expected	Variance		
Previous MI	12	1345/9984 (13.5%)	1708/10 022 (17.0%)	−159.8	567.6		25 (4)
Acute MI	15	1007/9658 (10.4%)	1370/9644 (14.2%)	−181.5	519.2		30 (4)
Previous stroke/transient ischemic attack	21	2045/11 493 (17.8%)	2464/11 527 (21.4%)	−152.1	625.8		22 (4)
Acute stroke	7	1670/20 418 (8.2%)	1858/20 403 (9.1%)	−94.6	795.3		11 (3)
Other high-risk	140	1638/20 359 (8.0%)	2102/20 543 (10.2%)	−222.3	737.0		26 (3)
Subtotal: all except acute stroke	188	6035/51 494 (11.7%)	7644/51 736 (14.8%)	−715.7	2449.6		25 (2)
All trials	195	7705/71 912 (10.7%)	9502/72 139 (13.2%)	−810.3	3244.9		22 (2)

Heterogeneity of odds reductions between:
five categories of trial: $\chi^2 = 21.4$, df = 4; $p = 0.0003$
acute stroke vs other: $\chi^2 = 18.0$, df = 1; $p = 0.00002$

Figure 27.2
Proportional effects of antiplatelet therapy on vascular events (myocardial infarction (MI), stroke, or vascular death) in five main high-risk categories. The stratified odds ratio of of an event in treatment groups compared with that in control groups plotted for each group of trials (black square) along with its 99% confidence interval (CI: horizontal line). The meta-analysis of results for all trials (and 95% CI) is represented by an open diamond. (Reproduced from Antithrombotic Trialists' Collaboration.[9])

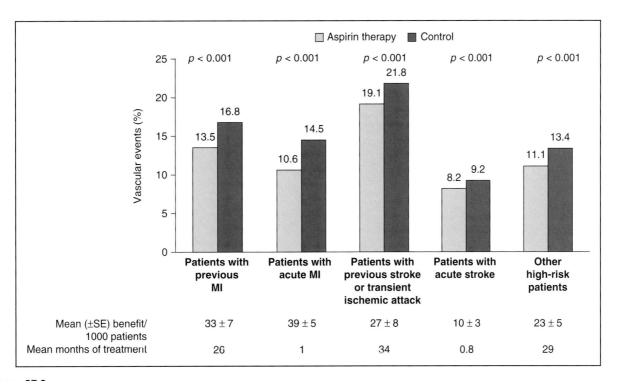

Figure 27.3
Absolute effects of aspirin monotherapy on the risk of vascular events (non-fatal myocardial infarction (MI), non-fatal stroke, or death from vascular causes) in five groups of high-risk patients. (Reproduced from Patrono C et al.[10])

They prevent platelet aggregation by selectively and irreversibly blocking the platelet adenosine diphosphate (ADP) $P2Y_{12}$ receptor. The two agents that have been most thoroughly studied are ticlopidine and clopidogrel.

Ticlopidine

Ticlopidine monotherapy (250 mg twice daily) reduces the risk of MI, stroke, or death about one-third or two-thirds in patients with PAD and claudication.[11,12] As a secondary prevention measure, one study of 1072 patients with prior transient ischemic attack (TIA) or stroke demonstrated that ticlopidine (500 mg daily) reduced the relative risk of stroke, MI, or vascular death by 23% compared with placebo at 2 years' follow-up.[13] Another similar study demonstrated that in 3069 patients with TIA or minor stroke, ticlopidine reduced the relative risk of non-fatal stroke or death by 12% and of all strokes by 21% at 3 years' follow-up when compared with aspirin alone.[14] Despite this level of efficacy, ticlopidine has been plagued by side-effects, including diarrhea, rash, and serious hematologic derangements, including a 1–2% risk of neutropenia or thrombocytopenia and a 0.025–0.05% risk of thrombocytopenic thrombotic purpura (TTP).[15] Ticlopidine, therefore, has largely been supplanted by clopidogrel.

Clopidogrel

Clopidogrel has also been studied against aspirin as an alternate monotherapy in patients with PAD as a secondary prevention measure. In the CAPRIE (Clopidogrel versus Aspirin in Patients at Risk of Ischemic Events) trial, 19 185 patients with recent MI, recent TIA or stroke, or symptomatic PAD were randomized to aspirin 325 mg daily or clopidogrel 75 mg daily.[16] Over a median follow-up of nearly 2 years, there was an 8.7% relative and a 0.5% absolute risk reduction of MI, stroke, and vascular death in favor of clopidogrel.[16] The greatest benefit was seen in patients with PAD, in whom there was a 23.8% relative and a 1.2% absolute risk reduction of MI, stroke, and vascular death. It therefore appears that clopidogrel may provide superior antiplatelet monotherapy in high-risk patients compared with aspirin. However, given the cost of clopidogrel, it has not replaced aspirin as a first-line agent in these patients.[17,18]

Picotamide

Picotamide, a drug that inhibits platelet thromboxane A_2 (TXA_2) synthase and antagonizes TXA_2 and prostaglandin endoperoxidase H_2 receptors, has demonstrated efficacy in clinical trials in the primary prevention of cardiovascular events in patients with PAD. One such trial, ADEP (Atherosclerotic Disease Evolution by Picotamide), recruited 2304 patients with PAD who were not taking any antiplatelet therapy. After a 1-month run-in period, the patients were randomly assigned to take either picotamide (300 mg three times daily) or placebo. After a mean follow-up of 18 months, the picotamide group experienced a risk reduction of 23% relative and 3% absolute for the composite endpoint of major and minor cardiovascular events, but these differences were not statistically significant.[19] A more recent study of 1209 patients from the DAVID (Drug Evaluation in Atherosclerotic Vascular Disease in Diabetics) study group in Italy demonstrated that in patients with type 2 diabetes and documented or symptomatic PAD, picotamide (600 mg twice daily) reduced overall mortality by 2.5% compared with aspirin 320 mg every other day.[20] While the availability of picotamide is limited, it has significant antiplatelet activity and may still prove useful in primary prevention in high-risk patients. Investigation of the application of this agent remains ongoing.

Dual antiplatelet therapy

The role of dual antiplatelet therapy in high-risk patients for primary prevention has been hotly debated. Active disease in extracoronary vascular beds provides support for the concept that dual antiplatelet therapy may provide greater reduction in ischemic events than aspirin alone. Two combinations have been studied carefully: aspirin plus clopidogrel and aspirin plus dipyridamole.

Aspirin plus clopidogrel

The enthusiasm for combining aspirin with clopidogrel therapy has emerged from a series of small studies and subgroup analyses of large clinical trials in the arena of percutaneous coronary intervention (PCI). For example, in a substudy of the CREDO (Clopidogrel for the Reduction of Events during Observation) study in which aspirin alone or aspirin and clopidogrel were administered to patients scheduled for PCI, patients with extracoronary atherosclerosis (PAD or CVD) had twice the relative risk reduction from subsequent death, MI, or stroke as those without extracoronary atherosclerosis when both groups received dual antiplatelet therapy (47.9% vs 18%).[21] Two large randomized controlled clinical trials have directly addressed the combination of aspirin and clopidogrel in high-risk patients. The first was the MATCH (Management of Atherothrombosis with Clopidogrel in High-risk patients) trial.[22] In this trial, the addition of aspirin (75 mg daily) to clopidogrel (75 mg daily) was assessed in a double-blind, placebo-controlled fashion in nearly 7600 patients with recent ischemic stroke or TIA and one additional risk factor over a mean duration of treatment and follow-up of 18 months. The study demonstrated a non-significant 1% absolute risk reduction of vascular events (defined as a composite of ischemic stroke, MI, vascular death, or rehospitalization for acute ischemia) with dual antiplatelet therapy compared with clopidogrel alone. The modest benefit came at the expense of a non-significant increase in life-threatening bleeding in the dual antiplatelet therapy group.

The role of dual antiplatelet therapy was further investigated in the CHARISMA (Clopidogrel for High Atherothrombotic Risk and Ischemic Stabilization, Management, and Avoidance) trial, which enrolled 15 603 patients aged 45 years or greater with either stable symptomatic atherosclerosis or those at high risk without previous symptomatic disease.[23] The primary efficacy endpoint was the first occurrence of cardiovascular death, MI, or stroke. The primary safety endpoint was severe bleeding, using the GUSTO definition. The secondary efficacy endpoint was the first occurrence of cardiovascular death, MI, stroke, or hospitalization for unstable MI, TIA, or revascularization. At enrollment, patients were randomized to aspirin 75–162 mg daily and clopidogrel 75 mg daily or matching placebo. During a median follow-up of 28 months, the incidence of the primary endpoint was 7.3% in the placebo group and 6.8% in the clopidogrel group, yielding a 7% relative risk reduction that was not statistically significant. The secondary efficacy endpoint, which included the primary endpoint plus hospitalization for unstable angina, TIA, or revascularization, was 17.9% in the placebo group and 16.7% in the clopidogrel group, generating an 8% relative risk reduction that was statistically significant ($p=0.04$). Severe bleeding trended higher with active therapy, and was 1.3% in the placebo group and 1.7% in the clopidogrel group: a 25% relative risk increase that did not reach statistical significance. Similarly, the rate of moderate bleeding was increased significantly with clopidogrel therapy from 1.3% in the placebo arm to 2.1% in the clopidogrel arm ($p < 0.001$). Intracranial hemorrhage did not vary between the two treatment arms.

A prespecified subgroup analysis was then conducted comparing those subjects enrolled for symptomatic disease and those were enrolled for asymptomatic disease or with multiple risk factors. In the latter group, 10.4% had a prior MI, 5.8% had a prior stroke, and 9.8% had undergone coronary artery bypass grafting. Among the 3284 designated asymptomatic patients enrolled, there was a non-significant 20% increase in the rate of primary events in patients in the clopidogrel arm compared with placebo (6.6% vs 5.5%). In the symptomatic subgroup of 12 153, there was a borderline reduction in primary events in the clopidogrel arm compared with placebo (6.9% vs 7.9%;

$p = 0.046$). More troubling still was an increase in all-cause mortality in the asymptomatic patients randomized to clopidogrel compared with placebo (5.4% vs 3.8%; $p = 0.04$) as well as an increase in cardiovascular death (3.9% vs 2.2%; $p = 0.01$). There was no effect of clopidogrel on death in the symptomatic group. Taken together, the CHARISMA data do not support the use of dual antiplatelet therapy with clopidogrel and aspirin in stable high-risk patients. In light of the negative finding of the primary endpoint, the prespecified subgroup analyses may require cautious interpretation. The risk and benefit of dual antiplatelet therapy in these groups must be weighed carefully prior to initiation (or cessation) of therapy with aspirin and clopidogrel.

Aspirin plus dipyridamole

In the prevention of stroke, the combination of aspirin with dipyridamole has been studied in large randomized controlled clinical trials. Dipyridamole is a pyridopyrimidine derivative inhibiting platelet activation by increasing platelet levels of cyclic adenosine monophosphate (cAMP) and cyclic guanosine monophosphate (cGMP). Dipyridamole also vasodilates coronary resistance vessels. In ESPS-2 (European Stroke Prevention Study 2), 6602 patients with recent stroke or TIA were randomized to one of four treatments: aspirin alone (50 mg daily), modified-release dipyridamole alone (400 mg daily), the two agents combined, or placebo.[24] Over 2 years of follow-up, stroke risk was reduced by 18% with aspirin alone, 16% with dipyridamole alone, and 37% with combination therapy when compared with placebo. Moreover, the risk of stroke or death was reduced by 13% with aspirin alone, 15% with dipyridamole alone, and 24% with the combination.

More recently, the role of aspirin with dipyridamole was revisited after meta-analyses of these two agents with different formulations and in different combinations suggested little or no benefit in the prevention of vascular events.[15] In ESPRIT (European/Australasian Stroke Prevention in Reversible Ischemia Trial), more than 2700 patients were randomly assigned to aspirin (30–325 mg daily) with or without dipyridamole (200 mg twice daily) within 6 months of a TIA or minor stroke of presumed arterial origin.[25] The study measured a primary composite endpoint of death from all vascular causes, non-fatal stroke, non-fatal MI, or major bleeding. Over a mean follow-up of 3.5 years, there was a reduction in the composite endpoint favoring the combination therapy of 20% relative and 3% absolute. The median dose of aspirin was 75 mg and extended-release dipyridamole was used 83% of the time. Taken together, the ESPS-2 and ESPRIT results support the role of aspirin combined with dipyridamole in the secondary prevention of ischemic cerebrovascular disease.

Antithrombin and oral anticoagulation therapy

In sharp contrast to the many studies of antiplatelet agents in high-risk patients with extracoronary cardiovascular disease, antithrombin and oral anticoagulation (OA) therapies have not found a significant role in primary or secondary prevention of major adverse cardiovascular events. In this section, we will review some of the data that have resulted in a limited role for these agents in these high-risk patients.

Antithrombin therapy with heparinoids has long been employed for the management of acute ischemic events in the cerebrovascular, peripheral arterial, and coronary circulations. However, the efficacy of these agents in primary or secondary prevention has been offset by bleeding risk and inconvenience in parenteral administration. One typical study is the TAIST (Tinzaparin in Acute Ischemic Stroke) trial.[26] This randomized double-blind aspirin-controlled trial randomized 487 patients to high-dose tinzaparin (175 anti-Xa IU/kg daily), 508 patients to medium-dose tinzaparin (100 anti-Xa IU/kg daily), and 491 patients to aspirin (300 mg daily) arms within 48 hours of an acute ischemic stroke. The primary endpoint was a Rankin Scale score of 0–2 at 6 months versus dependence or death (Rankin Scale scores of 3–6). All three treatment groups fared similarly, with a trend towards increased bleeding in the high-dose tinzaparin group. Similar meta-analysis data since the TAIST trial have reiterated the lack of efficacy of antithrombin agents in acute ischemic stroke[27] and have tempered the enthusiasm for their use in chronic stable patients with CVD.

With respect to OA therapy, two extensive meta-analyses have informed our understanding of the role of OA comprising largely coumarin derivatives such as warfarin superimposed upon aspirin therapy in coronary artery disease (CAD). A meta-analysis by Anand and Yusuf[28] synthesized 31 clinical trials and found that in patients with CAD, high- and moderate-intensity OA reduced recurrent MI and stroke, but at the expense of bleeding. Specifically, when compared with control, high-intensity (International Normalized Ratio (INR)>2.8) OA reduced mortality by 22%, MI by 42%, and thromboembolic complications including stroke by 63%, but with a 6.0-fold increase in major bleeding in over 10 000 patients. Compared with control, moderate-intensity (INR 2–3) OA similarly reduced mortality by 18%, MI by 52%, and stroke by 53%, with a 7.7-fold increase in major bleeding in over 1500 patients. When compared with aspirin, both high- and moderate-intensity OA did not reduce death, MI, or stroke, at the expense of a 2.4-fold excess in major bleeding in over 3500 patients. When moderate- to high-intensity OA and aspirin were compared with aspirin alone, the combination therapy reduced the composite endpoint of death, MI, or stroke by 56%, with a 1.9-fold increase in major bleeding in only 480 patients. Finally, low-intensity (INR<1.5–2) OA offered no benefit over aspirin alone in over 8400 patients. Thus, these data suggested a possible benefit to combination therapy of OA with aspirin with modest bleeding risk, albeit in a limited number of patients. Subsequently, the same group revisited the role of OA and aspirin, expanding the dataset.[29] This analysis demonstrated that moderate- to high-intensity OA and aspirin reduced major cardiovascular events including cardiovascular death, MI, or stroke by 12%, with an increase in bleeding of 1.7-fold in over 12 000 patients. These two studies therefore led to a large randomized controlled clinical trial of OA in patients with PAD, the WAVE (Warfarin Antiplatelet Vascular Evaluation) trial that has recently been completed.[30]

The WAVE trial sought to determine whether moderate-intensity (INR 2–3) OA combined with aspirin was superior to aspirin alone in preventing cardiovascular events such as death, MI, or stroke (primary endpoint) or severe ischemia in the coronary or peripheral circulation (secondary endpoint) while quantifying bleeding risk (safety endpoint). In total, more than 2100 patients were enrolled with documented PAD by ankle–brachial index (ABI). There was no significant difference between the two groups in either the primary composite endpoint of CV death, MI, or stroke or the secondary ischemia endpoint.[30] However, a significant increase in bleeding (4.0% vs 1.2%) emerged between the combination-therapy group and the antiplatelet group.[30] Thus, at present, there is no compelling evidence that OA with or without aspirin reduces atherothrombotic events in high-risk patients to a greater degree than aspirin alone.

Primary prevention of stroke

Finally, we will review the data on antithrombotic therapy for the primary prevention of stroke. The risk of first stroke can be estimated with a variety of risk prediction models. The Framingham Stroke Profile is perhaps most widely cited;[31] however, no clear consensus exists on a model to predict stroke risk.[32] Therefore, the risk profile of each individual patient must include a review of all non-modifiable and modifiable risk factors (Table 27.1).[32] Once the risk of stroke has been assessed, treatment centers upon risk factor modification.[32]

Several meta-analyses have reviewed the role of aspirin in primary prevention. The US Preventive Services Task Force (USPSTF) performed an important meta-analysis studying the role of aspirin in the primary prevention of cardiovascular disease events.[33] In this meta-analysis involving over 55 000 patients, aspirin reduced the incidence of first MI in patients without prior atherosclerotic vascular disease, but did not decrease the incidence of first stroke.[33] The USPSTF

Table 27.1 *Risk factors for first stroke*

Non-modifiable
- Age
- Race (Blacks>Hispanics>Whites)
- Sex (Men>Women)
- Low Birth Weight
- Family History of Stroke/TIA

Modifiable
- Cardiovascular disease:
  - Coronary heart disease
  - Heart failure
  - Peripheral Arterial disease
- Hypertension
- Diabetes
- Atrial fibrillation (non-valvular)
- Dyslipidemia
- Physical inactivity
- Metabolic syndrome
- Hyperhomocysteinemia
- Hypercoagulability
- High Lp(a)
- Sleep-disordered breathing.
- Inflammatory Processes
  - *Chlamydia pneumoniae*
  - *Helicobacter pylori*
  - Elevated C-reactive protein
  - Periodontal disease
  - Cytomegalovirus
  - Acute Infection
- Cigarette smoking
- Asymptomatic carotid stenosis
- Sickle cell disease
- Obesity
- Postmenopausal hormone therapy
- Alcohol abuse
- Drug abuse
- Oral contraceptive use
- Migraine
- High Lp-PLA$_2$

Adapted from Goldstein LB et al. Circulation 2006;113:e873–923.[32]

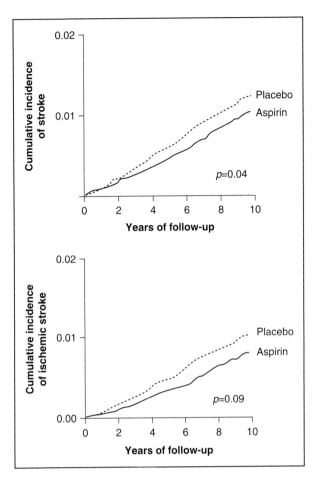

Figure 27.4
Cumulative incidence of stroke, especially ischemic stroke, is reduced by aspirin 100 mg daily in women. (Reproduced from Ridker PM et al.[34])

study noted that the benefit of aspirin would increase with increasing cardiovascular risk.[33]

As most of the patients in the USPSTF meta-analysis were men, the Women's Health Study sought to address the role of aspirin in primary prevention of atherothrombotic events in women. In this study, nearly 40 000 women without prior cardiovascular disease were randomized to aspirin 100 mg daily and/or vitamin E over 10 years of follow-up. The primary endpoint was a composite of MI, stroke, or death from cardiovascular causes, with prespecified secondary endpoints, including the individual endpoints of fatal or non-fatal MI, fatal or non-fatal stroke, ischemic stroke, hemorrhagic stroke, and death from cardiovascular causes. Additional analyses included the incidence of death from any cause, TIA, and the need for coronary revascularization. In this study, women on aspirin were found to have a significant 17% relative risk reduction of all strokes, a significant 24% reduction in the incidence of ischemic stroke, and a non-significant increase in hemorrhagic stroke (Figure 27.4). Based in large part upon these findings, the guidelines for the primary prevention of stroke

from the American Heart Association and American Stroke Association Stroke Council endorse the role of aspirin in the primary prevention of stroke in women with sufficiently high risk of stroke.[32]

Conclusions

Patients with extracoronary atherosclerosis are at the highest risk for coronary heart disease-related morbidity and mortality. Antithrombotic therapy in these high-risk patients centers on primary and secondary prevention of atherothrombosis. Individual antiplatelet agents, led by aspirin and clopidogrel, comprise the bulk of the therapeutic armamentarium. Dual antiplatelet therapy has failed to definitively show benefit except in acute coronary syndrome/PCI and secondary prevention of stroke. Novel antiplatelet agents such as picotamide may develop a larger role in clinical management with further study and wider availability. In sharp contrast, antithrombin and oral anticoagulant therapies have largely failed to find a role in the

Table 27.2 *Summary of antithrombotic therapy for high-risk patients with extracoronary atherosclerotic vascular disease*

- Aspirin 75 mg daily is effective for primary and secondary prevention of atherothrombotic events in high-risk patients
- Clopidogrel 75 mg daily is superior to aspirin >75 mg daily in preventing cardiovascular events in high-risk patients
- Picotamide shows promise as a potential antiplatelet agent in high-risk patients
- Aspirin + clopidogrel has no clear role in prevention of atherothrombosis in high-risk patients in the absence of acute coronary syndromes or endovascular stent placement[35]
- Aspirin + dipyridamole is effective in prevention of recurrent stroke
- Antithrombin and anticoagulation therapy have little role in prevention of atherothrombosis in high-risk patients
- Aspirin therapy is recommended for primary prevention of stroke in women

management of high-risk patients due to a failure to demonstrate both greater efficacy than and equal safety to antiplatelet therapy. Moreover, primary stroke prevention recognizes the importance of overlapping cardiovascular risk factors, with aspirin being the sole treatment that has to date proven to be effective in the primary prevention of stroke in women. New antithrombotic agents such as oral direct thrombin inhibitors and anti-factor IIa and Xa agents are currently under development. However, none has yet found a niche in the prevention of major cardiovascular events in extracoronary atherosclerotic vascular disease. Future research and development of these agents may hold new promise. A summary of recommended antithrombotic therapies for this high-risk patient population is presented in Table 27.2.

References

1. Criqui MH, Langer RD, Fronek A et al. Mortality over a period of 10 years in patients with peripheral arterial disease. N Engl J Med 1992;326:381–6.
2. Rothwell PM, Coull AJ, Silver LE et al. Population-based study of event-rate, incidence, case fatality, and mortality for all acute vascular events in all arterial territories (Oxford Vascular Study). Lancet 2005;366:1773–83.
3. Hirsch AT, Haskal ZJ, Hertzer NR et al. ACC/AHA 2005 Practice Guidelines for the management of patients with peripheral arterial disease (lower extremity, renal, mesenteric, and abdominal aortic): a collaborative report from the American Association for Vascular Surgery/Society for Vascular Surgery, Society for Cardiovascular Angiography and Interventions, Society for Vascular Medicine and Biology, Society of Interventional Radiology, and the ACC/AHA Task Force on Practice Guidelines (Writing Committee to Develop Guidelines for the Management of Patients With Peripheral Arterial Disease): endorsed by the American Association of Cardiovascular and Pulmonary Rehabilitation; National Heart, Lung, and Blood Institute; Society for Vascular Nursing; TransAtlantic Inter-Society Consensus; and Vascular Disease Foundation. Circulation 2006;113:e463–654.
4. Halliday A, Mansfield A, Marro J et al. Prevention of disabling and fatal strokes by successful carotid endarterectomy in patients without recent neurological symptoms: randomised controlled trial. Lancet 2004;363:1491–502.
5. Caro J, Migliaccio-Walle K, Ishak KJ, Proskorovsky I. The morbidity and mortality following a diagnosis of peripheral arterial disease: long-term follow-up of a large database. BMC Cardiovasc Disord 2005;5:14.
6. Fuster V, Moreno PR, Fayad ZA et al. Atherothrombosis and high-risk plaque: Part I: Evolving concepts. J Am Coll Cardiol 2005;46:937–54.
7. Hackam DG, Eikelboom JW. Antithrombotic therapy for peripheral arterial disease. Heart 2007;93:303–8.
8. Antiplatelet Trialists' Collaboration. Collaborative overview of randomised trials of antiplatelet therapy – I: prevention of death, myocardial infarction, and stroke by prolonged antiplatelet therapy in various categories of patients. BMJ 1994;308:81–106 [Erratum 1540].
9. Antithrombotic Trialists' Collaboration. Collaborative meta-analysis of randomised trials of antiplatelet therapy for prevention of death, myocardial infarction, and stroke in high risk patients. BMJ 2002;324:71–86.
10. Patrono C, Garcia Rodriguez LA, Landolfi R, Baigent C. Low-dose aspirin for the prevention of atherothrombosis. N Engl J Med 2005;353:2373–83.
11. Janzon L, Bergqvist D, Boberg J et al. Prevention of myocardial infarction and stroke in patients with intermittent claudication; effects of ticlopidine. Results from STIMS, the Swedish Ticlopidine Multicentre Study. J Intern Med 1990;227:301–8.
12. Blanchard J, Carreras LO, Kindermans M. Results of EMATAP: a double-blind placebo-controlled multicentre trial of ticlopidine in patients with peripheral arterial disease. Nouv Rev Fr Hematol 1994;35:523–8.
13. Gent M, Blakely JA, Easton JD et al. The Canadian American Ticlopidine Study (CATS) in thromboembolic stroke. Lancet 1989;i:1215–20.
14. Hass WK, Easton JD, Adams HP et al. A randomized trial comparing ticlopidine hydrochloride with aspirin for the prevention of stroke in high-risk patients. Ticlopidine Aspirin Stroke Study Group. N Engl J Med 1989;321:501–7.
15. Tran H, Anand SS. Oral antiplatelet therapy in cerebrovascular disease, coronary artery disease, and peripheral arterial disease. JAMA 2004;292:1867–74.
16. CAPRIE Steering Committee. A randomised, blinded, trial of clopidogrel versus aspirin in patients at risk of ischaemic events (CAPRIE). Lancet 1996;348:1329–39.
17. Gaspoz JM, Coxson PG, Goldman PA et al. Cost effectiveness of aspirin, clopidogrel, or both for secondary prevention of coronary heart disease. N Engl J Med 2002;346:1800–6.
18. Clagett GP, Sobel M, Jackson MR et al. Antithrombotic therapy in peripheral arterial occlusive disease: the Seventh ACCP Conference on Antithrombotic and Thrombolytic Therapy. Chest 2004;126(3 Suppl):609S–26S.

19. Balsano F, Violi F. Effect of picotamide on the clinical progression of peripheral vascular disease. A double-blind placebo-controlled study. The ADEP Group. Circulation 1993;87:1563–9.

20. Neri Serneri GG, Coccheri S, Marubini E, Violi F. Picotamide, a combined inhibitor of thromboxane A2 synthase and receptor, reduces 2-year mortality in diabetics with peripheral arterial disease: the DAVID study. Eur Heart J 2004;25:1845–52.

21. Mukherjee D, Topol EJ, Moliterno DJ et al. Extracardiac vascular disease and effectiveness of sustained clopidogrel treatment. Heart 2006;92:49–51.

22. Diener HC, Bogousslavsky J, Brass LM et al. Aspirin and clopidogrel compared with clopidogrel alone after recent ischaemic stroke or transient ischaemic attack in high-risk patients (MATCH): randomised, double-blind, placebo-controlled trial. Lancet 2004;364:331–7.

23. Bhatt DL, Fox KA, Hacke W et al. Clopidogrel and aspirin versus aspirin alone for the prevention of atherothrombotic events. N Engl J Med 2006;354:1706–17.

24. Diener HC, Cunha L, Forbes C et al. European Stroke Prevention Study. 2. Dipyridamole and acetylsalicylic acid in the secondary prevention of stroke. J Neurol Sci 1996;143:1–13.

25. Halkes PH, van Gijn J, Kappelle LJ et al. Aspirin plus dipyridamole versus aspirin alone after cerebral ischaemia of arterial origin (ESPRIT): randomised controlled trial. Lancet 2006;367:1665–73.

26. Bath PM, Lindenstrom E, Boysen G et al. Tinzaparin in acute ischaemic stroke (TAIST): a randomised aspirin-controlled trial. Lancet 2001;358:702–10.

27. Paciaroni M, Agnelli G, Micheli S, Caso V. Efficacy and safety of anticoagulant treatment in acute cardioembolic stroke. A meta-analysis of randomized controlled trials. Stroke 2007;38:423–30.

28. Anand SS, Yusuf S. Oral anticoagulant therapy in patients with coronary artery disease: a meta-analysis. JAMA 1999;282: 2058–67.

29. Anand SS, Yusuf S. Oral anticoagulants in patients with coronary artery disease. J Am Coll Cardiol 2003;41(4 Suppl S):62S–9S.

30. Anand S, Yusuf S, Xie C et al. The WAVE Investigators. Oral anticoagulant and antiplatelet therapy and peripheral arterial disease. N Engl J Med 2007;357:217–27.

31. Wolf PA, D'Agostino RB, Belanger AJ, Kannel WB. Probability of stroke: a risk profile from the Framingham Study. Stroke 1991;22:312–18.

32. Goldstein LB, Adams R, Albert MJ et al. Primary prevention of ischemic stroke: a guideline from the American Heart Association/American Stroke Association Stroke Council: cosponsored by the Atherosclerotic Peripheral Vascular Disease Interdisciplinary Working Group; Cardiovascular Nursing Council; Clinical Cardiology Council; Nutrition, Physical Activity, and Metabolism Council; and the Quality of Care and Outcomes Research Interdisciplinary Working Group. Circulation 2006;113:e873–923.

33. Hayden M, Pignone M, Phillips C, Mulrow C. Aspirin for the primary prevention of cardiovascular events: a summary of the evidence for the U.S. Preventive Services Task Force. Ann Intern Med 2002;136:161–72.

34. Ridker PM, Cook NR, Lee I-M et al. A randomized trial of low-dose aspirin in the primary prevention of cardiovascular disease in women. N Engl J Med 2005;352:1293–304.

35. Steinhubl SR, Berger PB, Mann JT et al. Early and sustained dual oral antiplatelet therapy following percutaneous coronary intervention: a randomized controlled trial. JAMA 2002;288:2411–20.

28

Dual antiplatelet strategies in patients requiring vitamin K antagonists

Giulia Renda, Marco Zimarino, and Raffaele De Caterina

Current indications for vitamin K antagonists

The clinical effectiveness of vitamin K antagonists (VKAs) in the treatment of a variety of disease conditions has been established by well-designed clinical trials. VKAs are effective for the primary and secondary prevention, as well as the therapy, of venous thromboembolism, for the prevention of systemic embolism in patients with prosthetic heart valves or atrial fibrillation, and for the prevention of stroke, recurrent infarction, or death in patients with acute myocardial infarction (AMI).

Prevention and therapy of venous thromboembolism

Prevention of venous thromboembolism

The rationale for the use of thromboprophylaxis with VKAs is based on solid principles and scientific evidence, centered on the consideration that virtually any hospitalized patient has one or more risk factors for venous thromboembolism (VTE), which are generally cumulative. For example, patients with fractures of the hip are at particularly high risk for VTE because of their usually advanced age, the presence of a proximal lower extremity injury as well as its operative repair, and the frequent marked reduction in mobility for weeks after surgery. If cancer is also present, the risk is even greater. Without prophylaxis, the incidence of objectively confirmed, hospital-acquired deep venous thrombosis (DVT) is approximately 10–40% among medical or general surgical patients, and 40–60% following major orthopedic surgery.[1] In this setting, anticoagulation with unfractioned heparin (UFH) at low dose or a low-molecular-weight heparin (LMWH) is recommended.[1] Adjusted-dose VKAs (International Normalized Ratio (INR) range 2.0–3.0) is also recommended, instead of heparins, in higher-risk conditions such as elective total hip or knee arthroplasty or hip fracture surgery for at least 10 days, or for rehabilitation following acute spinal cord injury.[1]

Therapy of venous thromboembolic events

Antithrombotic therapy with UFH or LMWH followed by VKAs is the cornerstone of treatment of VTE, such as DVT and pulmonary embolism (PE).[2] After initial treatment with UFH or LMWH, long-term therapy with VKAs, at a dose titrated to achieve an INR of 2.0–3.0, is required to prevent recurrent VTE, reducing the risk of recurrence by 90% compared with placebo.[2]

Long-term treatment with adjusted doses of UFH or therapeutic doses of LMWH is indicated only for selected patients in whom VKAs are contraindicated (e.g., pregnancy) or impractical, or in patients with concurrent cancer, for whom LMWH regimens have been shown to be more effective and safer.[3]

The optimal duration of anticoagulant treatment is a matter of debate because of the need to balance the risk of recurrence and the risk of bleeding, taking into account (if known) the provoking factors of VTE. The results of randomized trials[4,5] have indicated that patients who received treatment for 3–6 months had a low rate of recurrent VTE during the following 1–2 years, while a reduced duration of treatment is associated with an increased incidence of recurrent VTE. Moreover, the result of a recent double-blind trial[6] suggest that if VTE was caused by a transient risk factor (such as those shown in Table 28.1), patients should receive at least 3 months of VKAs for secondary prevention of VTE. After this period, the risk of recurrence off treatment becomes lower than the risk of fatal hemorrhage with VKAs (0.15% vs 0.3% per year).[2]

The optimal duration of therapy for patients with idiopathic events or who have continuing risk factors (such as malignancy) remains controversial. Patient with a first episode of idiopathic VTE, treated for 3 months, have an

Table 28.1 *Recommendations for duration of anticoagulant therapy*

Setting	Examples	Recurrent risk in year after discontinuation	Duration
Major transient risk factor	Major surgery, major medical illness, leg casting	3%	3 months
Minor risk factor, no thrombophilia:	Oral contraceptive or hormone replacement therapy		
Risk factor avoided		<10%	6 months
Risk factor persistent		>10%	At least 6 months or until factor resolves
Unprovoked, no or low-risk thrombophilia	Heterozygosity for factor V Leiden or prothrombin gene mutations	<10%	6 months
Unprovoked, high-risk thrombophilia	Antithrombin, protein C, or protein S deficiency		
	Homozygosity for factor V Leiden or prothrombin gene mutations		
	Double heterozygosity for these abnormalities	>10%	Indefinite
	Positivity for antiphospholipid antibodies		
More than one unprovoked event		>10%	Indefinite
Malignancy, other ongoing risks		>10%	Indefinite

increased risk of recurrence (10–27%) in the year after discontinuing VKAs compared with patients with a transient risk factor.[7,8] Randomized trials in patients with idiopathic DVT[7–9] indicate that extended treatment for 1–2 years with VKAs is highly effective in reducing the incidence of recurrent VTE compared with the conventional duration of treatment for 3–6 months. However, results of follow-up studies after VKAs have been discontinued indicate that the benefit in reducing recurrent VTE is not maintained after treatment is withdrawn:[7] the lower risk of recurrence obtained with 6 months of therapy does not decrease further when therapy is extended beyond 6 months. On the other hand, the benefit of extended treatment with VKAs is partially offset by the risk of major bleeding.[10] Extended anticoagulation (>6 months) should be considered for patients with unprovoked VTE or a continuing risk factor with a low risk of major bleeding.[10]

Some data suggest that patients with PE have a higher risk of recurrent VTE after discontinuation of therapy[7,10] and an higher risk of death[11,12] than those with DVT only. Therefore, it has been suggested that prolongation of anticoagulant therapy is useful in patients with PE, but this hypothesis requires more validation. Likewise, the presence of thrombophilic abnormalities, such as deficiency of antithrombin or of protein C or S, persistently positive antiphospholipid antibodies, or homozygosity for factor V Leiden mutation or for prothrombin mutation, increases the risk of recurrence and might justify prolongation of therapy, but the available data are still inconsistent.[13]

It has also been suggested that residual DVT[14] and elevated D-dimer levels[15] are helpful in the determination of anticoagulant duration, but since data are not conclusive, this issue also remains controversial.

Current recommendations for duration of anticoagulant therapy in the treatment of VTE[16] are summarized in Table 28.1.

Atrial fibrillation

The first use of VKAs for prevention of thromboembolism in patients with atrial fibrillation was mainly limited to patients with rheumatic heart disease and prosthetic heart valves,[17] in whom the high risk of thromboembolism has long been appreciated. VKAs were later evaluated in randomized trials of patients with non-valvular atrial fibrillation[18–22] and patients who had survived a non-disabling stroke or transient cerebral ischemic attack.[23] A meta-analysis of these trials showed that adjusted-dose VKAs are highly efficacious for the prevention of all strokes (both ischemic and hemorrhagic), with a risk reduction of 61% compared with placebo and of 33% compared with aspirin.[24] An INR range between 2.0 and 3.0 clearly conferred the best risk/benefit ratio,[22,25] and the incremental risk of serious bleeding was <1% per year among patients participating in these clinical trials. However, all of these trials excluded patients considered at high risk of bleeding, and, since patients' age and the intensity of anticoagulation are the two most powerful predictors of major bleeding[26] and trial participants have an average age of 69 years, it is unclear whether the relatively low rates of major hemorrhage also apply to older and less closely controlled patients with atrial fibrillation encountered in clinical practice.[27] The problem with very elderly patients is that they have a higher risk of stroke, but the benefit of anticoagulation therapy is potentially offset by an elevated risk of bleeding.[28] Therefore, targeting the lowest adequate intensity of anticoagulation to minimize the risk of bleeding is particularly important for these patients: low-intensity anticoagulation (target INR 2.0) may be as effective and safer in patients over 75 years.[22] Contemporary reports indicate that, despite current anticoagulation of more elderly patients with atrial fibrillation, rates of intracerebral hemorrhage are considerably lower than in the past (between 0.1% and 0.6%): this may reflect lower anticoagulation intensity, more careful dose regulation, or better control of hypertension.[29] Other than for dose intensity, advanced age, and hypertension, the importance of taking care of other factors related to higher rates of intracerebral hemorrhage during anticoagulant therapy, including associated cerebrovascular disease, concomitant antiplatelet therapy, tobacco or alcohol consumption, ethnicity, genotype, and certain vascular abnormalities, has been highlighted.[29]

Although VKAs clearly have the greatest efficacy in preventing stroke in atrial fibrillation among the treatments commonly available, and although the risk of major bleeding may be reduced by careful dose regulation, the dose–response relationship of these drugs is clearly variable, making it difficult for patients to remain within the ideal INR range. This results is a need for frequent, assiduous and unpleasant monitoring of the INR in order to reduce the risk of serious

bleeding on the one hand and the risk of under-treatment on the other.[30] For these reasons, criteria for the selection of an antithrombotic regimen in atrial fibrillation should be guided by the patient's overall risk profile, which is defined by the patient's thromboembolic profile and hemorrhagic profile, and also by the feasibility of an adequate monitoring of VKAs and the patient's preferences. Nowadays, the only alternative to VKAs in the prevention of thromboembolism in patients with atrial fibrillation is aspirin, which is safer and more handy, but less efficacious, and therefore indicated only in patients with low thromboembolic risk or with contraindications to VKAs.

A risk-based approach to antithrombotic therapy in patients with atrial fibrillation, according to the latest guidelines of the American College of Cardiology/American Heart Association/European Society of Cardiology (ACC/AHA/ESC),[31] is summarized in Table 28.2.

Prosthetic heart valves

It is generally agreed that all patients with mechanical prosthetic heart valves require anticoagulation for life, and there is no doubt that this is the safest approach under most circumstances.[32,33] Given the increasing risk of bleeding with increasing anticoagulation intensity, the ideal INR for patients after valve surgery is the lowest INR that achieves effective reduction in the incidence of thromboembolic events. Evidence from laboratory and clinical studies both in patients with non-valvular atrial fibrillation[34,35] and in patients with prosthetic valves[36] indicate that an INR in the range 2.0–2.5 is the minimum requirement for adequate prophylaxis against thrombosis occurring under conditions of relative stasis, but many

Table 28.2   *Risk-based approach to antithrombotic therapy in patients with atrial fibrillation (latest ACC/AHA/ESC guidelines)*

Patient features	Antithrombotic therapy	Class of recommendation
Age < 60 years, no heart disease (lone atrial fibrillation)	Aspirin (81–325 mg/day) or no therapy	I
Age < 60 years, heart disease but no risk factors[a]	Aspirin (81–325 mg/day)	I
Age 60–74 years, no risk factors[a]	Aspirin (81–325 mg/day)	I
Age 65–74 years with diabetes mellitus or coronary artery disease	VKAs (INR 2.0–3.0)	I
Age ≥ 75 years, women	VKAs (INR 2.0–3.0)	I
Age ≥ 75 years, men, no other risk factors[a]	VKAs (INR 2.0–3.0) or aspirin (81–325 mg/day)	I
Age ≥ 65 years, heart failure,	VKAs (INR 2.0–3.0)	I
Left ventricular ejection fraction ≤ 35% or fractional shortening ≤ 25%, and hypertension	VKAs (INR 2.0–3.0)	I
Rheumatic heart disease (mitral stenosis)	VKAs (INR 2.0–3.0)	I
Prosthetic heart valves	VKAs (INR 2.0–3.0 or higher)	I
Prior thromboembolism		I
Persistent atrial thrombus on transesophageal echocardiogram		IIa

[a]Risk factors for thromboembolism include heart failure, left ventricular ejection fraction <35% and hypertension.

patients will require a higher INR if adverse intra cardiac conditions or a more thrombogenic prosthesis impose a greater risk of thrombosis.

A unified approach to anticoagulation management, helpful for anticoagulation clinics, does not benefit individual patients who may be exposed to the risks of unnecessarily high anticoagulation intensity. In contrast, the trend in recent years has been towards lower-intensity anticoagulation, prosthesis- and patient-specific anticoagulation,[37] and greater concentration on the management of patient risk factors.[38] Table 28.3 shows recently proposed recommendations for anticoagulation after valve replacement, taking into account both patient-related and prosthesis-related factors.[39]

Myocardial infarction

Current VKA therapy in MI is mainly aimed at inhibition of the formation of coagulation factors involved in the generation and propagation of coronary thrombosis. The combination of VKAs with the standard antiplatelet regimen for secondary prevention after MI (low-dose aspirin) has been evaluated with the aim of achieing the highest possible antithrombotic benefit with an acceptable haemorragic risk. In patients who have survived an MI, it has been shown that the combination of warfarin at intermediate intensity (INR 2.0–2.5) and aspirin reduced death, reinfarction, and stroke by 30% compared with aspirin alone. This also compared favorably with full-intensity VKAs (INR 2.8–4.2), with an acceptable rate of bleeding.[40] Cerebral hemorrhage, the most dangerous complication of VKAs in combination with aspirin, is not significantly increased, while ischemic stroke

is considerably reduced by this combination. However, it is unclear whether the controlled conditions and the results of this clinical trial can be achieved in routine clinical practice, especially in particular settings such as patients undergoing percutaneous coronary intervention (PCI) and needing other antithrombotic drugs, or patients of advanced age who are at increased risk for hemorrhagic complications. Therefore, the latest guidelines of the ACC/AHA for the management of patients with ST-segment-elevation myocardial infarction (STEMI)[41] indicate the use of VKAs in the place of aspirin only for aspirin-allergic patients and in addition to aspirin only for high-risk patients or for both high- and low-risk patients when meticulous INR monitoring is standard and routinely accessible (Table 28.4).

VKAs are considered particularly efficacious for high-risk patients with MI, such as those with an intracardiac thrombus visible on echocardiography and those with a history of a thromboembolic event, those with left ventricular aneurysm, and those with strong indication for VKAs such as prosthetic heart valves and/or atrial fibrillation.[42] Moreover, VKAs may be advised in patients with left ventricular dilation and/or clinical heart failure,[43] especially because an interaction of aspirin with the beneficial effects of angioternsin-converting enzyme inhibitors has sometimes been observed.[44]

The indications for long-term anticoagulation after MI remain controversial and are evolving. Although the use of warfarin has been demonstrated to be cost-effective compared with standard therapy without aspirin, the superior safety, efficacy, and cost-effectiveness of aspirin have made it the antithrombotic agent of choice for secondary prevention.[41]

Table 28.3 *VKAs after valve replacement*		
Adjust target INR to	Without risk factors	With risk factors
Intracardiac conditions		
	Sinus rhythm	Atrial fibrillation
	Left atrial 0	Left atrial > 50 mm
	Mitral valve gradient 0	Mitral valve gradient +
	Normal left ventricle	Ejection fraction < 35%
	Spontaneous echo contrast 0	Spontaneous echo contrast +
	Aortic valve replacement	Mitral valve replacement
		Tricuspid valve replacement
		Pulmonary valve replacement
Prosthesis thrombogenicity[a]		
Low	2.5	3.0
Medium	3.0	3.5
High	3.5	4.0

[a]*Low* = Medtronic Hall, St Jude Medical (without Silzone), Carbomedics AVR;
Medium = Bileaflet valves with insufficient data, Bjork-Shiley valves;
High = Lillehei Kaster, Omniscience, Starr Edwards.
Adapted from Butchart E et al. In: Kristensen S et al, eds. Therapeutic Strategies in Thrombosis. Oxford: Clinical Publishing, 2006:217–49.[39])

Table 28.4 *Current indications for VKAs in the management of patients with STEMI*

Patient features	INR	Class of recommendation
Alternative to aspirin in aspirin-allergic patients with indications for VKA:		
Without stent implanted	2.5–3.5	I
With stent implanted + clopidogrel 75 mg/day	2.0–3.0	I
Alternative to clopidogrel in aspirin-allergic patients who do not have a stent implanted	2.5–3.5	I
Adding to aspirin in persistent or paroxysmal atrial fibrillation	2.0–3.0	I
Adding to aspirin in patients with left ventricular thrombus noted on an imaging study for at least 3 months; indefinitely in patients without an increased risk of bleeding	2.0–3.0	I
No stent implanted and indications for VKAs:		
VKAs alone	2.5–3.5	I
VKAs + aspirin (75–162 mg)	2.0–3.0	I
Less than 75 years of age without specific indications for VKAs who can have their level of anticoagulation monitored reliably:		
VKAs alone	2.5–3.5	IIa
VKAs + aspirin (75–162 mg)	2.0–3.0	IIa
Left ventricular dysfunction and extensive regional wall-motion abnormalities	2.0–3.0[a]	IIa
Severe left ventricular dysfunction, with or without congestive heart failure	2.0–3.0[a]	IIb

[a]Recommendation not included in current guideline and suggested by the authors.
From Antman EM et al. Circulation 2004;110:e82–292.[41]

Antithrombotic prevention of ischemic events after ACS and PCI

The term 'acute coronary syndromes' (ACS) encompasses a large constellation of clinical symptoms that are caused by acute myocardial ischemia, and comprises STEMI, unstable angina (UA) and non ST-segment elevation MI (NSTEMI). UA and MI are different clinical presentations of ACS resulting from a common underlying pathophysiological mechanism: atherosclerotic plaque rupture or erosion, with differing degrees of superimposed thrombosis and distal embolization.[45,46] Antithrombotic therapy is essential to modify the disease process and its progression to death, MI, or recurrent MI. Most recurrent cardiac events occur within a few months following the initial presentation. Initial stabilization of a patient's clinical conditions does not imply that the underlying pathological process has stabilized.

Percutaneous coronary intervention (PCI) for the treatment of coronary plaques, performed either with stand-alone balloon angioplasty or with stent implantation, while re-establishing myocardial perfusion, provokes endothelial denudation and increases the risk of early local mural thrombosis, since either plaque components – collagen and tissue factor above all (in the case of balloon angioplasty) – or the metallic struts of the stent (in the case of stent implantation) are suddenly exposed, at PCI, to flowing blood.[47]

Dual antiplatelet therapy with aspirin and a thienopyridine (ticlopidine or clopidogrel) reduces the occurrence of adverse events subsequent to coronary thrombus formation in both ACS and PCI; recommended dosages and duration of such therapy are summarized in Table 28.5.

In the setting of ACS, anticoagulation is achieved with either UFH or an LMWH during the hospital phase. Long-term anticoagulation with VKAs, in combination with aspirin or given alone, has been documented as being superior to aspirin alone in reducing the incidence of composite events after acute MI, but was associated with a higher risk of bleeding.[40] In a wide range of patients with acute MI – both NSTEMI and STEMI – the adjunctive long-term administration of clopidogrel reduced the risk of death, non-fatal MI, or stroke compared with aspirin alone.[48,49] To date, although there are no large-scale clinical trials comparing VKAs with a thienopyridine as adjunctive therapy versus aspirin, the better safety profile of dual antiplatelet therapy has made it become the standard treatment for secondary prevention after an episode of ACS.

In the setting of PCI, there is compelling evidence that the combination of aspirin and a thienopyridine reduces acute and subacute stent thrombosis compared with aspirin or aspirin plus an oral anticoagulant in the first 30 days after stent implantation. Moreover, the incidence of severe hemorrhagic and peripheral vascular events is significantly lower with antiplatelet drugs than with VKAs.[50,51] The efficacy of antiplatelet therapy derives from the key role of platelet activation after ACS and stent-PCI: patients who received anticoagulant agents showed a progressive activation of platelets, while the surface expression of activated

Table 28.5 *Recommended utilization of oral antiplatelet drugs in ACS and PCI*

Drug	Clinical situation	Initial dose (mg)	Maintenance Daily dose (mg)	Suggested duration
Aspirin	ACS–PCI	160–320	75–160	Indefinitely
Ticlopidine	PCI		500	30 days after bare metal stent implantation
Clopidogrel	ACS	300	75	9–12 months
	PCI	600	75	30 days after bare metal stent implantation 6–12 months after drug-eluting stent implantation

fibrinogen receptors decreased in patients given combined antiplatelet therapy.[52]

Among thienopyridines, clopidogrel is at least as effective as ticlopidine, but shows a better safety profile.[53] Therefore clopidogrel has now become the standard thienopyridine in the antiplatelet cocktail after stent-PCI.

For patients unable to take aspirin because of intolerance or hypersensitivity, clopidogrel alone should be administered at the standard dose.[54]

Based on their ability to prevent ischemic complications following PCI, glycoprotein (GP) IIb/IIIa inhibitors should be administered in high-risk patients with NSTEMI.[55] Although similar effects have been noted with the various GPIIb/IIIa inhibitors available (abciximab, eptifibatide, and tirofiban), the timing of PCI should be determined before an agent is selected. Available data favor the use of abciximab or accelerated-dose eptifibatide if PCI is to be performed soon after presentation (≤4 hours), reserving tirofiban and eptifibatide for patients treated medically during the first 48 hours.[56]

Stent PCI – bare metal stents versus drug-eluting stents

More recently, in the search of ways to reduce neointimal formation leading to restenosis, stents have been used as vehicles for local drug delivery. Drug-eluting stents (DES) are coated stents capable of releasing antiproliferative agents into the surrounding tissues.

Clinical trials have documented a three- to fourfold reduction in the rate of in-stent restenosis after PCI with DES compared with bare-metal stents (BMS).[57–59] In clinical trials using sirolimus- or paclitaxel-eluting stents, the risk of late thrombosis initially appeared to be unrelated to the presence of the drug, and was documented within the usual range of ≤1% at 9 months. However, the drugs eluting from the stent inhibit strut endothelialization, making the vascular surface thrombogenic for longer time periods than with BMS.[60] In consecutive series of patients receiving BMS, stent thrombosis was reported infrequently (0.8–2.8%). Stent thrombosis is, however, a catastrophic event, leading to

sudden death or major MI in the majority of cases.[61] Histological characterization of tissue responses to DES in animals indicates that healing is delayed, with sustained (up to 6 months) presence of inflammatory cells.[62] Until now, the duration of antithrombotic treatment after DES has been determined empirically (Table 28.6). In major clinical trials, combined therapy has been recommended for 2–3 months after sirolimus-eluting stents[58,63,64] and for 3–6 months after paclitaxel-eluting stents.[59,65–67] Thrombosis of a DES may occur intraprocedurally or – more insidiously – later on. Acute intraprocedural stent thrombosis is rare (0.7%), and has been related to stent length.[68] In the first month after PCI, subacute DES thrombosis was identified in 1.1% of patients. Smaller balloon diameters and clopidogrel discontinuation were risk factors for such adverse events.[69] Patients who received DES and prematurely (<30 days) discontinued thienopyridine therapy showed a ninefold risk of 1-year death (7.5%) compared with those who did not (0.7%; $p < 0.001$).[70] Very late (>1 year) acute DES occlusion has been reported in close temporal relationship to clopidogrel discontinuation, often for major non-cardiac surgery.[71] A general consensus is rapidly growing on long-term (≥ 1 year) double antiplatelet therapy with aspirin and clopidogrel after DES-PCI.[72]

Overlapping indications for VKAs and dual antiplatelet therapy: relevance of the problem and strategies to minimize complications

Concomitant VKA therapy may be necessary in patients undergoing PCI for the possible coexistence of atrial fibrillation, left ventricular mural thrombus, prosthetic heart valves, and previous atheroembolic events. In patients with atrial fibrillation at high risk of embolic events, dual antiplatelet therapy with aspirin and clopidogrel is significantly less effective than oral anticoagulation with VKAs in

Table 28.6 Duration of clopidogrel therapy and the occurrence of late thrombosis in major clinical trials comparing drug-eluting with bare metal stents in PCI

	RAVEL[57]		TAXUS-II[65]		SIRIUS[58]		E-SIRIUS[63]		TAXUS-IV[59,67]		RESEARCH[64]		ELUTES[66]	
Eluted drug	Rapamycin		Paclitaxel		Rapamycin		Rapamycin		Paclitaxel		Rapamycin		Paclitaxel	
Clopidogrel after DES[a]	2 months		6 months		3 months		2 months		6 months		3 (^{b}) months		3 months	
Follow-up	1 year		1 year		9 months		8 months		1 year		1 year		1 year	
Stent type	DES	BMS	DES	BMS	DES	BMS	DES	BMS	DES	BMS	DES	BMS	DES	BMS
Study population (n)	120	118	266	270	533	525	175	177	662	652	508	450	81	39
Late thrombosis (%)	0	0	0	0.7	0.4	0.8	1.1	0	0.6	0.8	0.4	1.6	0	0

RAVEL, RAndomized study with the sirolimus-coated bx Velocity balloon-Expandable stent in the treatment of patients with de-novo native coronary artery Lesions); TAXUS, Randomized double-blind trial to assess Taxus Paclitaxel-eluting stents in the treatment of high-risk de novo coronary lesions; SIRIUS, Multicenter, randomized, double-blind study of the SIRolimUS-eluting balloon-expandable stent in the treatment of patients with de novo native coronary-artery lesions; E-SIRIUS, European SIRIUS; RESEARCH, Rapamycin-Eluting Stent Evaluated At Rotterdam Cardiology Hospital registry; DES, drug-eluting stent; BMS, bare metal stent.

^{a}Standard 4-week clopidogrel administration was recommended after BMS in all trials.

^{b}After PCI with multiple DES implantation, in chronic total occlusion, and in bifurcations.

the prevention of vascular events (stroke, systemic embolus, MI, or vascular death), and therefore cannot be considered a valuable alternative to VKAs.[73] On the other hand, VKAs cannot be considered substitutes for thienopyridines as adjuncts to aspirin after stent-PCI, because a 30-day increased risk of ≥ 50% of death or MI (from approximately 0.8–1.5% to ≥2.5%) would be expected, due to subacute stent thrombosis (Figure 28.1).

The American College of Chest Physicians (ACCP) suggests that patients anticoagulated with VKAs and undergoing surgery or other invasive procedures should be managed according to their risk of thromboembolic events[74] (Table 28.7). Patients at high risk of thromboembolic events who require percutaneous diagnostic or interventional cardiovascular procedures are exposed to an increased risk of vascular access site complication, in which case full anticoagulation is recommended. In such patients, either the radial artery has been proposed for access, with the aim of minimizing the risk of bleeding; where femoral access is preferred, effective hemostasis may be achieved with closure devices.[75,76]

The concomitant use of VKAs (mostly warfarin) and antiplatelet therapy with aspirin and thienopyridines has to be carefully evaluated, because of the variability of anticoagulant response and its potential relation to excess bleeding complications. Data regarding patients treated with such a triple-drug combination after PCI are sparse, mainly because this group represents a limited percentage (<3%) of both populations of patients undergoing PCI and those requiring VKAs. Orford et al[77] performed a retrospective analysis of the Mayo Clinic PCI database and identified 66 consecutive patients who were discharged after PCI between January 2000 and August 2002 receiving a combination of dual antiplatelet therapy and systemic anticoagulation; a

bleeding event was reported in 9.2% and blood transfusion was required in 3% s. Porter et al,[78] in the largest currently available experience, analyzed a population of 180 patients who received 30 days of triple therapy after PCI with BMS implantation. During the triple-therapy period, bleeding complications occurred in 11% of subjects, in 90% minor hematomas. For a median follow-up of 16 months, subjects were kept primarily under warfarin and aspirin, and 10% newer bleeding complications were recorded, 95% being minor hematomas. During the study period, the INR was carefully kept between 2 and 3, and the aspirin dose was 100 mg/day; in this INR range, bleeding occurrence was not related to the INR.

Tentative recommendations

The issue of triple antithrombotic therapy in patients requiring both intensive antiplatelet treatment with aspirin plus clopidogrel and VKAs is a gray area of current therapeutic indications because of the limited data available. Registry data are being accumulated at present, and will likely shed more light on the optimal risk–benefit ratio. The issue is mostly confined to the increasing population of patients requiring a stent-PCI because of coronary artery disease and already having an indication for VKAs because of an underlying comorbid condition, such as atrial fibrillation or the presence of an artificial prosthetic valve. Other indications for dual antiplatelet therapy, such as ACS (both non-ST-segment-elevation ACS and STEMI) pose lesser problems, because, in such conditions, VKAs have been proven effective, and the need of triple-drug combination therapy appears here less pressing.

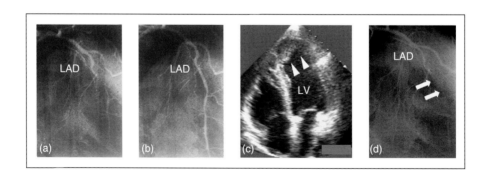

Figure 28.1
In a patient admitted for ST-segment-elevation myocardial infarction (STEMI) after 5 hours from symptom onset, an urgent coronary angiogram (a) showed that the left anterior descending (LAD) coronary artery was occluded in its distal segment (asterisk). A successful primary percutaneous coronary intervention (PPCI) was performed, with implantation of a bare metal stent (b). An echocardiogram (c) documented a left ventricular (LV) apical aneurysm with a thrombotic formation (arrowheads). The patient was discharged with aspirin (100 mg) indefinitely, clopidogrel (75 mg) for 30 days and warfarin for 6 months, aiming at an INR in the range 2–3. The patient prematurely discontinued clopidogrel after 14 days, and was admitted after further 7 days for a recurrent episode of STEMI (on day 21 from the first episode). Repeat angiography documented a thrombotic occlusion (arrows) of the previously deployed stent (d).
(see color plate)

Table 28.7 *Recommendations of the American College of Chest Physicians (ACCP) for patients anticoagulated with VKAs and undergoing surgery or other invasive procedures*

Condition	Description
Low risk of thromboembolism[a]	Stop warfarin therapy approximately 4 days before surgery, allow the INR to return to near normal, briefly use postoperative prophylaxis (if the intervention itself creates a higher risk of thrombosis) with a low dose of UFH (5000 U SC) or a prophylactic dose of LMWH and simultaneously begin warfarin therapy; alternatively, a low dose of UFH or a prophylactic dose of LMWH can also be used preoperatively
Intermediate risk of thromboembolism	Stop warfarin approximately 4 days before surgery, allow the INR to fall, cover the patient beginning 2 days preoperatively with a low dose of UFH (5000 U SC) or a prophylactic dose of LMWH and then commence therapy with low-dose UFH (or LMWH) and warfarin postoperatively; some individuals would recommend a higher dose of UFH or a full dose LMWH in this setting
High risk of thromboembolism[b]	Stop warfarin approximately 4 days before surgery, allow the INR to return to normal; begin therapy with a full dose of UFH or a full dose of LMWH as the INR falls (approximately 2 days preoperatively); UFH can be given as an SC injection as an outpatient, and can then be given as a continuous IV infusion after hospital admission in preparation for surgery and discontinued approximately 5 hours before surgery with the expectation that the anticoagulant effect will have worn off at the time of surgery; it is also possible to continue with SC UFH or LMWH and to stop therapy 12–24 hours before surgery with the expectation that the anticoagulant effect will be very low or have worn off at the time of surgery
Low risk of bleeding	Continue warfarin therapy at a lower dose and operate at an INR of 1.3–1.5, an intensity that has been shown to be safe in randomized trials of gynecologic and orthopedic surgical patients; the dose of warfarin can be lowered 4 or 5 days before surgery; warfarin therapy can then be restarted postoperatively, supplemented with a low dose of UFH (5000 U SC) or a prophylactic dose of LMWH if necessary

[a]Low risk of thromboembolism includes no recent (<3 months) venous thromboembolism, atrial fibrillation without a history of stroke or other risk factors, and bileaflet mechanical cardiac valve in aortic position.
[b]Examples of a high risk of thromboembolism include recent (<3 months) history of venous thromboembolism, mechanical cardiac valve in mitral position, and an old model of cardiac valve (ball/cage).
From Ansell J et al. Chest 2004;126:204S–33S.[80]

The following advice appears to be dictated more by commonsense than by rigorous data at the time of writing:

Patients at low thromboembolic risk
- Consider the suspension of VKAs.
- Do not use drug-eluting stents.
- Use the radial approach during PCI.
- For medium-term prophylaxis, use an aspirin plus clopidogrel combination for 4 weeks.
- For long-term prophylaxis, resume medium-intensity INR (2.0–3.0) anticoagulation with VKAs plus aspirin (≤100 mg/day).

Patients at high thromboembolic risk
- During the PCI procedure, do not stop anticoagulation, but use bridging therapy with UFH/LMWH at full dose.

- Do not use drug-eluting stents.
- Use the radial approach during PCI.
- For medium-term prophylaxis:
  - Try to limit the duration of overlap between dual antiplatelet therapy and VKAs as much as possible. There is, therefore, a strong case for advocating the use of BMS rather than DES in such conditions, limiting the time of overlap to 4 weeks after stenting.
  - Use the lowest effective aspirin dose. In the CURE population, a clear relationship between aspirin dosages and bleeding was observed, even within the narrow dose range of 75–325 mg/day allowed by the protocol.[79] Therefore, aspirin doses should not exceed 100 mg/day.
  - Target the lower end of the effective INR range (2–3 in most cases) in these patients. This requires more frequent assessment of the INR and close

monitoring of patients' variables affecting the response to VKAs;

- Decide in all cases bearing in mind the different time-course of stent-related thrombosis (quickly decreasing – with BMS – after the first week and practically disappearing after 4 weeks) against the persistent risk of thromboembolic events (e.g., in a patient implanted with a mechanical prosthetic valve).

- For long-term prophylaxis, use VKAs at intermediate intensity (INR 2.0–3.0) plus aspirin at doses ≤100 mg/day.

References

1. Geerts WH, Pineo GF, Heit JA et al. Prevention of venous thromboembolism: the Seventh ACCP Conference on Antithrombotic and Thrombolytic Therapy. Chest 2004;126:338S–400S.

2. Buller HR, Agnelli G, Hull RD et al. Antithrombotic therapy for venous thromboembolic disease: the Seventh ACCP Conference on Antithrombotic and Thrombolytic Therapy. Chest 2004;126:401S–28S.

3. Lee AY, Levine MN, Baker RI et al. Low-molecular-weight heparin versus a coumarin for the prevention of recurrent venous thromboembolism in patients with cancer. N Engl J Med 2003;349:146–53.

4. Levine MN, Hirsh J, Gent M et al. Optimal duration of oral anticoagulant therapy: a randomized trial comparing four weeks with three months of warfarin in patients with proximal deep vein thrombosis. Thromb Haemost 1995;74:606–11.

5. Schulman S, Rhedin AS, Lindmarker P et al. A comparison of six weeks with six months of oral anticoagulant therapy after a first episode of venous thromboembolism. Duration of Anticoagulation Trial Study Group. N Engl J Med 1995;332:1661–5.

6. Kearon C, Ginsberg JS, Anderson DR et al. Comparison of 1 month with 3 months of anticoagulation for a first episode of venous thromboembolism associated with a transient risk factor. J Thromb Haemost 2004;2:743–9.

7. Agnelli G, Prandoni P, Santamaria MG et al. Three months versus one year of oral anticoagulant therapy for idiopathic deep venous thrombosis. Warfarin Optimal Duration Italian Trial Investigators. N Engl J Med 2001;345:165–9.

8. Kearon C, Gent M, Hirsh J et al. A comparison of three months of anticoagulation with extended anticoagulation for a first episode of idiopathic venous thromboembolism. N Engl J Med 1999;340:901–7.

9. Ridker PM, Goldhaber SZ, Danielson E et al. Long-term, low-intensity warfarin therapy for the prevention of recurrent venous thromboembolism. N Engl J Med 2003;348:1425–34.

10. Kearon C. Long-term management of patients after venous thromboembolism. Circulation 2004;110(9 Suppl 1):I10–8.

11. Heit JA, Silverstein MD, Mohr DN et al. Predictors of survival after deep vein thrombosis and pulmonary embolism: a population-based, cohort study. Arch Intern Med 1999;159:445–53.

12. Murin S, Romano PS, White RH. Comparison of outcomes after hospitalization for deep venous thrombosis or pulmonary embolism. Thromb Haemost 2002;88:407–14.

13. Margaglione M, D'Andrea G, Colaizzo D et al. Coexistence of factor V Leiden and factor II A20210 mutations and recurrent venous thromboembolism. Thromb Haemost 1999;82:1583–7.

14. Prandoni P, Lensing AW, Prins MH et al. Residual venous thrombosis as a predictive factor of recurrent venous thromboembolism. Ann Intern Med 2002;137:955–60.

15. Eichinger S, Minar E, Bialonczyk C et al. D-dimer levels and risk of recurrent venous thromboembolism. JAMA 2003;290:1071–4.

16. Bates S, O'Donnell M, Hirsh J. Antithrombotic therapy in venous thrombosis and pulmonary embolism. In: Kristensen S, De Caterina R, Moliterno D, eds. Therapeutic Strategies in Thrombosis. Oxford: Clinical Publishing, 2006:217–49.

17. Wolf PA, Abbott RD, Kannel WB. Atrial fibrillation as an independent risk factor for stroke: the Framingham Study. Stroke 1991;22:983–8.

18. Petersen P, Boysen G, Godtfredsen J et al. Placebo-controlled, randomised trial of warfarin and aspirin for prevention of thromboembolic complications in chronic atrial fibrillation. The Copenhagen AFASAK study. Lancet 1989;i:175–9.

19. The Boston Area Anticoagulation Trial for Atrial Fibrillation Investigators. The effect of low-dose warfarin on the risk of stroke in patients with nonrheumatic atrial fibrillation. N Engl J Med 1990;323:1505–11.

20. Stroke Prevention in Atrial Fibrillation Study. Final results. Circulation 1991;84:527–39.

21. Connolly SJ, Laupacis A, Gent M et al. Canadian Atrial Fibrillation Anticoagulation (CAFA) study. J Am Coll Cardiol 1991;18:349–55.

22. Ezekowitz MD, Bridgers SL, James KE et al. Warfarin in the prevention of stroke associated with nonrheumatic atrial fibrillation. Veterans Affairs Stroke Prevention in Nonrheumatic Atrial Fibrillation Investigators. N Engl J Med 1992;327:1406–12.

23. EAFT (European Atrial Fibrillation Trial) Study Group. Secondary prevention in non-rheumatic atrial fibrillation after transient ischaemic attack or minor stroke. Lancet 1993;342:1255–62.

24. Hart RG, Benavente O, McBride R, Pearce LA. Antithrombotic therapy to prevent stroke in patients with atrial fibrillation: a meta-analysis. Ann Intern Med 1999;131:492–501.

25. Risk factors for stroke and efficacy of antithrombotic therapy in atrial fibrillation. Analysis of pooled data from five randomized controlled trials. Arch Intern Med 1994;154:1449–57.

26. Hylek EM, Singer DE. Risk factors for intracranial hemorrhage in outpatients taking warfarin. Ann Intern Med 1994;120:897–902.

27. Feinberg WM, Blackshear JL, Laupacis A et al. Prevalence, age distribution, and gender of patients with atrial fibrillation. Analysis and implications. Arch Intern Med 1995;155:469–73.

28. Palareti G, Legnani C, Cosmi B et al. Predictive value of D-dimer test for recurrent venous thromboembolism after anticoagulation withdrawal in subjects with a previous idiopathic event and in carriers of congenital thrombophilia. Circulation 2003;108:313–18.

29. Hart RG, Tonarelli SB, Pearce LA. Avoiding central nervous system bleeding during antithrombotic therapy: recent data and ideas. Stroke 2005;36:1588–93.

30. Albers GW, Dalen JE, Laupacis A et al. Antithrombotic therapy in atrial fibrillation. Chest 2001;119:194S–206S.

31. Fuster V, Ryden LE, Cannom DS et al. ACC/AHA/ESC 2006 guidelines for the management of patients with atrial fibrillation: a report of the American College of Cardiology/American Heart Association Task Force on Practice Guidelines and the European Society of Cardiology Committee for Practice Guidelines (Writing Committee to Revise the 2001 Guidelines for the Management of Patients With Atrial Fibrillation): developed in collaboration with the European Heart Rhythm Association and the Heart Rhythm Society. Circulation 2006;114:e257–354.

32. Borow RO, Carabello B, de Leon AC Jr et al. ACC/AHA guidelines for the management of patients with valvular heart disease. A report of the American College of Cardiology/American Heart Association. Task Force on Practice Guidelines (Committee on Management of Patients with Valvular Heart Disease). J Am Coll Cardiol 1998;32:1486–588.

33. Salem DN, Stein PD, Al-Ahmad A et al. Antithrombotic therapy in valvular heart disease – native and prosthetic: the Seventh ACCP Conference on Antithrombotic and Thrombolytic Therapy. Chest 2004;126:457S–82S.

34. Stroke Prevention in Atrial Fibrillation Investigators. Adjusted-dose warfarin versus low-intensity, fixed-dose warfarin plus aspirin for high-risk patients with atrial fibrillation: Stroke Prevention in Atrial Fibrillation III randomised clinical trial. Lancet 1996;348:633–8.

35. Feinberg WM, Cornell ES, Nightingale SD et al. Relationship between prothrombin activation fragment F1.2 and international normalized ratio in patients with atrial fibrillation. Stroke Prevention in Atrial Fibrillation Investigators. Stroke 1997;28:1101–6.

36. van Wersch JW, van Mourik-Alderliesten CH, Coremans A. Determination of markers of coagulation activation and reactive fibrinolysis in patients with mechanical heart valve prosthesis at different intensities of oral anticoagulation. Blood Coagul Fibrinolysis 1992;3:183–6.

37. Butchart E. Prosthesis-specific and patient-specific anticoagulation. In: Butchart E, Bodnar E, eds. Current Issues in Heart Valve Disease: Thrombosis, Embolism and Bleeding. London: ICR Publishers, 1992:293–317.

38. Butchart EG, Ionescu A, Payne N et al. A new scoring system to determine thromboembolic risk after heart valve replacement. Circulation 2003;108(Suppl 1):II68–74.

39. Butchart E, Gohlke-Baerwolf C, De Caterina R. Antithrombotic management in patients with prosthetic valves. In: Kristensen S, De Caterina R, Moliterno D, eds. Therapeutic Strategies in Thrombosis. Oxford: Clinical Publishing, 2006:217–49.

40. Hurlen M, Abdelnoor M, Smith P et al. Warfarin, aspirin, or both after myocardial infarction. N Engl J Med 2002;347:969–74.

41. Antman EM, Anbe DT, Armstrong PW et al. ACC/AHA guidelines for the management of patients with ST-elevation myocardial infarction: a report of the American College of Cardiology/American Heart Association Task Force on Practice Guidelines (Committee to Revise the 1999 Guidelines for the Management of Patients with Acute Myocardial Infarction). Circulation 2004;110:e82–292.

42. Brouwer MA, Verheugt FW. Oral anticoagulation for acute coronary syndromes. Circulation 2002;105:1270–4.

43. Loh E, Sutton MS, Wun CC et al. Ventricular dysfunction and the risk of stroke after myocardial infarction. N Engl J Med 1997;336:251–7.

44. Massie B. The Warfarin and Antiplatelet Therapy in Heart Failure trial (WATCH). Presented at American College of Cardiology, New Orleans, March 2004.

45. Davies MJ. The composition of coronary-artery plaques. N Engl J Med 1997;336:1312–14.

46. Goldstein JA, Demetriou D, Grines CL et al. Multiple complex coronary plaques in patients with acute myocardial infarction. N Engl J Med 2000;343:915–22.

47. Orford JL, Selwyn AP, Ganz P, Popma JJ, Rogers C. The comparative pathobiology of atherosclerosis and restenosis. Am J Cardiol 2000;86:6H–11H.

48. Chen ZM, Jiang LX, Chen YP et al. Addition of clopidogrel to aspirin in 45,852 patients with acute myocardial infarction: randomised placebo-controlled trial. Lancet 2005;366:1607–21.

49. Yusuf S, Zhao F, Mehta SR et al. Effects of clopidogrel in addition to aspirin in patients with acute coronary syndromes without ST-segment elevation. N Engl J Med 2001;345:494–502.

50. Leon MB, Baim DS, Popma JJ et al. A clinical trial comparing three antithrombotic-drug regimens after coronary-artery stenting. Stent Anticoagulation Restenosis Study Investigators. N Engl J Med 1998;339:1665–71.

51. Schomig A, Neumann FJ, Kastrati A et al. A randomized comparison of antiplatelet and anticoagulant therapy after the placement of coronary-artery stents. N Engl J Med 1996;334:1084–9.

52. Gawaz M, Neumann FJ, Ott I et al. Platelet activation and coronary stent implantation. Effect of antithrombotic therapy. Circulation 1996;94:279–85.

53. Bertrand ME, Rupprecht HJ, Urban P, Gershlick AH. Double-blind study of the safety of clopidogrel with and without a loading dose in combination with aspirin compared with ticlopidine in combination with aspirin after coronary stenting: the clopidogrel aspirin stent international cooperative study (CLASSICS). Circulation 2000;102:624–9.

54. CAPRIE Steering Committee. A randomised, blinded, trial of clopidogrel versus aspirin in patients at risk of ischaemic events (CAPRIE). Lancet 1996;348:1329–39.

55. Gluckman TJ, Sachdev M, Schulman SP, Blumenthal RS. A simplified approach to the management of non-ST-segment elevation acute coronary syndromes. JAMA 2005;293:349–57.

56. Zimarino M, De Caterina R. Glycoprotein IIb–IIIa antagonists in non-ST elevation acute coronary syndromes and percutaneous interventions: from pharmacology to individual patient's therapy: Part 2: When and how to use various agents. J Cardiovasc Pharmacol 2004;43:477–84.

57. Morice MC, Serruys PW, Sousa JE et al. A randomized comparison of a sirolimus-eluting stent with a standard stent for coronary revascularization. N Engl J Med 2002;346:1773–80.

58. Moses JW, Leon MB, Popma JJ et al. Sirolimus-eluting stents versus standard stents in patients with stenosis in a native coronary artery. N Engl J Med 2003;349:1315–23.

59. Stone GW, Ellis SG, Cox DA et al. A polymer-based, paclitaxel-eluting stent in patients with coronary artery disease. N Engl J Med 2004;350:221–31.

60. Gallo R, Padurean A, Jayaraman T et al. Inhibition of intimal thickening after balloon angioplasty in porcine coronary arteries by targeting regulators of the cell cycle. Circulation 1999;99:2164–70.

61. Cutlip DE, Baim DS, Ho KK et al. Stent thrombosis in the modern era: a pooled analysis of multicenter coronary stent clinical trials. Circulation 2001;103:1967–71.

62. Drachman DE, Edelman ER, Seifert P et al. Neointimal thickening after stent delivery of paclitaxel: change in composition and arrest of growth over six months. J Am Coll Cardiol 2000;36:2325–32.

63. Schofer J, Schluter M, Gershlick AH et al. Sirolimus-eluting stents for treatment of patients with long atherosclerotic lesions in small coronary arteries: double-blind, randomised controlled trial (E-SIRIUS). Lancet 2003;362:1093–9.

64. Lemos PA, Serruys PW, van Domburg RT et al. Unrestricted utilization of sirolimus-eluting stents compared with conventional bare stent implantation in the 'real world': the Rapamycin-Eluting Stent Evaluated At Rotterdam Cardiology Hospital (RESEARCH) registry. Circulation 2004;109:190–5.

65. Colombo A, Drzewiecki J, Banning A et al. Randomized study to assess the effectiveness of slow- and moderate-release polymer-based paclitaxel-eluting stents for coronary artery lesions. Circulation 2003;108:788–94.

66. Gershlick A, De Scheerder I, Chevalier B et al. Inhibition of restenosis with a paclitaxel-eluting, polymer-free coronary stent: the European evaLUation of pacliTaxel Eluting Stent (ELUTES) trial. Circulation 2004;109:487–93.

67. Stone GW, Ellis SG, Cox DA et al. One-year clinical results with the slow-release, polymer-based, paclitaxel-eluting TAXUS stent: the TAXUS-IV trial. Circulation 2004;109:1942–7.

68. Chieffo A, Bonizzoni E, Orlic D et al. Intraprocedural stent thrombosis during implantation of sirolimus-eluting stents. Circulation 2004;109:2732–6.

69. Jeremias A, Sylvia B, Bridges J et al. Stent thrombosis after successful sirolimus-eluting stent implantation. Circulation 2004;109:1930–2.

70. Spertus JA, Kettelkamp R, Vance C et al. Prevalence, predictors, and outcomes of premature discontinuation of thienopyridine therapy after drug-eluting stent placement: results from the PREMIER registry. Circulation 2006;113:2803–9.

71. McFadden EP, Stabile E, Regar E et al. Late thrombosis in drug-eluting coronary stents after discontinuation of antiplatelet therapy. Lancet 2004;364:1519–21.

72. Zimarino M, Renda G, De Caterina R. Optimal duration of antiplatelet therapy in recipients of coronary drug-eluting stents. Drugs 2005;65:725–32.

73. Connolly S, Pogue J, Hart R et al. Clopidogrel plus aspirin versus oral anticoagulation for atrial fibrillation in the Atrial fibrillation Clopidogrel Trial with Irbesartan for prevention of Vascular Events (ACTIVE W): a randomised controlled trial. Lancet 2006;367: 1903–12.

74. Ansell J, Hirsh J, Dalen J et al. Managing oral anticoagulant therapy. Chest 2001;119:22S–38S.

75. Hildick-Smith DJ, Walsh JT, Lowe MD, Petch MC. Coronary angiography in the fully anticoagulated patient: the transradial route is successful and safe. Catheter Cardiovasc Interv 2003;58:8–10.

76. Jessup DB, Coletti AT, Muhlestein JB et al. Elective coronary angiography and percutaneous coronary intervention during uninterrupted warfarin therapy. Catheter Cardiovasc Interv 2003;60:180–4.

77. Orford JL, Fasseas P, Melby S et al. Safety and efficacy of aspirin, clopidogrel, and warfarin after coronary stent placement in patients with an indication for anticoagulation. Am Heart J 2004;147:463–7.

78. Porter A, Konstantino Y, Iakobishvili Z et al. Short-term triple therapy with aspirin, warfarin, and a thienopyridine among patients undergoing percutaneous coronary intervention. Catheter Cardiovasc Interv 2006;68:56–61.

79. Peters RJ, Mehta SR, Fox KA et al. Effects of aspirin dose when used alone or in combination with clopidogrel in patients with acute coronary syndromes: observations from the Clopidogrel in Unstable angina to prevent Recurrent Events (CURE) study. Circulation 2003;108:1682–7.

80. Ansell J, Hirsh J, Poller L et al. The pharmacology and management of the vitamin K antagonists: the Seventh ACCP Conference on Antithrombotic and Thrombolytic Therapy. Chest 2004;126:204S–33S.

Appendix: Common anticoagulants in cardiovascular disease

Subclass	Drug	Indications	Dosing	Dose Comments	Antidote	Adverse Reactions	References
Heparins	Unfractioned heparin	ST elevation MI (when treated with fibrinolytic)	60 u/kg (max 4000 u) IV bolus + 12 u/kg/hr IV (max 1000 u/hr)		Protamine 1–1.5 mg IV per 100 u heparin	HITT	2004 ACC/AHA guidelines
		ST elevation MI (when treated with PCI)	70–100 u/kg IV bolus (when given alone), 50–70 u/kg IV bolus (with GP IIb/IIIa inhibitors)	Target to ACT 250–350 (or > 200 when used with GP IIb/IIIa inhibitors)			2005 ACC/AHA guidelines
		Unstable Angina/Non ST elevation MI	60–70 u/kg (max 5000 u) IV bolus + 12–15 u/kg/ hr IV (max 1000 u/hr)				2002 ACC/AHA guidelines
		Percutaneous Coronary Intervention	70–100 u/kg IV bolus (when given alone), 50–70 u/kg IV bolus (with GP IIb/IIIa inhibitors)	Target to ACT 250–350 (or > 200 when used with GP IIb/IIIa inhibitors)			2005 ACC/AHA guidelines
		DVT prophylaxis	5000 u SC q8–12hrs				
		DVT/PE	80 IU/kg IV bolus, then maintenance infusion of 18 IU/kg/hour IV continuous infusion to maintain PTT 1.5–2.3 × of normal				

(Continued)

Antithrombotics (Continued)

Subclass	Drug	Indications	Dosing	Dose Comments	Antidote	Adverse Reactions	References
	Low Molecular Weight heparin (Enoxaparin)	ST elevation MI (when treated with fibrinolytic)	30 mg IV bolus + 1 mg/kg SC BID (no bolus and 0.75 mg/kg SC BID if age >75)	Maximum 100 mg if age >75 or 75 mg if age >75, Given only if CrCl < 2.5 (men) and < 2.0 (women), if GFR < 30, change to 1 mg/kg SC q 24hrs	Protamine 1 mg per 1 mg of LMWH	HITT	Extract TIMI 25 N Engl J Med 2006; 354:1477–88.
		ST elevation MI (when treated with PCI)	1 mg/kg SC (given in previous 8hrs), additional 0.3 mg/kg IV if > 8hrs since last dose				2005 ACC/AHA guidelines
		Unstable Angina/Non ST elevation MI	1 mg/kg SC BID				SYNERGY JAMA. 2004;292:45–54 + 2007 ESC guidelines
		Percutaneous Coronary Intervention	1 mg/kg SC (given in previous 8hrs), additional 0.3 mg/kg IV if > 8hrs since last dose				2005 ACC/AHA guidelines
		DVT prophylaxis	1 mg/kg SC daily				
		DVT/PE	1 mg/kg SC every 12 hours or 1.5 mg/kg SC every 24 hours				

Direct Thrombin Inhibitors				
	Bivalirudin	ST elevation MI	0.25 mg/kg IV bolus + 0.5 mg/kg/h for 12hrs then 0.25 mg/kg/h for 36hrs	As adjunctive to streptokinase in patient with HITT	2004 ACC/AHA guidelines
		Unstable Angina/Non ST elevation MI	0.1 mg/kg IV bolus + 0.25 mg/kg/h, with 0.5 mg/kg IV bolus + increase infusion to 1.75 mg/kg/h before PCI		ACUITY NEJM 2006;355: 2203–2216
		Percutaneous Coronary Intervention	0.75 mg/kg IV bolus + 1.75 mg/kg/hr	If GFR <30 ml/ min, reduce infusion to 1 mg/kg/hr; in dialysis dependent patients reduce infusion to 0.25 mg/kg/hr	REPLACE 2 JAMA. 2003;289:853–863.
Pentasaccharides	Fondaparinux	Unstable Angina/Non ST elevation MI without PCI	2.5 mg SC daily for 8 days or until discharge		OASIS-5 NEJM 2006;354: 1464–1476
		Unstable Angina/Non ST elevation MI with PCI	2.5 mg SC daily for 8 days or until discharge + 2.5 mg IV (if < 6hrs since last dose and no 2b–3a inhibitor) or 5 mg IV (if > 6hrs since last dose and no 2b–3a inhibitor) or 2.5 mg IV (if > 6hrs and 2b–3a inhibitor is used)		OASIS-5 NEJM 2006;354: 1464–1476

(Continued)

Antithrombotics (Continued)

Subclass	Drug	Indications	Dosing	Dose Comments	Antidote	Adverse Reactions	References
		DVT prophylaxis following orthopedic surgery	2.5 mg SC daily (starting 6–8 hrs after surgery) for up to 24 days				Arch Intern Med 2003;163: 1337–42.
		DVT/PE	5 mg SC once daily for weight < 50 kg; 7.5 mg SC once daily for weight 50–100 kg; or 10 mg SC once daily for weight > 100 kg				N Engl J Med 2003;349: 1695–1702

Antiplatelets

Subclass	Drug	Indications	Dosing	Dose Comments	Antidote	Adverse Reactions	References
COX-1 inhibitor	Aspirin						
		Primary and secondary prevention CAD	75–325 mg PO daily				
		ST elevation MI	162–325 mg PO				2004 ACC/AHA guidelines
		Unstable Angina/Non ST elevation MI	162–325 mg PO				2002 ACC/AHA guidelines
		Percutaneous Coronary Intervention	100–325 mg PO (2–24hrs before procedure) then 325 mg PO daily thereafter (3–6 months) then 75–162 mg PO daily				2005 ACC/AHA guidelines

		Indication	Dose	Adverse effects	Reference
Thienopyridines	Clopidogrel (Plavix)	ST elevation MI (when treated with fibrinolytic)	300 mg PO load + 75 mg PO daily (up to 8 days or discharge, whichever day comes first)		TIMI 28 Clarity NEJM 2005;352: 2647–2648
		ST elevation MI (when treated with PCI)	300–600 mg PO load + 75 mg PO daily (for those undergoing DES PCI 12 months, BMS PCI 1 month)		
		Unstable Angina/Non ST elevation MI	300–600 mg PO load + 75 mg PO daily for at least 1 year		2007 ACC/AHA guidelines
		Percutaneous Coronary Intervention	300–600 mg PO load + 75 mg PO daily × 1 year (for those undergoing DES PCI at least 12 months, BMS PCI at least 1 month)		ARMYDA 2 Circulation. 2005;111: 2099–2106/ESC 20065 guidelines
	Ticlopidine	ST elevation MI	250 mg PO BID	Neutropenia, thrombo- cytopenia, TTP	Knudsen et al. Thromb Haemost 1985;53:332–6.
		Unstable Angina/Non ST elevation MI	250 mg PO BID (500 mg PO load is optional)		2002 ACC/AHA guidelines
		Percutaneous Coronary Intervention	250 mg PO BID		Schomig et al. N Engl J Med 1996; 334:1084–9.

(Continued)

Antiplatelets (Continued)

Subclass	Drug	Indications	Dosing	Dose Comments	Antidote	Adverse Reactions	References
Glycoprotein IIb/IIIa Inhibitors	Abciximab (Reopro)	ST elevation MI	0.25 mg/kg IV bolus + 0.12 mcg/kg/min for 12hrs	Can be considered with half dose Tenectaplase or Reteplase in patients with anterior infarct and age <75		Hypersensitivity, thrombocytopenia	ADMIRAL NEJM 2001;344: 1895–903
		Unstable Angina/Non ST elevation MI	0.25 mg/kg IV bolus + 10 mcg/min IV 18–24h before PCI until 1 hr afterward	As adjunctive in patients in whom PCI is performed			2002 ACC/AHA guidelines
		Percutaneous Coronary Intervention	0.25 mg/kg IV bolus given 10–60 minutes before the start of the PCI + 0.125 mcg/kg/min (max = 10 mcg/min) for 12 hours				ISAR-REACT N Engl J Med 2004;350:232–8.
	Eptifibatide (Integrilin)	ST elevation MI	180 mcg/kg IV (max: 22.6 mg) bolus + 2 mcg/kg/min (max: 15 mg/hour) IV for 18–24hrs	Can be considered with half dose Tenectaplase or Reteplase in patients with anterior infarct and age <75			2004 ACC/AHA guidelines
		Unstable Angina/Non ST elevation MI	180 mcg/kg IV (max: 22.6 mg) bolus + 2 mcg/kg/min (max: 15 mg/hour) IV for 18–24hrs	As adjunctive in patients in whom PCI is performed			2002 ACC/AHA guidelines

Drug	Indications	Dosing	Dose Comments	References
	Percutaneous Coronary Intervention	180 mcg/kg IV (max: 22.6 mg) bolus + 180 mcg/kg IV bolus (2nd bolus 10min after 1st bolus) + 2 mcg/kg/min (max: 15 mg/hour) IV for 18–24hrs	In patients with an estimated clearance <50 mL/min, reduce the dose by 50%.	2005 ACC/AHA guidelines
Tirofiban (Aggrastat)	Unstable Angina/Non ST elevation MI	0.4 mcg/kg/min IV for 30 minutes + 0.1 mcg/kg/min IV up to 18–24hrs	In patients with an estimated clearance <30 mL/min, reduce the dose by 50%.	
	Percutaneous Coronary Intervention	10 ug/kg in 3 mins IV bolus + 0.1 mcg/kg/min IV for a minumum of 12 hrs and up to 18–24hrs (standard dose regimen)		
		25ug/kg in 3 mins IV bolus + 0.1 mcg/kg/min IV for a minumum of 12 hrs and up to 18–24hrs (high bolus regimen)		

Drugs for Peripheral Vascular Disease

Subclass	Drug	Indications	Dosing	Dose Comments	Antidote	Adverse Reactions	References
	Cilostozol	PAD	100 mg PO BID				2006 ACC/AHA guidelines
	Dipyrimidole/Aspirin	Secondary stroke prevention	200 mg/25 mg PO daily				

Index

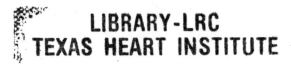